Alzheimer's Disease

DEMENTIA REVIEWS

Series Editors

JOHN P. BLASS, M.D.
Cornell University Medical Center at
Burke Medical Research Institute
White Plains, New York

ZAVEN S. KHACHATURIAN, PH.D.
National Institute on Aging
National Institutes of Health
Bethesda, Maryland

1. Alzheimer's Disease: New Treatment Strategies, *edited by Zaven S. Khachaturian and John P. Blass*

Additional Volumes in Preparation

Alzheimer's Disease

NEW TREATMENT STRATEGIES

edited by

ZAVEN S. KHACHATURIAN
National Institute on Aging
National Institutes of Health
Bethesda, Maryland

JOHN P. BLASS
Cornell University Medical College at
Burke Medical Research Institute
White Plains, New York

Marcel Dekker, Inc. **New York • Basel • Hong Kong**

Library of Congress Cataloging-in-Publication Data

Alzheimer's disease : new treatment strategies / edited by Zaven S. Khachaturian, John P. Blass.

p. cm.

Includes bibliographical references and index.

ISBN 0-8247-8620-3 (alk. paper)

1. Alzheimer's disease--Chemotherapy. 2. Alzheimer's disease--Treatment. I. Khachaturian, Zaven S. II. Blass, John P.

[DNLM: 1. Alzheimer's Disease. WM 220 A4788]

RC523.A3975 1992

616.8'31061--dc20

DNLM/DLC

for Library of Congress 91-46936

CIP

This book is printed on acid-free paper.

MARCEL DEKKER, INC.
270 Madison Avenue, New York, New York 10016

Current printing (last digit):
10 9 8 7 6 5 4 3 2 1

PRINTED IN THE UNITED STATES OF AMERICA

Series Introduction

This volume is the first in a planned series reviewing topics on the cutting edge of new knowledge of Alzheimer's disease and other dementing disorders of the elderly. Fifteen years ago, planning such a series would have been chimeral, since there was little new knowledge in these areas. The last decade and a half have, however, seen an exponential growth in research on these topics. The knowledge generated has become vast. Some of it is theoretical and some practical, some laboratory and some clinical, some oriented to the care of individual patients and caregivers and some dealing with broad epidemiological and public policy issues. Indeed, the scientific literature now contains bemused comments that "Dementology" and even "Alzheimerology" have become recognized, specialized fields within the neurosciences. In 1991, the question is not "Why a book on dementias?" Rather the question is "Why another one?"

The aim of this series is to present convenient summaries of topics that have not yet joined the mainstream of research on dementias but that seem likely to do so. Recognition of the immensity of the practical problems posed by these disorders and of the fascination of the scientific problems they pose has led to a steady stream of congresses, focused symposia, and review publications on areas of current research interest. It is already difficult to keep up with the reviews, let alone the original articles. On the other hand, there are topics related to the dementias on which a significant amount of exciting information has been gathered, but that have not yet received the visibility of the more popular topics. Some of these relatively neglected topics may turn out with time to have been justifiably neglected. The history of science suggests, however, that others of these currently less popular topics will turn out to be the bases of future waves of research.

This book and its successors in the Dementia Reviews series attempts to make knowledge of potentially important but as yet relatively unexplored areas conveniently available to the growing population of scholars and others interested in the dementias.

John P. Blass
Zaven S. Khachaturian

Preface

This book discusses the scientific bases of innovative approaches to the treatment of Alzheimer's disease. It derives from a conference sponsored by the National Institute on Aging and held at the National Institutes of Health. This book is the first in a planned series on current aspects of Alzheimer's disease and related dementing disorders.

The fact that a book can be put together on the treatment of Alzheimer's disease is a tribute to the explosion of knowledge in this area during the last fifteen years. In the early 1970s, discussions of dementia in the elderly tended to become philosophical disquisitions on whether or not dementia was an inevitable consequence of aging. Ground-breaking studies at the National Hospital for Neurological Diseases at Queen Square in London then demonstrated that the techniques of modern chemistry could be applied to human brain obtained at autopsy and led to the report in 1976 by three English groups of a deficiency of the acetylcholine system in Alzheimer brain. Realization that this disease could be studied meaningfully by the techniques of modern cellular and molecular biology and recognition of the magnitude of the public health problem it poses led to a progressive increase in support for research on Alzheimer's disease and related disorders. The resulting exponential expansion of knowledge has led to a relatively complete description of the neurotransmitter lesions in Alzheimer's disease and of the nature of some of the materials that characteristically accumulate in Alzheimer brain, notably Alzheimer amyloid and its precursor protein. Active research continues on these topics, as well as on the compelling questions of why and how the affected brain cells degenerate. The development of the innovative approaches to therapy described in this book is based on this continuingly expanding basis of scientific knowledge.

There are, at the present time, four broad approaches to the treatment of Alzheimer's disease. One attempts to identify medications that ameliorate the deficit in acetylcholine or other neurotransmitters. This approach is analogous to the use of L-dopa to treat Parkinson's disease. A second attempts to identify medications that alter the mechanisms of nerve cell degeneration and thereby slow or stop premature nerve cell degeneration. Medications based on these approaches are already in clinical trial, and others are being developed. A third approach involves dramatically innovative techniques that are still in the stage of animal experimentation. These include, for instance, neural transplantation or the use of growth factors such as NGF. All three of these approaches are discussed in this book. Although symptomatic management using psychotropic drugs and behavioral techniques is a mainstay of current clinical practice in this area, it is not discussed in any detail in this volume, which concentrates instead on innovative approaches to treating the disease process itself.

We wish to thank all the contributors, whose independent scientific contributions make this volume worthwhile. We also wish to thank Mr. Paul Dolgert and his colleagues at Marcel Dekker, Inc., for their inspiring leadership in this project. Ms. Elsie Brierly at the NIA and Ms. Carol Montanaro at the Burke Medical Research Institute provided the editors with administrative, secretarial, and moral support without which this book would not have been completed.

John P. Blass
Zaven S. Khachaturian

Contents

Series Introduction *iii*
Preface *v*
Contributors *xi*

Introduction 1
John P. Blass and Zaven S. Khachaturian

PART I. NEW TREATMENT-ORIENTED DRUGS—STATE OF THE ART

1. **Current Treatments for Alzheimer's Disease and Problems in the Conduct of Clinical Drug Trials** 9
Leon J. Thal

2. **Clinical Trials in Alzheimer's Disease: State of the Art and Future Directions** 15
Peter J. Whitehouse

3. **Strategies for the Treatment of Multi–Neurotransmitter Deficits in Alzheimer's Disease** 23
Kenneth L. Davis and Vahram Haroutunian

PART II. NEW APPROACHES TO DRUG DEVELOPMENT

4. **Brain-Enhanced Drug Delivery Systems for the Treatment of Dementia** 37
James W. Simpkins and Nicholas Bodor

5. **Strategies for the Treatment of Alzheimer's Disease: Cholinergic Agonists** 57
Lincoln T. Potter

6. **The Use of Molecular Modeling in Alzheimer's Research: Cholinergic Toxins, Amyloid Inhibitors–Diagnostics, and NMDA Agonists and Antagonists** 67
Donald J. Abraham

PART III. NEUROTROPHIC AGENTS—GROWTH FACTORS

7. **Growth Factors and Neurotrophic Factors in Neurodegenerative Diseases** 87
Franz Hefti, Paul A. Lapchak, and Timothy L. Denton

8. **Functional Effects of Chronic Nerve Growth Factor Infusions on Adult and Aged Basal Forebrain Cholinergic Neurons** 103
Karen S. Chen, Mark H. Tuszynski, Gerald A. Higgins, and Fred H. Gage

9. **The Potential Use of Neurotrophic Factors in the Treatment of Alzheimer's Disease** 125
Lars Olson and Barry J. Hoffer

PART IV. ANTI-INFLAMMATORY DRUGS

10. **Human Antibodies to Alzheimer's Disease and Normal Neural Elements** 137
Felicia Gaskin

11. **Immune-Related Mechanisms of Alzheimer's Disease Pathogenesis** 147
Joseph Rogers, Patrick L. McGeer, W. Harold Civin, and Scot D. Styren

12. **Does Anti-Inflammatory Treatment Protect Against Alzheimer's Disease?** 165
Patrick L. McGeer, Joseph Rogers, Edith G. McGeer, and John Sibley

PART V. OTHER INNOVATIVE APPROACHES

13. **A Cell Biological Approach to the Therapy of Alzheimer-Type Cerebral β/A4-Amyloidosis** 175
Samuel E. Gandy, Joseph D. Buxbaum, and Paul Greengard

14. **Phosphomonoesters, Phospholipids, and High-Energy Phosphates in Alzheimer's Disease: Alterations and Physiological Significance** 193
Jay W. Pettegrew, Williams E. Klunk, Richard J. McClure, Kanagasabai Panchalingam, and Sandra Strychor

15. **Abnormal Phospholipid Metabolism and the Pathophysiology of Alzheimer's Disease** 213
Jan Krysztof Blusztajn, He-Chong Lee, John H. Growdon, Mary Logue, Mordechai Loscovitch, Ignacio Lopez G-Coviella, Charlotte Mauron, U. Ingrid Richardson, Richard J. Wurtman, and Ismail Ulus

16. **Acetyl-L-Carnitine: Its Role in Neuronal Metabolism** 223
Menotti Calvani and Angelico Carta

Index 229

Contributors

Donald J. Abraham, Ph.D. Department of Medicinal Chemistry, Medical College of Virginia, Virginia Commonwealth University, Richmond, Virginia

John P. Blass, M.D. Cornell University Medical College at Burke Medical Research Institute, White Plains, New York

Jan Krzysztof Blusztajn, Ph.D. Department of Pathology and Psychiatry, Boston University School of Medicine, Boston, Massachusetts

Nicholas Bodor, Ph.D., D.Sc. Center for Drug Discovery, University of Florida, Gainesville, Florida

Joseph D. Buxbaum, Ph.D. Laboratory of Molecular and Cellular Neuroscience, The Rockefeller University, New York, New York

Menotti Calvani, M.D. Department of Neurological Research, Sigma Tau Pharmaceutical Industries, Rome, Italy

Angelico Carta, M.D. Department of Neurological Research, Sigma Tau Pharmaceutical Industries, Rome, Italy

Karen S. Chen Department of Neurosciences, University of California, San Diego, La Jolla, California

W. Harold Civin, M.D. Institute for Biogerontology Research, Sun City, Arizona

Kenneth L. Davis, M.D. Department of Psychiatry, Mount Sinai School of Medicine/Medical Center, New York, New York

Timothy L. Denton, Ph.D. Andrus Gerontology Center, University of Southern California, Los Angeles, California

Fred H. Gage, Ph.D. Department of Neurosciences, University of California, San Diego, La Jolla, California

Samuel E. Gandy, M.D., Ph.D. Laboratory of Molecular and Cellular Neuroscience, The Rockefeller University, New York, New York

Felicia Gaskin, Ph.D. Department of Behavioral Medicine, and Psychiatry and Neuroscience, University of Virginia School of Medicine, Charlottesville, Virginia

Paul Greengard, Ph.D. Laboratory of Molecular and Cellular Neuroscience, The Rockefeller University, New York, New York

John H. Growdon, M.D. Department of Neurology, Massachusetts General Hospital, Boston, Massachusetts

Vahram Haroutunian, Ph.D. The Bronx Veterans Affairs Medical Center, Bronx, New York

Franz Hefti, Ph.D. Department of Gerontology and Biological Sciences, University of Southern California, Los Angeles, California

Gerald A. Higgins Molecular Neurobiology Section, Laboratory of Biological Chemistry, Gerontology Research Center, National Institute on Aging, National Institutes of Health, Bethesda, Maryland

Barry J. Hoffer, M.D., Ph.D. Department of Pharmacology, Health Sciences Center, University of Colorado, Denver, Colorado

Zaven S. Khachaturian, Ph.D. Neuroscience and Neuropsychology of Aging Program, National Institute on Aging, National Institutes of Health, Bethesda, Maryland

William E. Klunk, M.D., Ph.D. Department of Psychiatry, Western Psychiatric Institute and Clinic, University of Pittsburgh School of Medicine, Pittsburgh, Pennsylvania

Paul A. Lapchak, Ph.D. Andrus Gerontology Center, University of Southern California, Los Angeles, California

He-Chong Lee Boston University School of Medicine, Boston, Massachusetts

Mordechai Liscovitch Department of Hormone Research, Weizmann Institute of Science, Rehovot, Israel

Mary Logue Massachusetts General Hospital, Boston, Massachusetts

Ignacio Lopez G-Coviella, M.D., Ph.D. Department of Cognitive Sciences, Massachusetts Institute of Technology, Cambridge, Massachusetts

Charlotte Mauron Massachusetts Institute of Technology, Cambridge, Massachusetts

Richard J. McClure, Ph.D. Neurophysics Laboratory, Western Psychiatric Institute and Clinic, University of Pittsburgh School of Medicine, Pittsburgh, Pennsylvania

Edith G. McGeer Kinsmen Laboratory of Neurological Research, University of British Columbia, Vancouver, British Columbia, Canada

Patrick L. McGeer, M.D., Ph.D., F.R.C.P. Department of Psychiatry, Kinsmen Laboratory of Neurological Research, University of British Columbia, Vancouver, British Columbia, Canada

Lars Olson Department of Histology and Neurology, Karolinska Institute, Stockholm, Sweden

Kanagasabai Panchalingam Department of Psychiatry, Western Psychiatric Institute and Clinic, University of Pittsburgh School of Medicine, Pittsburgh, Pennsylvania

Jay Pettegrew, M.D. Department of Psychiatry, Western Psychiatric Institute and Clinic, University of Pittsburgh School of Medicine, Pittsburgh, Pennsylvania

Lincoln T. Potter, M.D. Department of Molecular and Cellular Pharmacology, University of Miami School of Medicine, Miami, Florida

Donald L. Price, M.D. Department of Pathology, The Johns Hopkins University School of Medicine, Baltimore, Maryland

U. Ingrid Richardson Massachusetts Institute of Technology, Cambridge, Massachusetts

Joseph Rogers, Ph.D. Institute for Biogerontology Research, Sun City, Arizona

John Sibley Department of Internal Medicine, University of Saskatchewan, Saskatoon, Canada

James W. Simpkins, Ph.D. Department of Pharmacodynamics, University of Florida, Gainesville, Florida

Sandra Strychor, M.P.H. Department of Clinical Pharmacology, Western Psychiatric Institute and Clinic, Graduate School of Public Health, University of Pittsburgh School of Medicine, Pittsburgh, Pennsylvania

Scot D. Styren, Ph.D. Department of Electronmicroscopy, Institute for Biogerontology Research, Sun City, Arizona

Leon J. Thal, M.D. Department of Neurosciences, University of California, San Diego, La Jolla, California, and Neurology Service, San Diego Veterans Affairs Medical Center, San Diego, California

Mark H. Tuszynski, M.D., Ph.D. Department of Neurosciences, University of California, San Diego, La Jolla, California

Ismail Ulus Uldag University Medical School, Bursa, Turkey

Peter J. Whitehouse, M.D., Ph.D. Department of Neurology, University Hospitals of Cleveland, Cleveland, Ohio

Henry M. Wisiewski, M.D., Ph.D. New York State Institute for Basic Research in Developmental Disabilities, Staten Island, New York

Richard J. Wurtman, M.D. Department of Brain and Cognitive Science, Massachusetts Institute of Technology, Cambridge, Massachusetts

Alzheimer's Disease

Introduction

John P. Blass
Cornell University Medical College at Burke Medical Research Institute, White Plains, New York
Zaven S. Khachaturian
National Institute on Aging, National Institutes of Health, Bethesda, Maryland

The aim of this volume is to summarize, in a convenient form, currently promising avenues to the treatment of Alzheimer's disease. This disease is widely recognized to be a major public health problem in the United States and, indeed, in the whole world. It is estimated that as many as 4 million or perhaps even more individuals in the United States have this disorder (1). Not only they but their families and other caregivers are appropriately considered victims of this dreadful, disabling, often lingering disease (2). The cost of care is variously estimated, depending on the assumptions used and the number of "opportunity costs" included, but even on conservative assumptions the *current* annual cost in the United States exceeds 20 billion dollars (3). Although the annual budget for biological research on this disorder is less than 1% of that figure, research is already yielding hopeful new therapies which are being tested in pilot and multicenter trials in the United States and abroad. The immediate, annual market for an effective medication for Alzheimer's disease has been estimated to be between 2 and 8 billion dollars a year. The newspapers and other news media have reflected the interest of the general public and of the pharmaceutical and financial communities in the development of a possible treatment for Alzheimer's disease. In addition, the controversies that have swirled about the reviews by the Food and Drug Administration of some of the tested medications have been the subject of extensive public comment. A review of potential avenues to treatment of Alzheimer's disease therefore seems timely.

This volume is based on a conference held at the National Institutes of Health on January 8–10, 1990. The conference was sponsored by the National Institute on Aging, the Alzheimer's Association, the International Society for the Diagnosis and Treatment of Senile Dementias, and the Sigma-Tau Foundation. The conference title was New Strategies for the Treatment of Alzheimer's Disease. The focus of the conference was not only to review medications already in or near the stage of clinical trial, but also and primarily to stimulate imaginative new approaches to therapy based on current biological research. This volume does not include all of the presentations at the conference. Participants were asked to speculate freely so as to stimulate new ideas, and a number of the participants felt that speculations which were appropriate in the framework of a closed "brainstorming" conference could not be well documented and therefore were not appropriate for a formal, printed format.

Emphasis should be placed on certain topics relevant to the treatment of Alzheimer's disease which were not discussed in detail either in this volume or in the conference from which it was derived. There was no discussion of symptomatic management by behavioral or other techniques. There was limited discussion of symptomatic management by psychotropic drug use or other currently available medications. The organizers and participants were deeply aware of the major role of symptomatic care for the patients and of the vital role of support for the caregivers, under the present circumstances where an effective neurobiological treatment is not yet available. Indeed many of the participants were also physicians who spend an important fraction of their time caring for these patients and their families. However, the belief that underlay the organization of this meeting was that the greatest benefit to the patients and their caregivers, and the most cost-effective approach for government and the society, is to find an effective means to slow or halt the neurobiological ravages of this disorder and make symptomatic treatment relatively unnecessary.

This volume is divided into five parts:

I. NEW TREATMENT-ORIENTED DRUGS—STATE OF THE ART

Part I focuses on current approaches to the treatment of Alzheimer's disease. Dr. Leon J. Thal (Chapter 1) reviews both the range of agents which have been tested and the problems with clinical trials in this potentially heterogeneous disease. Many of the treatments tried so far focus on amelioration of the well-established deficit incholinergic systems in this disorder, and Dr. Thal reviews in some detail the results of trials with agents designed to ameliorate the resultant deficit in acetylchiline. Dr. Peter J. Whitehouse (Chapter 2) reviews the same issues from the viewpoint of a director of a large academic program. Among other points, he deals with the problem of recognizing pharmacological subgroups of patients with Alzheimer's disease, whose responsiveness to a medication may not be detected if one averages them in with a larger group of patients unresponsive to that drug. Drs. Kenneth L. Davis and Vahram Haroutunian (Chapter 3) discuss the practical problems in trying to design treatments for deficits of more than one neurotransmitter, and the statistical problems in trying to determine the efficacy of such treatments, in experimental animals as well as in human patients. These are very practical issues in therapeutic trials in Alzheimer's disease, which has been clearly shown to involve other neurotransmitters as well as acetylcholine.

II. NEW APPROACHES TO DRUG DEVELOPMENT

Part II deals with some of the new approaches to the development of drugs, primarily with agents acting on neurotransmitter systems. Drs. James W. Simpkins and Nicholas Bodor (Chapter 4) discuss the chemical modifications of existing medications to make them more suitable for treatment of a brain disorder, specifically including linkage to a steroid or other lipid-soluble molecule to enhance the penetration of these drugs into the brain. Dr. Lincoln T. Potter (Chapter 5) reviews newer and more selective approaches to the development of cholinergic therapies, based on increasing knowledge of the nature of the different acetylcholine receptors in the mammalian brain. Dr. Donald J. Abraham (Chapter 6) illustrates the potential use of molecular modeling techniques to design new drugs for the treatment of Alzheimer's disease, using as his examples cholinergic toxins, potential inhibitors of the formation of Alzheimer's disease, using as his examples cholinergic toxins, potential inhibitors of the formation of Alzheimer amyloid, and agonists and antagonists for the NMDA receptor.

III. NEUROTROPHIC AGENTS—GROWTH FACTORS

One of the most exciting potential areas of treatment of neurodegenerative diseases in general and of Alzheimer's disease in particular is the recognition of "neurotrophic" factors which are needed not only for the development but also for the maintenance of neurons. The best known of these factors, nerve growth factor (NGF), is now known to affect the maintenance of cholinergic cells of the nucleus basalis complex which are known to be affected in Alzheimer's disease. The potential uses of neurotrophic factors in neurodegenerative diseases including Alzheimer's disease are reviewed in Chapter 7 by Drs. Franz Hefti, Paul A. Lapchak, and Timothy L. Denton and in Chapter 9 by Drs. Lars Olson and Barry Hoffer. In Chapter 8, Dr. Karen Chen and her co-workers present intriguing and hopeful data on the functional effects of infusions of NGF in experimental animals.

IV. ANTI-INFLAMMATORY DRUGS

While concern that Alzheimer's disease may have an autoimmune component has existed for many years, a recent innovative proposal is that there is an active inflammatory component to the disorder which can be treated effectively by aspirin and perhaps other common anti-inflammatory medications. This proposal is discussed in this section. In Chapter 10, Drs. Joseph Rogers, Patrick L. McGeer, and co-workers present evidence that the components of an autoimmune reaction exist in the brain. Dr. Gaskin (Chapter 11) presents evidence for the existence of antibrain antibodies in Alzheimer's disease. Finally, in Chapter 12, Drs. McGeer and Rogers and their co-workers present retrospective epidemiological evidence that conditions such as theumatism which are associated with chronic use of anti-inflammatory medications are associated with a lower-than-expected incidence of the diagnosis of Alzheimer's disease. The prospect of treatment of Alzheimer's disease with a medicine as relatively safe and inexpensive as aspirin is, of course, very exciting. One caveat which must, however, be borne in mind is that aspirin has been reported to retard the development of mental impairment due to strokes (4), and it can be difficult to distinguish clinically with certainty between degenerative dementia due to Alzheimer's disease and dementia due to cerebrovascular disease.

V. OTHER INNOVATIVE APPROACHES

The final part deals with a number of other potential approaches. Drs. Samuel E. Gandy, Joseph D. Buxbaum, and Paul Greengard (Chapter 13) discuss the possibility of preventing the development of Alzheimer's disease by reducing the accumulation of the characteristic Alzheimer's amyloid, by ameliorating the abnormal processing of this protein which appears to occur in this disorder. This proposal is in accord with a major line of current research on Alzheimer's disease, which focuses on the possibility that the amyloid protein or its precursors are important agents in triggering the premature neuronal dysfunction and damage in this disease. Dr. Jay W. Pettegrew and his colleagues (Chapter 14) and Dr. Jan Krzysztof Blusztajn and his colleagues (Chapter 15) review the evidence for a defect in membranes, particularly in cells in the nervous system, which is evident in an abnormality in phospholipids. They also discuss some of the potential implications for possible avenues of therapy. In the final chapter, Drs. Menotti Calvani and Angelico Carta from Sigma Tau Pharmaceuticals discuss evidence for a cerebral metabolic abnormality in Alzheimer's disease and review evidence including preliminary clinical studies that acetyl-L-carnitine may ameliorate it.

The editors wish to reemphasize that the aim of this volume is not to recommend for or against any particular avenue of therapy, and certainly not for or against any particular medication produced by any particular company. However, testing actual treatments rather than theories requires using real medications, which are typically manufactured by specific companies which are therefore in a position to make a profit if the medication is successful. Indeed, a major aim of research is to bring new information to bear which will allow the development of effective therapy, which can be applied on a widespread, practical, and therefore potentially commercial level. It is our hope that this book will help to stimulate thought, laboratory experimentation, and clinical trials, so that more effective means may be found to reduce or abolish the ravages of this terrible disease on the patients and their families.

REFERENCES

1. Schoenberg BS, Kokmen E, Okazaki H. Alzheimer's disease and other dementing illneses in a defined United States population: Incidence rates and clinical features. Ann Neurol 22:724–729, 1987.
2. Katzman R, Brown T, Thal LJ, et al. Comparison of rate of annual change of mental status score in four independent studies of patients with Alzheimer's disease. Ann Neurol 24:384–389, 1988.
3. Huang LF, Cartwright WS, Hu TW. The economic cost of senile dementia in the United States, 1985. Public Health Rep. 103:3–7, 1988.
4. Meyer JS, Rogers RL, McClintic K, et al. Randomized clinical trial of daily aspirin therapy in multi-infarct dementia. J Am Geriatr Soc 37:549–555, 1989.

PART I

New Treatment-Oriented Drugs—State of the Art

1

Current Treatments for Alzheimer's Disease and Problems in the Conduct of Clinical Drug Trials

Leon J. Thal
University of California, San Diego, La Jolla, and San Diego Veterans Affairs Medical Center, San Diego, California

I. INHERENT PROBLEMS IN CLINICAL TRIALS

The momentum for clinical drug trials in Alzheimer's disease (AD) stems from a number of findings. These include: 1) the realization that memory loss is not an inevitable consequence of aging, 2) the aging of the population, 3) the realization that AD and senile dementia of the Alzheimer type (SDAT) are one and the same entity, and 4) the great strides made regarding the basic neurochemistry of AD during the last 14 years.

However, there are a number of difficulties in carrying out clinical AD drug research. The first is the issue of diagnosis. A biological marker for this disease is not available. Although several putative markers have been recently described (1,2), none have adequate sensitivity and specificity to serve as useful markers in biologically available material in the living patient. In addition to the absence of a marker, the AD population is heterogenous. There are innate differences of cognition, memory, language, and intelligence. The disease progresses differently in each patient. While all patients with AD have a memory disorder, many patients also have disturbances of language, visuospatial relations, mood, and behavior. These symptoms are often as important as the memory disorder itself.

The accuracy of clinical diagnosis based on standardized criteria such as the National Institute of Neurological Communicative Disorders and Stroke/Alzheimer's Disease and Related Disorders Association (NINCDS/ADRDA) (3) criteria, approach an accuracy of approximately 85% when verified pathologically (4). The main difficulty facing the clinician is the differentiation of AD from individuals who have both AD and vascular dementia. Using the NINCDS/ADRDA criteria for probable AD, overall diagnostic accuracy approaching 90% can be obtained for clinical drug trials. However, this means that each clinical drug trial will still contain about 10% of patients with other disorders.

Clinical drug trials tend to utilize strict inclusion and exclusion criteria to develop homogenous populations for testing. Screening for inclusion in clinical drug trials results in the selection of only about one patient out of every 7–10 screened individuals. Nevertheless, once the drug is marketed, patients excluded from clinical drug trials will receive the drug. Therefore, the patients in clinical drug trials are not completely representative of the patient population that will ultimately be receiving these agents, and extrapolation of safety and efficacy from clinical drug trials to the total population may not be accurate. As development of a drug continues, it is therefore extremely useful to liberalize the entrance criteria and to expose as broad a range of patients to the drug as possible.

In addition to the memory disorder, many patients with AD have behavioral disturbances. At the San Diego Alzheimer's Disease Research Center, a survey of the AD population revealed that at the time of evaluation, 36% of patients had paranoid delusions. Additionally, another 24% had had paranoid delusions at some point in the past after the onset of their dementing illness. Thus, 60% of this AD cohort had paranoid delusions at some point during their dementing illness. For the majority of AD patients, memory loss per se is not the reason for institutionalization. Institutionalization usually occurs when families can no longer care for an individual because of either physical problems such as incontinence or because of prominent behavioral disturbances such as aggression, wandering, or nighttime misdemeanors.

II. CURRENT APPROACHES TO TREATMENT

Treatment for AD would be simpler if the cause were known. Epidemiological investigations have attempted to identify risk factors that may predispose to this disorder. The major risk factors identified at present are: age (5) female sex (6,7) and a history of familial AD (8,9). More recently suggested risk factors found in two studies also include low levels of education (10) and silent myocardial infarcts (11). However, the latter two risk factors have not been confirmed by other investigators. Given the lack of knowledge regarding the cause of this disorder, treatments have been aimed primarily at improving symptoms.

Specific symptom complexes in AD patients require treatment. These include depression, anxiety, agitation, delusions, and insomnia. These symptoms are extremely important in the overall treatment of the disorder, since they occur commonly and give rise to significant comorbidity. Unfortunately, to date, very few well-controlled pharmacological studies have been carried out to help the practitioner decide which agents are most effective in treating these secondary symptoms.

The second level of treatment is aimed at improving memory—the core symptom of AD. The majority of clinical trials in AD during the past three decades have approached this aspect of treatment.

While many current drug trials are attempting to produce acute improvements in cognition, future drug trials will attempt to alter the rate of decline in this disease. However, it is necessary to understand the natural history of the disorder to know if one has altered the rate of decline. The natural rate of decline has been determined for several simple mental status tests. On the Blessed Information-Memory-Concentration Test (BIMC), the average rate of decline in four separate populations was 4.4 ± 3.6 (mean $\pm$ standard deviation) points per year (12). Furthermore, the rate of decline was independent of stage of dementia, site of population studied, and age of onset. Rate of decline, for the Mini-Mental State Exam (MMSE) and Dementia Rating Scale of Mattis (DRS) has also been determined. In general, the rate of decline over 1 year was approximately equal to the standard deviation for the rate of decline. These rates and their standard deviations are essential for the calculation of group sizes needed to demonstrate efficacy for drugs altering the natural rate of decline.

A fourth approach to the treatment of AD would be to delay the onset of appearance of the disease. Since AD is a disorder of late life, the delay of the disease for one or two decades might be sufficient to reduce its impact on public health. Even if the disease is genetically determined, there must be some degree of environmental control. This must be the case, since at least one pair of monozygotic twins developed AD 10 years apart (13).

The most important way of treating AD would, of course, be prevention. However, our ability to prevent the disease awaits the development of additional information regarding either the pathogenesis or etiology of this illness.

III. DRUGS TESTED

Over the past decades many different classes of drugs have been tested in patients with AD. Some were tested before it was realized that AD is a neurodegenerative disorder responsible for the majority of patients with so-called "senility" in the Untied States. Early trials of vasodilators were based on the mistaken premise that AD is secondary to "cerebral atherosclerosis." Drugs for this indication did not improve cognition in AD patients and are no longer marketed for this indication. The second class of agents tested were nootropic agents. The rationale for the use of many of these agents in AD was weak. Several large-scale, adequately controlled studies of nootropics have been carried out; the overall results are negative (14). A number of neuropeptides have also been tested in AD. Most were small-scale trials. However, a recent large-scale, multicenter trial involving 115 patients convincingly demonstrated the lack of efficacy of vasopressin in AD (15). Results with most other neuropeptides remain uncertain. Administration of neuropeptides is fraught with many difficulties, including peripheral degradation and failure to cross the blood-brain barrier. For example, a somatostatin analog was administered to six patients with AD (16). The results were negative. More importantly, however, there was no evidence of somatostatin in the cerebrospinal fluid of any of these patients (16).

During the last decade, a great deal of time and energy has been focused on drugs designed to alter cholinergic functioning. This focus has occurred because, although many other neurotransmitters are disordered in AD, the deficit in cholinergic neurotransmission is the most robust of all the neurotransmitters studied. In addition, changes in the cholinergic system correlate best with changes in mental status test scores. Adequate testing using the acetylcholine precursors choline and lecithin now exist. Results from the well-controlled double-blind studies are uniformly negative (14). In addition, results from the majority of studies utilizing cholinergic agonists are also negative. However, many of the cholinergic agonists chosen were inappropriate agents and should not have been utilized to treat AD patients (see Chapter 5). Most agonists tested were actually mixed agonists-antagonists. Many produced unacceptable peripheral toxicity and lacked adequate selectivity for the central nervous system.

The third main category of cholinomimetic agents examined are the cholinesterase inhibitors. Most double-blind, placebo-controlled studies utilizing the intravenous cholinesterase inhibitor physostigmine reported positive results. Studies utilizing orally administered physostigmine are mixed, with about one half reporting positive results while the remainder are negative. Approximately 125 patients have received immediate-release physostigmine, and approximately 30–40% of these individuals have shown improvement in verbal memory (14). However, the pharmacokinetic profile of immediate-release physostigmine is suboptimal, since peak plasma levels are reached within 30 minutes, followed by complete disappearance of the drug within 2 hours. More recently, a number of longer-acting, controlled-release physostigmine preparations have been developed. These are currently in clinical trials.

A second cholinesterase inhibitor, tetrahydroaminoacridine (THA), has received considerable attention following an earlier report claiming remarkable improvement in 16 of 17 AD patients treated with THA (17). This study, however, has been criticized on methodological grounds. Two additional studies have since been completed in Canada (19) and France (20). Both reported negative results in crossover design trials. The largest THA trial, a multicenter trial in the United States, was completed during the latter portion of 1990 but is not available at this time.

While 10 or 15 years ago very few drugs were being developed for AD, we now have the opposite situation. At the present time, 15–20 drugs for AD are either in, or about to enter, human clinical trials. Using very restrictive criteria for inclusion and exclusion of subjects into clinical trials, the readily available supply of patients meeting inclusion criteria may soon be exhausted. Two major questions that will be faced in the future are 1) should this large a number of drugs enter clinical trials, given the major cost, time, and effort involved in the conduct of these trials, and 2) do we need to alter the inclusion/exclusion criteria to make experimental drugs available to a larger, more representative, cohort of subjects? These are all very real, perplexing, and complex issues that need to be dealt with during the next decade.

REFERENCES

1. Wolozin B, Davies P. Alzheimer-related neuronal protein A68: specificity and distribution. Ann Neurol 22:521–526, 1987.
2. Ghanbari HA, Miler BE, Haigler HJ, et al. Biochemical assay of Alzheimer's disease-associated protein(s) in human brain tissue. JAMA 263:2907-2910, 1990.
3. McKhann G, Drachman D, Folstein MF, et al. Clinical diagnosis of Alzheimer's disease: report of the NINCDS-ADRDA work group. Neurology 34:939–944, 1984.
4. Wade JPH, Mirsen TR, Hachinski VC, et al. The clinical diagnosis of Alzheimer's disease. Arch Neurol 44:24–29, 1987.
5. Evans DA, Funkenstein HH, Albert MS, et al. Prevalence of Alzheimer's disease in a community population of older persons. JAMA 262:2551–2556, 1989.
6. Molsa PK, Marttila RJ, Rinne UK. Epidemiology of dementia in a Finnish population. Acta Neurol Scand 65:541–552, 1982.
7. Schoenberg BS, Anderson DW, Haerer AF. Severe dementia: prevalence and clinical features in a biracial US population. Arch Neurol 42:740–743, 1985.
8. Nee LE, Polinsky RJ, Eldridge R, et al. A family with histologically confirmed Alzheimer's disease. Arch Neurol 40:203–208, 1983.
9. St George-Hyslop, Tanzi R, Polinsky RJ, et al. The genetic defect causing familial Alzheimer disease maps on chromosome 21. Science 235:885–890, 1987.
10. Zhang M, Katzman R, Salmon D, et al. The prevalence of dementia and Alzheimer's disease in Shanghai, China: Impact of age, gender, and education. Ann Neurol 27:428–437, 1990.
11. Aronson MK, Ooi WL, Morgenstern H, et al. Women, myocardial infarction, and dementia in the very old. Neurology 40:1102–1106, 1990.
12. Katzman R, Brown T, Thal LJ, et al. Comparison of rate of annual change of mental status score in four independent studies of patients with Alzheimer's disease. Ann Neurol 24:384–389, 1988.
13. Nee, LE, Elderidge R, Sunderland T, et al. Dementia of the Alzheimer type: clinical and family study of 22 twin pairs. Neurology 37:359–363, 1987.
14. Thal LJ. Pharmacological treatment of memory disorders. In Boller F, Grafman J, (eds). *Handbook of Neuropsychology*. Vol 3. Elsevier Science Publishers, Amsterdam, 1989, pp. 247–267.

15. Wolters ECh, Riekkinen P, Lowenthal A, et al. DGAVP (Org 5667) in early Alzheimer's disease patients: An international double-blind, placebo-controlled, multicenter trial. Neurology 40:1099–1101, 1990.
16. Cutler NR, Haxby JU, Narung PK, et al. Evaluation of an analogue of somatostatin (L363,586) in Alzheimer's disease. N Engl J Med 312:725, 1985.
17. Summers WK, Majovski LV, Marsh GM, et al. Oral tetrahydroaminoacridine in long-term treatment of senile dementia, Alzheimer type. N Engl J Med 315:1241–1245, 1986.
18. Gauthier S, Bouchard R, Lamontagne A, et al. Tetrahydroaminoacridine-lecithin combination treatment in patients with intermediate-stage Alzheimer's disease. N Engl J Med 322:1272–1276, 1990.
19. Chatellier G, Lacomblez L. Tacrine (tetrahydroaminoacridine; THA) and lecithin in senile dementia of the Alzheimer type: A multicentre trial. Br Med J 300: 395–399, 1990.

2

Clinical Trials in Alzheimer's Disease: State of the Art and Future Directions

Peter J. Whitehouse
University Hospitals of Cleveland, Cleveland, Ohio

The following discussion is organized into three categories: basic research, clinical studies, and societal perspectives. First, considerable advances in our understanding of the molecular biology and systems neuroscience of AD have been made. What do they contribute to the development of effective therapy? Second, several natural history studies and multicenter clinical trials have been conducted over the last several years. How can they be used to improve the design of future studies? Third, attempts to develop effective therapies for AD are occurring in an increasingly active public policy arena concerned with health-care reform. How will the behavior of policy makers influence our future work in this area?

I. BASIC RESEARCH

The major focus for developing AD therapies has been the basal forebrain cholinergic system, since dysfunction in this cell population relates more closely to the degree of intellectual impairment in AD than in any other single neurotransmitter system affected in the disorder. It is equally clear, however, that other neurotransmitter systems are affected in the disease. What types and degree of cognitive impairment are due to cholinergic dysfunction remain empirical questions. In many ways, the ultimate answer to these questions will depend on whether a drug that acts through the cholinergic system is efficacious enough to be approved for use in AD or related disorders that demonstrate loss of cholinergic markers. Most current effort is directed at developing cholinesterase inhibitors or selective muscarinic cholinergic agonists.

We have also learned more about how other neurotransmitters, such as γ-aminobutyric acid (GABA) and galanin, regulate basal forebrain neurons, which suggest indirect ways of modifying cholinergic neuron function. For example, antagonists of the inhibitory galaninergic inputs to basal forebrain might improve cognition (1). Moreover, some of the neurons in the basal forebrain that are not cholinergic may play a role in cognition (2).

Studies of cholinergic neurons may also lead to the development of strategies to actually slow disease progression. In my opinion, the major central question that we need to understand in AD—and degenerative disorders in general—is why neurons die. One reasonable hypothesis is that the death of neurons in disease may be due to dysfunction in the normal mechanisms that promote cell viability. Nerve growth factor (NGF), the first neurotrophic factor identified in the 1960s, has been found necessary for normal development of cholinergic neurons in the basal forebrain in cell culture and in in vivo animal models. Intraventricular NGF or one of the related trophic factors, such as brain-derived neurotrophic factor or neurotropin-3, may be tested in this country if animal safety and efficacy studies suggest its use. Human recombinant NGF has apparently already been given intraventricularly to at least one AD patient in Sweden. Even if growth factors are not effective therapeutically, understanding their mechanisms of action may lead to other clues about maintaining cell health in AD. In our laboratory, Dr. Gary Landreth and others are focusing on the mechanisms of action of NGF (3) and have recently characterized some of the kinases in the second messenger cascade activated by NGF. With his colleague, Dr. Jeffrey Twiss, he has also recently identified, and is in the process of cloning, genes that are specifically activated by NGF (unpublished observations).

As other speakers discussed, another critical research area in AD is the development of a biological marker that allows more accurate premortem diagnosis. Dr. Robert Friedland of our center, in collaboration with investigators in St. Louis and Boston, is attempting to use positron emission tomography to label β-amyloid markers in blood vessels. Dr. Steven Younkin in our group has recently reported alterations in the ratios of the different products of the amyloid precursor protein in CSF which seem to discriminate AD patients from controls (7). Moreover, these changes in the ratio of the 105 kilodalton to 25 kilodalton segments of the amyloid precursor protein appear to correlate with the severity of dementia. Many other investigators and commercial companies are attempting to develop a diagnostic test based on detecting either neurofibrillary tangle or senile plaque components in cerebrospinal fluid.

Another area of development of diagnostic tests relies on detecting disease markers outside the nervous system, either in biopsy of tissue or blood products.

We have recently discovered abnormalities in membrane fluidity restricted to the internal membrane fragments (4). This finding builds on previous work suggesting that abnormalities in membranes may occur in peripheral and central nervous system cells in AD (5,6). The development of a more specific diagnostic test of AD would clearly help in the process of designing drug studies by ensuring greater homogeneity of diagnoses in the study. However, these approaches may be limited by overlap in distributions of measured variables between normal aging and AD.

II. CLINICAL STUDIES

Through the 20 National Institute on Aging Alzheimer's Disease Research Centers and other centers, thousands of Alzheimer's patients have been followed and observed carefully as studies of natural history and drug intervention are performed. As Dr. Leon J. Thal has pointed out (Chapter 1), we now known more about the rate of the decline in cognitive abilities over time in AD. These studies will allow us to measure the effects of drugs designed to slow the progression of the disease against the backdrop of a greater understanding of the natural history of the disorder. Unfortunately, these studies demonstrate that the rate of decline is quite variable, and this problem of clinical heterogeneity will continue to vex AD pharmacologists. For example, several authors have claimed that AD has subtypes based on factors such as age of onset, family history, associated neurological and psychiatric symptoms, and even rate of decline; the term "benign" AD has even been suggested (8-10). The issue that continues to surface in the design of new studies is the range of severity properly included in the drug protocol. Many continue to believe that patients with mild AD are more likely to respond to drugs, since less neuronal loss has occurred and more flexibility of neuronal response to drugs is likely. Understanding the relationship between responsiveness and disease stage can clearly be enhanced by reviewing current protocols, such as those involving cholinesterase inhibitors, to see if such a correlation exists. My own belief is that we ought to consider expanding the entrance criteria for studies to include patients that are more severely demented. I also believe that a trend occurring over the past several years to include patients with more concurrent medications and illnesses will continue. Although broadening entrance criteria might increase the error variance, changes in exclusion criteria would enhance subject eligibility and might alleviate some of the practical problems in recruitment mentioned by Dr. Thal and others. One also needs to be creative about where to find patients. For example, the new day-care program adjacent to our Alzheimer Center may enable us to study drug effects in patients in an environment in which patients are present for a considerable period during the day. We are also starting drug studies in special-care units in nursing homes; research on these units has shown that their patients tend to be less severely demented and have less concomitant medical illnesses than patients in regular nursing home wards.

A frequently cited subtype of patient is the one that appears to respond to a particular medication. When study results indicate that a small subgroup of individuals benefits from the drug, the investigator will often claim that a "drug responder" subtype exists. However, identifying the characteristics of a patient who is going to be drug responsive prior to entering the study has proven difficult. "Drug responders" may, in many cases, represent the tail of a distribution reflecting chance improvements occurring in relation to testing the drug. A test of whether a patient is really a drug responder or not is to stop the drug, rechallenge, and compare the patient with others who had not responded previously. The so-called enriched design used in the HP 029, oral physostigmine, and Tacrine studies can be examined retrospectively to see whether the design allowed patients who were more likely to respond to a drug to enter the study. In the oral physostigmine trial, both those who did and did not appear to respond in an initial dose-finding phase are being entered into the double-blind phase. In this protocol, the investigators will be able to determine whether this initial dose-finding phase did, in fact, enrich the double-blind phase with patients who were more likely to respond to the drug.

It also seems reasonable that if one can identify a specific patient or a small group of patients who do respond particularly dramatically to a drug, this population of patients should be studied more intensively to determine for example, which particular neuropsychological or global assessment instrument is most sensitive to drug effects. This information could then be taken to a larger population of patients. As Dr. Gamzu said, and I concur, we have not made tremendous advances in the ability of our assessment instruments to detect drug effect. It seems reasonable to develop tests based on animal models of cognition, such as delayed matched-to-sample. In addition, computerized testing will have potentially great advantage, particularly as computers become cheaper and more portable. Computer testing can be made ecologically valid, for example, by having patients watch a television screen of people's faces that they are supposed to remember or actually use a telephone in recalling telephone numbers. Computerization also allows the measurement of reaction time, which may be more sensitive than error measurements to drug effect. Expanded computerized testing outside the experimental site where nonprofessionals can be asked to record data will be explored. Finally, the computerization of data allows more efficient information management, which will be increasingly important in future multicenter international studies.

As a final clinical studies comment, I again agree with Dr. Thal that a major area that has not been addressed is the behavioral and psychiatric aspect of Alzheimer's disease. Studies such as those performed in Cleveland by Mendez et al. (11) and Patterson et al. (12) show that the major sources of caregiver stress are, in fact, the agitation, wandering, hallucinations, and delusions, or what Dr. Drachman calls "obstreperous behaviors." Clinicians use antidepressants and major and minor tranquilizers with little empirical data to guide their use. Some of these drugs may have specific effects in AD since, for example, bioaminergic nuclei in the brainstem, namely, the locus ceruleus and raphe, have distinct pathology in AD and neuropsychiatric drugs may act through these neural systems.

III. SOCIETAL PERSPECTIVES

AD's most important societal perspective is its epidemiology. Recent estimates suggest that almost 50% of people over the age of 85 develop AD and demonstrate that the risk of getting AD increases dramatically as one ages (13)—potentially making AD an even greater problem in countries whose life expectancy is higher, such as Japan. The evaluation of drugs in AD is taking on an increasingly international perspective. With the rapid changes occurring in the pharmaceutical industry in Japan and with the formation of the European economic community, more standardization of studies is likely to occur, and more studies will cross national boundaries.

Society also needs better education of professionals and the lay public in AD and the process of drug development. As drugs for this disorder come on the market, professionals need to understand their use as well as the diagnostic evaluation necessary to ensure appropriateness for a patient. Educating the public about the process of drug development is perhaps our most pressing task. The Alzheimer's Association plays an important role in the dissemination of information about drug studies. We have to avoid the shattered expectations that occur when breakthroughs are reported in the press which turn out to be less important than originally portrayed. The complexities of the drug development process need to be explained so that the costs involved are understood. We also need to stress the critical role of the Food and Drug Administration (FDA). Under Dr. Paul Leber's leadership, his Division is providing guidance to the pharmaceutical industry in this difficult area of drug development. Their group will soon issue general guidelines resulting from a July 1989 meeting. As the number of drug studies continues to rise, it will become increasingly difficult for the already understaffed FDA to provide assistance and to evaluate all this data; the public must recognize that more resources are needed to keep up with the activity in this field.

A final important issue is conflict of interest. To my mind, this holds two opposing dangers. Too much concern results in restrictive regulation that decreases productive science, while too little attention to this problem leads to untrustworthy science. Difficulties can be avoided if relationships between industry and academia are identified in appropriate places, such as journal articles. Potentially conflicting motivations are of more concern to people when they are not disclosed. Academic investigators should continue to consult and collaborate with pharmaceutical companies, even if they are involved in studying a drug: preclinical consultation is key to bringing the latest in academic basic research to the applied drug research arenas and impeding such collaboration will delay production of effective therapies. Clinical consulting allows investigators and companies to develop relationships that permit selecting the best drugs and testing sites for the later stages of drug development. To support our center's educational and research activities, I consult for and receive some financial support from Warner Lambert/Parke-Davis and Bristol-Myers/Squibb (as well as others). Although I do not personally evaluate patients in the studies, our group is currently testing their products. I do believe, however, that academics should not evaluate a medication if they could benefit directly from the approval of that medication. Thus, ownership of a company or its stock should preclude someone from participating in a study evaluating that company's drugs. No contracts between companies and evaluation sites should include royalties based on a successful approval process. The greatest area of difficulty is *perception* of conflict of interest, where conflict is in the eye of the beholder, e.g., policy makers, the Securities and Exchange Commission, or members of a regulatory body. Whether some relationship is perceived to be a conflict depends on the history of the relationship between that observer and the individuals in question and relates to the degree of trust already present in that relationship. Scientists, clinicians, regulators, and companies involved in drug development need to improve communication of the importance of our collaborations and to avoid real conflicts of interest when they exist. I believe that it would be foolish if we allowed every *possibility* of perception of conflict of interest to preclude establishing working relationships between academics and industry.

IV. CONCLUSION

We are entering an exciting phase of drug development in AD. Tacrine has been submitted for consideration for approval by the FDA. More multicenter studies are underway than ever before involving companies around the world. Basic research is allowing hopes, not only for palliative therapy but for therapies to slow the progression of the disease. It will remain, however, a daunting goal to develop medication to improve the ability of a human being to think.

REFERENCES

1. Crawley JN, Wenk GL. Co-existence of galanin and acetylcholine: is galanin involved in memory processes and dementia? Trend Neurosic 12(8):278–282, 1989.
2. Wenk GL, Markowska AL, Olton DS. Basal forebrain lesions and memory: Alterations in neurotensin, not acetylcholine, may cause amnesia. Neurosci 103(4):765–769, 1989.

3. Landreth GF, Smith DS, McCabe C, Gittinger C. Characterization of a nerve growth factor-stimulated protein kinase in PC12 cells which phosphorylates microtubule-associated protein 2 and pp250. Neurochem 55(2):514-523, 1990.
4. Piletz JE, Sarasua M, Whitehouse PJ, Chotani M. Increased intracellular membrane fluidity in platelets from Alzheimer's disease patients. Arch Neurol (Submitted for publication).
5. Pettegrew JW, Minshew NJ, Cohen MM, Kopp SJ, Glonek T. P-31 NMR changes in Alzheimer's and Huntington's disease brain. Neurology 34:281, 1984.
6. Zubenko GS, Cohen BM, Reynolds CF III, Boller F, Malinakova I, Keefe N. Platelet membrane fluidity in Alzheimer's disease and major depression. Am J Psychiatr 144:860-868, 1987.
7. Palmert MR, Usiak M, Mayeux R, Raskind M, Tourtellotte WW, Younkin SG. Soluble derivatives of the β amyloid protein precursor in cerebrospinal fluid: Alterations in normal aging and in Alzheimer's disease. Neurology 40:1028-1034, 1990.
8. Friedland RP, Koss E, Haxby JV, Grady CL, Luxenberg J, Schapiro MB, Kaye J. Alzheimer disease: clinical and biological heterogeneity. Ann Intern Med 109:298-311, 1988.
9. Jorn AF. Subtypes of Alzheimer's dementia: A conceptual analysis and critical review. Psychol Med 15:543-553, 1985.
10. Mayeux R, Stern Y, Spanton S. Heterogeneity in dementia of the Alzheimer type: Evidence of subgroups. Neurology 35:453-461, 1985.
11. Mendez MF, Martin RJ, Smyth KA, Whitehouse PJ. Psychiatric symptoms associated with Alzheimer's disease. J Neuropsych Clin Neurosci 2:28-33, 1990.
12. Patterson MB, Schnell AH, Martin RJ, Mendez MF, Smyth KA, Whitehouse PJ. Assessment of behavioral and affective symptoms in Alzheimer's disease. J Geriatr Psychiatr Neurol 3:21-30, 1990.
13. Evans DA, Funkenstein HH, ALbert MS, Scherr PA, Cook NR, Chown MJ, Hebert LE, Hennekens CH, Taylor JO. Prevalence of Alzheimer's disease in a community population of older persons: Higher than previously reported. JAMA 262:2551-2556, 1989.

3

Strategies for the Treatment of Multi-Neurotransmitter Deficits in Alzheimer's Disease

Kenneth L. Davis
Mount Sinai School of Medicine/Medical Center, New York, New York
Vahram Haroutunian
The Bronx Veterans Affairs Medical Center, Bronx, New York

The focus of this paper is the question of whether animal models can teach us anything about the basis for the heterogeneous response to cholinesterase inhibitors. Table 1 (1-14) summarizes the literature on cholinesterase treatments in Alzheimer's disease. The table clearly suggests a heterogeneity of responsivity to these inhibitors. Some of the variance is due to problems in pharmacokinetics, such as the drug simply not getting absorbed or not getting into the brain (3,5,15). However, other reasons for this heterogeneity presumably could be due to the numerous neurotransmitter deficits that exist in Alzheimer's disease (16-21) and are not directly affected by a cholinesterase inhibitor.

Animal models can be used to study the effects of neurotransmitter deficits. By using a series of neurotoxins, such as ibotenic acid, quisqualic acid, N-methyl-D-aspartic acid, cysteamine, 6-hydroxydopamine, and parachloroamphetamine, it is possible to create multiple neurotransmitter deficits in a rodent's brain. Table 2 presents the typical results from a ibotenic acid lesion made by injecting the drug bilaterally into the nucleus basalis. By this method, we can produce a relatively selective cholinergic depletion of around 30-40%. The topographic distribution of this lesion is rather exquisite (Table 3); it is possible that in certain areas this deficiency is significantly greater than 30%, whereas in other areas it is significantly less, averaging 30-40% for the whole cortex.

As has been shown repeatedly, animals with a nucleus basalis lesion show a deficit in passive avoidance learning (22,23). Figure 1 displays the typical in-

Table 1 Cholinesterase Inhibitor Treatment in Patients With Alzheimer's Disease (AD)

Patients	Drug & doses	Mode of administration	Results	Ref.
8 (58–83 yr): Met *DSM-III* criteria for primary degenerative dementia	Physostigmine 0.5, 1.0, 2.0 mg q2h	Oral	Improvement in primary memory	1
8: Clinical diagnosis of Alzheimer's presenile dementia	Physostigmine 1.0 mg qid	Oral	No improvement in memory or behavior	2
12 (52–76 yr): Clinical history and current mental status consistent with AD disgnosis	Physostigmine 0.5, 1.0, 1.5, 2.0 mg qid	Oral	Cognitive improvement correlated with cortisol rise	3
22 (67 yr): Met *DSM-III* criteria for primary degenerative dementia	Physostigmine 2–4 mg q2h	Oral	No effect on memory	4
8 (55–78 yr): Clinical signs of AD	Physostigmine 0.5–2.5 mg q2h plus lecithin 10.8 g/day	Oral	Significant increase in verbal memory	5
16 (56–80 yr): Early stages of AD	Physostigmine 2.0, 3.0, 4.0 mg qid	Oral	Improvement in memory but not other areas of cognition	6
8 (59–70 yr): Clinically diagnosed mild to severe AD	Physostigmine 1–2 mg q2h plus lecithin 18 g/day	Oral	No improvement in praxis, language orientation or behavior	7

12 (54–68 yr): Progressing with memory disturbance before age 65	Physostigmine 0.75 mg	i.v.	Significant improvement in recognition and memory	8
11: Clinical diagnosis of Alzheimer presenile dementia	Physostigmine 0.25, 0.375, 0.75 mg	i.v.	Significant increases in picture recognition	9
10 (56–68 yr): Clinical diagnosis of AD	Physostigmine 0.125, 0.25, 0.5 mg	i.v.	Significant increases in recognition memory	10
6 (51–63 yr): Clinical diagnosis of presenile dementia of the Alzheimer type	Physostigmine 0.3–1.0 mg	i.v. or s.c.	3 of 6 showed improvement in praxis	11
5 (58–79 yr): Diagnosed from history of progressive decline in memory, spatial orientation and judgment	Physostigmine 0.005–0.015 mg/kg plus 3.6 g lecithin	s.c.	4 of 5 showed improvement in verbal learning	12
10 (51–71 yr): Met *DSM-III* diagnostic criteria for primary degenerative dementia	THA 30 mg plus lecithin	Oral	Significant increase in serial learning for least demented patients	13
12 (42–85 yr): Unselected cases of Alzheimer-like senile dementia	THA 0.25–1.5 mg/kg	i.v.	Significant improvement in orientation for some patients	14

DSM-III = *Diagnostic and Statistical Manual*, 3rd ed.

Table 2 Effects of Ibotenic Acid Lesions of the nbM on Cortical Values of Some Neurochemical Markers*

Marker	Sham	nbM	% Depletion
Choline acetyltransferase (nmol ACh/h/mg protein)	19.2 ± 0.3 (12)	14.1 ± 0.7 (14)	26.3†
Acetylcholinesterase (nmol/h/mg protein)	1512 ± 24 (12)	1070 ± 54 (14)	29.1†
Norepinephrine (ng/100 mg tissue)	30.1 ± 0.8 (12)	29.1 ± 0.9 (14)	3.2
Depamine (ng/100 mg tissue)	6.7 ± 0.2 (12)	6.4 ± 0.3 (14)	5.2
Serotonin (ng/100 mg tissue)	32.2 ± 0.8 (11)	29.0 ± 0.8 (12)	9.9
Somatostatin-LI (pg/mg tissue)	377.8 ± 11 (12)	387 ± 18 (12)	2.6
CRF (pg/mg tissue)	1.9 ± 0.1 (12)	1.8 ± 0.1 (12)	3.1

*Values expressed as mean ± SEM (n).
†nbM vs. Sham, $p < 0.01$.

Table 3 Regional Cortical Depletion of Choline Acetyltransferase (ChAT) Following NMDA-Induced Lesions of the nbM*

Site (distance from frontal pole)	ChAT (nM ACh/h/mg protein)	% of Sham
Frontal 0–2 mm	13.3 ± 1.2	42.8
Frontal 2–4 mm	10.1 ± 1.2	33.0
Frontal 4–6 mm	8 7 ± 0.6	31.0
Frontal 6–8	8.1 ± 0.3	27.1
Occipital 8–16 mm	23.0 ± 1.8	73.2

*Values expressed as mean ± SEM (n).

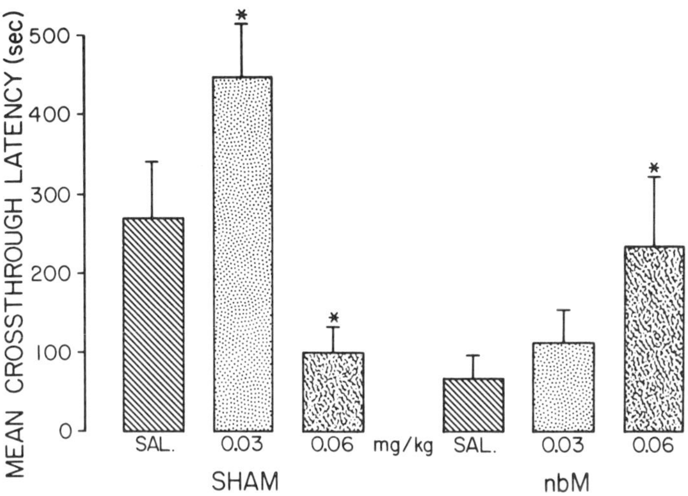

Figure 1 Effects of 0.0–0.06 mg/kg physostigmine on the 72-hour retention of one trial passive avoidance in nbM-lesioned and sham-operated rats. (Ns = 12.)

verted U-shaped curve, the effect of physostigmine on the ability of a group of animals to perform a passive avoidance task. In animals with a nucleus basalis lesion, a dose of 0.06 mg/kg of physostigmine normalizes their passive avoidance behavior. It is striking how easily cholinomimetic compounds normalize the behavior of animals with a nucleus basalis deficiency. Indeed, in our hands all cholinomimetic compounds tested (physostigmine, oxotremorine, 4-amino-pyridine) do so. These results are in stark contrast to what happens in Alzheimer's disease, where perhaps between 30–45% of patients have a modest improvement following treatment with cholinesterase inhibitors (Table 1).

As a consequence of the discrepancy between clinical experiments and laboratory results with nucleus basalis lesioned animals, subsequent experiments were designed to elucidate the basis for the difference between lesioned animals and Alzheimer's patients in responsivity to cholinomimetics. In these studies, it was decided to administer a series of other neurotoxic agents to produce the additional neurotransmitter deficiencies that exist in the brains of people with Alzheimer's disease.

The first focus of the studies was somatostatin depletion, because it is reported in the literature to be relatively ubiquitous in Alzheimer's patients (19,20). It was thought that the addition of a somatostatin depletion, through the use of cysteamine, may in fact produce a decrement in the efficacy of physostigmine in lesioned animals (24,25).

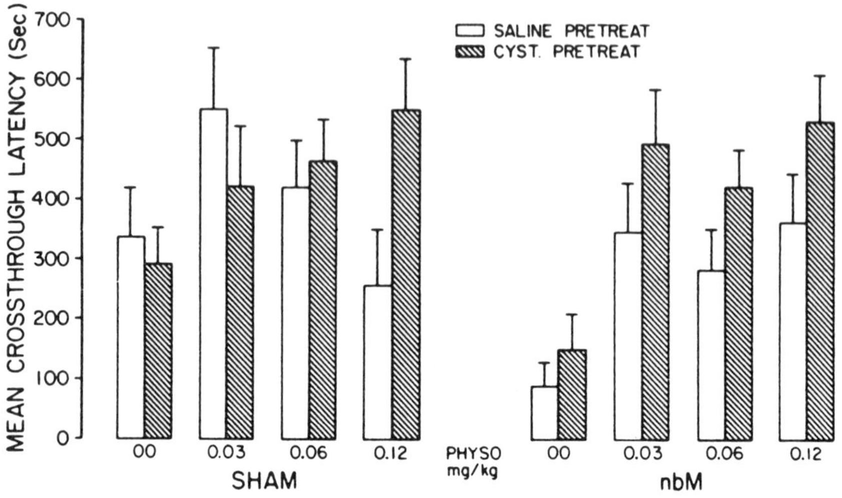

Figure 2 Effects of 0.0–0.12 mg/kg physostigmine on the passive avoidance retention test performance of nbM- or sham-lesioned rats pretreated for 3 consecutive days with 150 mg/kg cysteamine. (Ns = 10–12.) (From Ref. 25. Reproduced with permission of the publisher.

Figure 2 summarizes the results of studies in which somatostatin and cholinergic lesions were produced. Ibotenic acid-induced nucleus basalia-lesioned animals were pretreated with cysteamine, in a dose relatively selective for somatostatin depletion (150 mg/kg leading to a 48% depletion of cortical somatostatin levels). When such animals received physostigmine, their performance was indistinguishable from control animals. In other words, the addition of a somatostatin depletion to nucleus basalis-lesioned animals did not result in the loss of activity of the cholinergic agent to enhance performance on a passive avoidance task. Therefore, another deficiency must account for the lack of some efficacy of the cholinomimetic in Alzheimer's disease.

Noradrenergic lesions were produced both with DSP-4 or with 6-hydroxydopamine (26). When animals receive DSP-4, depletions like those reported in Table 4 were obtained. They are modest depletions; nonetheless, they are statistically significant and comparable to those seen in a subset of Alzheimer's patients. Animals treated with DSP-4 have a host of changes in their responsivity to cholinergic agents. For example, control animals, who receive a dose of oxotremorine of .2 mg/kg body weight display catalepsy. However, the effect of increasing doses of DSP-4 on the ability of oxotremorine to induce catalepsy is to obliterate the effect of oxotremorine to induce this cholinergic behavior. Here is a behavior, but not a cognitive behavior, that is dependent for its expression on the

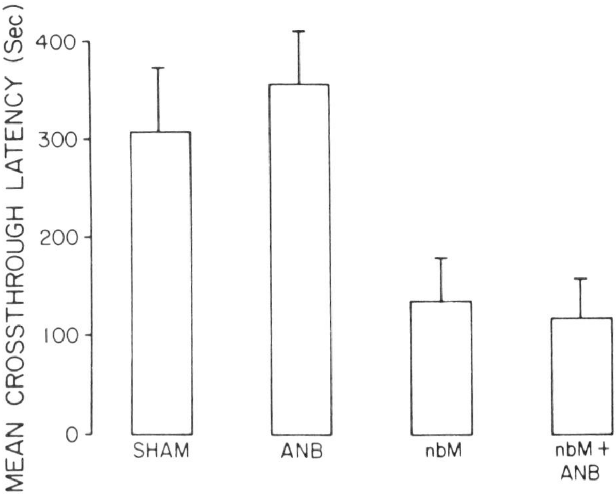

Figure 3 Effects of bilateral lesions of the nbM, ascending noradrenergic bundle (ANB), or nbM + ANB on the 72-hour retention of passive avoidance. (Ns = 8-10.)

intactness of the noradrenergic system. Obviously this result raises the question of whether the loss of the intactness of the noradrenergic system would alter the memory-enhancing properties of the cholinergic drugs.

The animals depicted in Figure 3 have a 6-hydroxydopamine-induced lesion in the ascending noradrenergic bundle (ANB) as well as an ibotenic acid-induced nucleus basalis lesion. A subset of animals has only a deficit in choline acetyl transferase (CAT) and cholinesterase activity. Other animals have only a norepinephrine deficit. Hence there are a series of animals with both noradrenergic and cholinergic lesions as well as cholinergic and noradrenergic lesions alone.

Table 4 Effects of Different Doses of DSP-4 on Forebrain Norepinephrine Levels (ng/mg Tissue)

DSP-4 dose	Frontal CTX	Hippocampus	Hypothalamus
0.0	52.9 ± 1.3	21.6 ± 1.9	24.5 ± 1.6
12.5	40.5 ± 2.9	19.1 ± 2.1	22.1 ± 1.9
25.0	24.1 ± 4.3	8.6 ± 2.0	19.0 ± 1.8
50.0	22.3 ± 3.8	8.7 ± 2.8	19.6 ± 2.2
75.0	7.1 ± 1.3	2.1 ± 0.2	15.9 ± 2.8

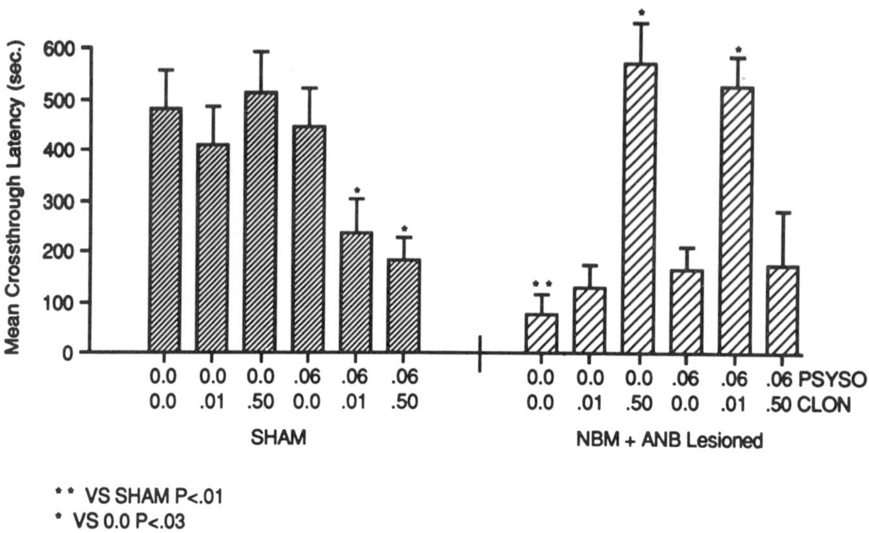

Figure 4 Effects of post-acquisition administrationof clonidine and physostigmine either alone or in combination on the 72-hour retention of passive avoidance in nbM + ANB-lesioned rats. (Ns = 11-12.) (From Ref. 26. Reproduced with permission of the publisher.)

Figure 4 displays the effect of physostigmine in increasing doses on controls and animals with nucleus basalis/ANB lesions. The sham controls respond, as do other animals in previous experiments, to increasing doses of physostigmine with the usual inverted U-shaped curve, with maximal improvement at 0.03 mg/kg. If these had been lesioned nucleus basalis animals, the ideal does would be .06 mg/kg. In contrast, the animals with the double lesion show no effect of drug over a broad dose range. The efficacy of the cholinergic agent to improve performance on a passive avoidance task, by adding a noradrenergic lesion to the nucleus basalis lesion has been completely lost.

Could the positive effect of the physostigmine be restored by treating these animals with a noradrenergic agent such as clonidine? Figure 4 displays the answer to this question. When animals who have the combined nucleus basalis/ANB lesion are treated with 0.06 mg/kg of physostigmine they are not improved, but when just 0.01 mg/kg of clonidine was added to the dose of physostigmine, passive avoidance behavior was again normalized. A very high dose of clonidine by itself also normalized the animals, but this is a dose that could not possibly be administered to humans because of the hypotention inducing effects. It is also a rather nonspecific dose, attacking numerous neurotransmitters. It is important to realize that these animals have such a profound noradrenergic lesion that clonidine's effect was postsynaptic. Consequently clonidine was enhancing noradrenergic activity.

These results encouraged the combining of cholinergic and noradrenergic agents in patients with Alzheimer's disease. However, such studies are exceedingly complex. Cholinomimetic plus adrenergic agents could provide complex interactions on the cardiovascular system; as a consequence, studies have proceeded with caution. Alpha-2 agonists combined with cholinesterase inhibitors are a rational first choice.

The α_2 agonists clonidine and guanfacine have been studied in old monkeys by Arnsten and Goldman-Rakic (27), as well as in humans by McEntee and Main (28). Those studies, have produced some really compelling evidence for the ability of the α_2 agonist to have favorable effects on delayed spatial matching to sample tasks.

The argument for a noradrenergic drug is also supported by numerous postmortem studies that document the loss of norepinephrine, MHPG, and locus coeruleus cells in Alzheimer's disease (16–18). However, this is a variable abnormality that occurs within the cholinergic system. There are in fact elderly patients with Alzheimer's disease who have a basically intact locus, whereas there are other people, generally younger and with a longer duration of illness, who have a profound deficit.

It is interesting to superimpose the results of post mortem studies on the noradrenergic system, with responsivity rates to cholinesterase inhibitors. It is noted that the number of patients who are relatively devoid of profound noradrenergic problems approximates the number of Alzheimer's patients who seem to have a modest response to cholinesterase inhibitors. The problem remains, then, to establish markers which will identify patients who will respond to cholinergic treatment. A recent report (29) suggests that blood pressure drop may be a possible predictor of response to cholinesterase inhibitor in Alzheimer's disease. Patients who did not respond to the cholinesterase inhibitor HP 029 showed a significantly greater decrease in postural blood pressure drop, perhaps due to an underlying autonomic dysfunction. Therefore, in the future, patients who show defects in sympathetic responsivity may be candidates for combined cholinomimetic and noradrenergic therapies.

REFERENCES

1. Beller SA, Overall JE, Swann AC. Efficacy of oral physostigmine in primary degenerative dementia. Psychopharmacology 87:147–151, 1985.
2. Caltagirone C, Gainotti G, Masullo C. Oral administration of chronic physostigmine does not improve cognitive or mnesic performance in Alzheimer's presenile dementia. Int J Neurosci 16:247–249, 1982.

3. Mohs RC, Davis BM, Johns CA, Mathe AA, et al. Oral physostigmine treatment of patients with Alzheimer's disease. Am J Psychiatr 142:28–33, 1985.
4. Stern Y, Sano M, Mayeux R. Effects of oral physostigmine in Alzheimer's disease. Ann Neurol 22: 306–310, 1987.
5. Thal LJ, Flud PA, Masur DM, et al. Oral physostigmine and lecithin improve memory in Alzheimer disease. Ann Neurol 13:491–496, 1983.
6. Thal LJ, Masur DM, Blau AD, et al. Chronic oral physostigmine without lecithin improves memory in Alzheimer disease. J Am Geriatr Soc 37:42–48, 1989.
7. Wettstein A. No effect from double-blind trial of physostigmine and lecithin in Alzheimer's disease. Ann Neurol 13:210–212, 1983.
8. Blackwood DHR, Christie JE. The effects of physostigmine on memory and auditory P300 in Alzheimer-type dementia. Biol Psychiatry 21:557–560, 1986.
9. Christie JE, Shering A, Ferguson J, et al. Physostigmine and arecoline: Effects of intravenous infusions in Alzheimer presenile dementia. Br J Psychiatr 138:56–50, 1981.
10. Davis KL, Mohs RC. Enhancement of memory processes in Alzheimer's disease with multiple-dose intravenous physostigmine. Am J Psychiatr 139:1421–1424, 1982.
11. Muramoto O, Sugishita M, Ando K. Cholinergic system and constructional praxis: a further study of physostigmine in lzheimer's disease. J Neurol Neurosurg Psychiatr 47:485–491, 1984.
12. Peters BH, Levin HS. Effects of physostigmine and lecithin on memory in ALzheimer disease. Ann Neurol 6:219–221, 1979.
13. Kaye WH, Sitaram N, Weingartner H, et al. Modest facilitation of memory in dementia with combined lecithin and anticholinesterase treatment. Biol Psychiatr 17:275–280, 1982.
14. Summers WK, Viesselman JO, Marsh GM, et al. Treatment of Alzheimer-like dementia: Pilot study in twelve patients. Biol Psychiatr 16:145–153, 1981.
15. Sherman KA, Kumar V, Ashford JW, et al. Effects of oral physostigmine in senile dementia patients: Utility of blood cholinesterase inhibition and neuroendocrine responses to define pharmacokinetics and pharmacodynamics. In Strong R (ed). *Central Nervous System Disorders of Aging: Strategies for Intervention.* Vol. 33, Raven Press, New York, 1987, pp. 71–90.
16. Arai H, Kosaka K, Iizuka R. Changes of biogenic amines and their metabolites in postmortem brains from patients with Alzheimer's-type dementia. J Neurochem 43:388–393, 1984.
17. Bondareff W, Mountjoy CQ, Roth M. Loss of neurons of origin of the adrenergic projection to cerebral cortex (nucleus locus ceruleus) in senile dementia. Neurology 32: 164–168, 1982.
18. Cross AJ. Serotonin in neurodegenerative disorders. In Osborn NN, Hamon M (eds.: *Neuronal Serotonin.* John Wiley & Sons, New York, 1987, pp. 231–254.
19. Davies P, Katzman R, Terry RD. Reduced somatostatin-like immunoreactivity in cerebral cortex from cases of Alzheimer's disease Alzheimer's senile dementia. Nature 288:279–280, 1980.
20. Davies P, Terry RD. Cortical somatostatin-like immunoreactivity in cases of Alzheimer's disease and senile dementia of Alzheimer's type. Neurobiol Aging 2:9–14, 1981.

21. DeSouza EB, Whitehouse PJ, Kuhar MJ, et al. Reciprocal changes in corticotropin-releasing factor (CRF)-like immunoreactivity and CRF receptors in cerebral cortex of Alzheimer's disease. Nature 319:593-595, 1986.
22. Haroutunian V, Kanof PD, Davis KL. Pharmacological alleviation of cholinergic lesion induced memory deficits in rats. Life Sci 37:945-952, 1985.
23. Olton DS, Wenk GL. In Meltzer HY (ed), Dementia: Animal models of the cognitive impairment produced by degeneration of the basal forebrain cholinergic system. *Psychopharmacology: The Third Generation of Progress.* Raven Press, New York, 1987, pp. 941-953.
24. Haroutunian V, Mantin R, Campbell GA, et al. Cysteamine-induced depletion of central somatostatin-like immunoactivity: Effects on behavior, learning, memory and neurochemistry. Brain Res 403:234-242, 1987.
25. Haroutunian V, Kanof PD, Davis KL. Interactions of forebrain cholinergic and somatostatinergic systems in the rat. Brain Res 496:98-104, 1989.
26. Haroutunian V, Kanof PD, Tsuboyama G, et al. Restoration of cholinomimetic activity by clonidine in cholinergic/noradrenergic lesioned rats. Brain Res 507:261-266, 1990.
27. Arnsten AFT, Goldman-Rakic PS. α_2-adrenergic mechanisms in prefrontal cortex associated with cognitive decline in aged nonhuman primates. Science 230:1273-1279, 1985.
28. McEntee WJ, Mair RG. Memory enhancement in Korsakoff's psychosis by clonidine: Further evidence for a noradrenergic deficit. Ann Neurol 7:466-470, 1980.
29. Pomar N, Deptual D, Singh RR. Postural blood pressure drop as a possible predictor of response to cholinergic therapy in Alzheimer's disease. Neurobiol Aging 11(3):343, 1990.

Part II

New Approaches to Drug Development

4

Brain-Enhanced Drug Delivery Systems for the Treatment of Dementia

James W. Simpkins and Nicholas Bodor
University of Florida, Gainesville, Florida

I. GENERAL PHARMACOTHERAPY CONSIDERATIONS

The pharmacotherapy of neurodegenerative diseases presents formidable problems which are both common to and distinct from the acute treatment of diseases of the brain. Therapeutic considerations which are common to both acute and chronic brain diseases are: 1) the innate efficacy of the drug for the disease state; 2) acute toxicity of the drug in the brain and in peripheral tissues; and 3) the capacity of the drug to cross the blood-brain barrier (BBB). For a drug to be effective in treatment of a brain disease, it must show innate efficacy, have an acceptably high therapeutic ratio (toxic dose ÷ effective dose), and reach the brain tissue by virtue of its ability to cross the BBB.

The literature is replete with examples of drugs of potential use in the treatment of brain disease which are ineffective because of their failure to meet one or more of the aforementioned criteria. Efficacy has been the foremost consideration in the development of drugs for the treatment of brain disease. In the preclinical evaluation of drugs, those compounds which exhibit the greatest efficacy for the targeted disease state, as assessed in animal models or in vitro systems, are given preference in subsequent preclinical evaluation of the compound (1).

The second pharmacotherapy consideration is the therapeutic ratio. For a compound to be a useful drug product, it must exert its beneficial effects at doses which are lower than doses at which toxic side effects are observed. Thus, the relationship between effective doses and toxic doses is a measure of the relative safety of the drug product. However, the extent of acceptable safety of a drug is dependent upon the severity of the disease state treated. For self-limiting disease, i.e., mild systemic infections, the therapeutic ratio of useful drugs is quite high. These diseases require that the drug product be completely safe, so that the chance of drug-induced toxicity is minuscle. By contrast, for life-threatening diseases, the small therapeutic ratio, while not optimal, is acceptable. Thus, anticancer agents are intrinsically cytotoxic and exhibit a very low therapeutic ratio. However, the benefits of therapy—i.e., remission of disease and/or extension of useful life—dictate use of these highly toxic agents (2).

As with systemic diseases, brain maladies are subject to the same considerations of a variable efficacy-toxicity relationship depending upon the severity of the disease under treatment. Minor analgesics commonly used in the treatment of headache and fever must show a large therapeutic ratio (3). As such, most of these drug products are extremely safe and can be dispensed as over-the-counter preparations. By contrast, drugs used to treat life-threatening brain diseases are administered despite concerns for toxicity. Viral or bacterial meningitis and brain edema are treated acutely with doses of antiviral, antimicrobial, and anti-inflammatory drugs which cause extreme peripheral toxicity (3). In these latter cases, the benefit to the patient far outweighs the risk of the outcome of the disease. As indicated below, the pharmacotherapy of neurodegenerative diseases will require a careful consideration of the therapeutic ratio of the drugs used.

Third, therapy of brain disease requires that the drug readily penetrate the BBB and gain access to the diseased tissue. As considered in more detail below, most drugs gain access to the brain by passive diffusion across the endothelial cells of brain capillaries (4). For now it should be indicated that the ability of drugs to cross the BBB affects their efficacy in treatment of brain disease and influences their toxicity. Obviously, drugs which have high efficacy for the biochemical defect which is the target of the brain therapy, but which do not gain access to the brain, will be completely ineffective. In the alternative case—drugs which are highly lyophilic and hence readily cross the BBB—the high lipophilicity also encourages their wide distribution in the body (4), and hence increases their chances of causing peripheral toxicity. Thus, design of drugs for brain delivery, based upon lipophilicity considerations alone, is limited by two concerns: 1) efficacy related to brain penetration, and 2) peripheral toxicity related to broad body distribution.

II. ALZHEIMER'S SPECIFIC PHARMACOTHERAPY CONSIDERATIONS

The pharmacotherapy of neurodegenerative diseases presents other problems which are not common to the acute treatment of brain diseases. Successful drug therapy of Alzheimer's disease will necessitate drug use for years, if not decades. By extending the life of the Alzheimer's patient, the duration of drug therapy will be long. As such, the effective Alzheimer's disease treatment will need to be relatively free of both acute and chronic toxicity, which may limit treatment. Chronic toxicity, often associated with long-term drug therapy, will be a major issue with the discovery of highly efficacious anti-Alzheimer's drugs. The effective anti-Alzheimer's drug should exhibit predictable biotransformation to metabolites which are nontoxic and which are cleared rapidly from brain and peripheral tissue.

A second issue in chronic drug therapy for Alzheimer's disease is the possibility of development of tolerance to the drug. Tolerance represents adaptive, compensatory responses of cells/tissues to drug effects. Typically, tolerance is handled by elevating dose to achieve the desired response or by programming "holidays" into the drug therapy to allow tissue/cell recovery from the therapy (5). With chronic therapy, progressive dose enhancement would reduce the therapeutic window and drug toxicity would be observed.

Third, the Alzheimer's patient would exhibit the expected age-related alterations in pharmacokinetic and pharmacodynamic responses to drugs (6); superimposed upon this is the late-stage, general physical debilitation of the advanced Alzheimer's patient. Thus, the Alzheimer's patient would be expected to exhibit toxic responses to lower doses of the drug than an age-matched control or a young patient.

Finally, the current major obstacle to effective therapy of Alzheimer's disease is our limited knowledge of the cause of the disease. Over the short term, elucidation of the cellular mechanism(s) responsible for the manifestation of the progressive cognitive decline which characterizes the disease will be required to develop the next generation of effective anti-Alzheimer's drugs. Inasmuch as the vast majority of current research on Alzheimer's disease is aimed at the determination of the cause of the disease and the cellular alteration associated with cognitive decline, it is safe to speculate that a drug with intrinsic efficacy for various defects in Alzheimer's disease will be discovered. Indeed, much of the research described in the present text represents novel approaches to the modification of observed cellular alterations in Alzheimer's brain tissue.

The remainder of this chapter deals with our efforts to solve problems associated with the selective delivery of drugs to the brain and the resulting effects on their efficacy and toxicity.

III. PROBLEMS OF DRUG DELIVERY TO THE BRAIN

It is now recognized that the BBB is a complex of morphological and enzymatic components which retard the passage of both large and small molecules which are not essential for cerebral function and specific transport system for essential molecules (4,7,8). Unlike systemic capillaries, the endothelial cells of cerebral capillaries are joined by tight junctions (8). These tight junctions form a zona occluda and provide, for large molecules, an absolute barrier. Structurally, the junctions consist of aligned intramembranous ridges and grooves which are in close opposition (9,10).

Systemic capillaries lack these close junctions; thus, there is nonspecific transport of nutrients and other compounds. In the brain, however, tight junctions severely restrict this type of nonspecific transport. Thus, to enter the brain, substances must utilize transcellular transport. Lipophilic compounds can readily pass through the phospholipoidal membranes, but hydrophilic compounds and high molecular weight substances are excluded.

Three additional aspects of cerebral capillaries contribute to the BBB. First cerebral endothelial cells have a paucity of vesicles and vesicular transport capacity (11). Second, astrocytic end feet may be involved in the regulation of amino acid flux and the absorption of protein (12). Third, the enzymatic component of the BBB may be vital in protecting the brain from a variety of blood-borne neurotransmitters (13,14).

The transport of essential into the brain is accomplished by carriers which are located in the endothelial cell of the cerebral vasculature. These proteinaceous carriers are bidirectional in nature and can be saturated (15). These systems are for hexose (16), neutral, acidic, and basic amino acids (17,18), monocarboxylic acids (19), choline (20), nucleosides (7), purines (21), thiamine, and thyroid hormones (15,22).

Once in the brain parenchyma, substance can be removed either actively at the choroid plexus or passively by bulk afflux of cerebrospinal fluid (CSF). Active transport systems for disposal of both anions (23–29) and cations (26) have been described which are energy-dependent. These systems are likely most important in the removal of metabolic acids and bases from the brain. Alternatively, CSF, which is produced at the choroid plexus, passes through the ventricular system, leaves at a constant rate, and carries with it dissolved polar substances. In this manner, substances which have no active transport system or passive carrier system can be eliminated from the brain.

Drugs can gain access to the brain through one of several routes. First, if a drug has affinity for one of the carrier systems, it can diffuse across the BBB in association with that carrier. Second, drugs with intrinsic lipophilicity can diffuse passively through the phospholipid cellular matrix of capillary endothelial cells. The lipophilicity correlates with their ability to penetrate the BBB for several classes of drugs, including narcotics (27), β-receptor antagonists (28), and barbiturates (29). Third, drugs which cannot penetrate the BBB can gain access to limited areas around the circumventricular organs.

IV. STRATEGIES FOR THE DELIVERY OF DRUG TO THE BRAIN

A. Prodrugs

The BBB excludes a number of pharmacological agents from the brain and limits concentrations of other compounds to levels which are subtherapeutic. To increase the effectiveness of drugs against central maladies, the concentrations and/or transit time of the drug in the brain should be increased. Further, if selective drug delivery to the brain is achieved, the therapeutic index of the drug should increase for two reasons: 1) the increase in concentration and/or residence time of the agent at its receptor, and 2) of equal importance, the peripheral concentration of the drug would be reduced, thus decreasing its peripheral toxicity.

A general approach to enhance delivery of drugs to the brain is the prodrug approach (30,31–38). Prodrugs are pharmacological agents which have been transiently modified to improve their lipophilicity. Ideally, the prodrug is biologically inactive but reverts to the active, parent compounds in vivo at or around the site of action. This transformation can be mediated by an enzyme or may occur chemically as a result of designed instability in the agent. By temporarily masking the polar groups of a drug, the lipophilicity of a drug can be increased and its ability to pass membranes is enhanced. This technique has been applied to a number of drugs (4,32,33).

By increasing the lipoid solubility of drugs nonspecifically by the prodrug approach, all tissues are exposed to a greater drug burden. This is a major limiting factor in the use of these prodrugs, particularly those with cytotoxic activity.

B. Redox-Based Chemical Delivery Systems

One approach to eliminate the problem of general toxicity associated with enhanced lipophilicity of prodrugs has been the application of redox-based technology to brain-targeted drugs. The most widely studied redox-delivery system is based upon the dihydropyridine ⇌ pyridinium salt redox reaction. In this system, the lipoidal dihydropyridine moiety (Fig. 1) is covalently attached to the drug, thus increasing its lipophilicity and its ability to penetrate the BBB. The reduced, noncharged dihydropyridine can be oxidized to the charge pyridinium ion in the brain and in systemic tissues (Fig. 1). The ubiquitous NADP ⇌ NADPH redox system catalyzes this oxidation reaction. The charged pyridinium-drug moiety is thus "locked" into the brain while the peripherally formed pyridinium-drug complex can be rapidly cleared by renal or biliary processes due to its increased hydrophilicity (Fig. 1). Sustained release of the active drug from the delivery system occurs in the brain as a result of enzymatic hydrolysis of the ester (or amide, etc.) linkage between the drug and the pyridinium moiety (Fig. 1). This redox-based chemical delivery system has been applied successfully to the brain-en-

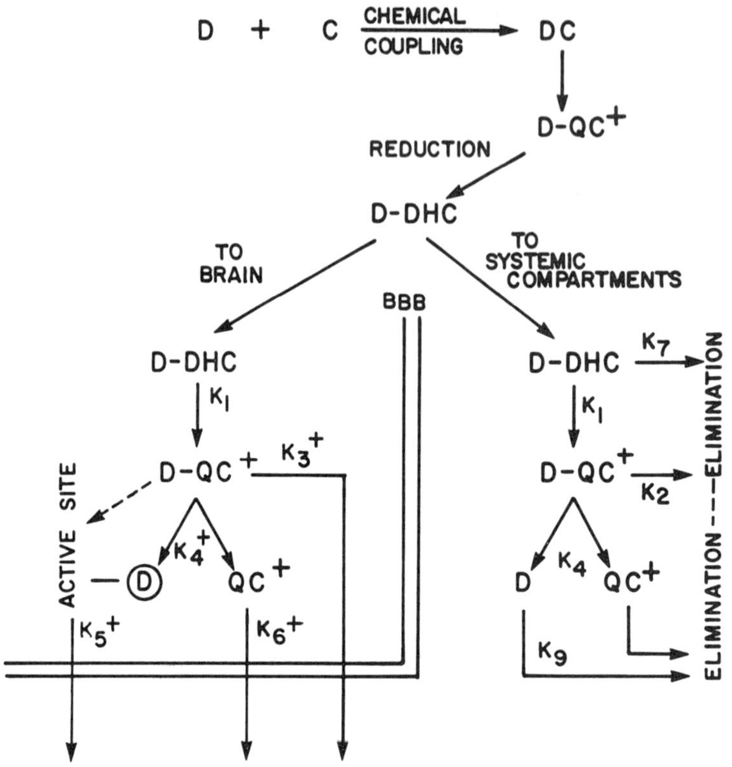

Figure 1 Schematic representation of the body distribution of a drug (D), which is attached to the dihydropyridine carrier (C). The drug is coupled via two reaction steps to the quaternary pyridinium form of the carrier resulting molecule (here indicated as D-QC⁺). This charged moiety must be reduced to the dihydropyridine carrier (here indicated as D-DHC). The reduced drug-carrier complex (D-DHC) is the lipophilic form administered to the animal. Following the intravenous administration of D-DHC, it can penetrate the blood-brain barrier (BBB) to partition into the brain or remain in the periphery. In both compartments, oxidation of D-DHC to the quaternary D-QC⁺ occurs. In the periphery, this process enhances its rate of elimination from the circulation; in the brain, the formation of the charged moiety serves to "lock-in" the drug-carrier complex. In the brain, hydrolysis of the D-QC⁺ to the drug and the carriers results in a sustained release of active drug. Also released is the small, inert carrier molecule, trigonelline (QC⁺), which is easily eliminated from the brain.

hanced delivery of a number of drugs which do not normally cross the BBB, including, phenylethylamine (34,35), dopamine (36,37), antitumor drugs (38,39), antiepileptic drugs (40), γ-aminobutyric acid (41), antiviral (42) and antibiotic agents (43), and cholinesterase inhibitors (44).

C. Brain-Enhanced Delivery of Steroids with a Redox Chemical Delivery System

An additional novel application of this redox chemical delivery system is to molecules with intrinsically high lipid solubility, which can themselves readily pass into and out of the brain. Their attachment to the dihydropyridine carrier encourages this brain-enhanced delivery by:

1. locking them into the brain following the oxidation in the brain of the dihydropyridine carrier to the charged pyridium moiety; and
2. enhancement of the rate of elimination of the lipoidal drug, a still inactive form, from the periphery following its oxidation to the charged compound (Fig. 2).

We have extensively evaluated the pharmacokinetic and pharmacodynamic behavior of one of these steroid delivery systems, an estradiol-chemical delivery system (E_2-CDS), for two important reasons. First, it is now recognized that E_2 can have broad modulatory effects on the central nervous system and that treatment of many brain maladies may be possible with the selective brain delivery of E_2. Second, we have now demonstrated that steroid delivery systems can be used to deliver neuroactive peptides to the brain. As such, the steroid delivery systems themselves or steroid delivery systems as carriers for neuropeptides may be useful in the treatment of neurodegenerative diseases, such as Alzheimer's disease.

1. Pharmacokinetic Studies

The predicted pharmacokinetic behavior of the E_2-CDS is depicted in Figure 2. After systemic administration of the E_2-CDS, it distributes throughout the body and the carrier moiety (E_2-CDS) is rapidly oxidized to the quaternary pyridinium ion (E_2-Q^+) in the brain and in peripheral tissues. The E_2-Q^+ is thus locked into the brain because of the BBB, while the charged E_2-Q^+ is rapidly cleared from the periphery, the result of the 40,000-fold decrease in lipophilicity during the oxidation of the E_2-CDS to the E_2-Q^+ (45). Sustained release of E_2 from E_2-Q^+ should result from the enzymatic hydrolysis of the bond linking the E_2 to the pyridinium moiety.

To evaluate the proposed biotransformation of E_2-CDS, we conducted pharmacokinetic evaluations of E_2-CDS for a single intravenous administration. The parent drug, E_2-CDS, was rapidly cleared from both the brain and periphery by oxidation to E_2-Q^+ (Fig. 3). E_2-CDS showed a $t_{1/2}$ in brain tissue of 29 minutes (45). By contrast, while E_2-Q^+ was rapidly cleared from plasma, brain levels of

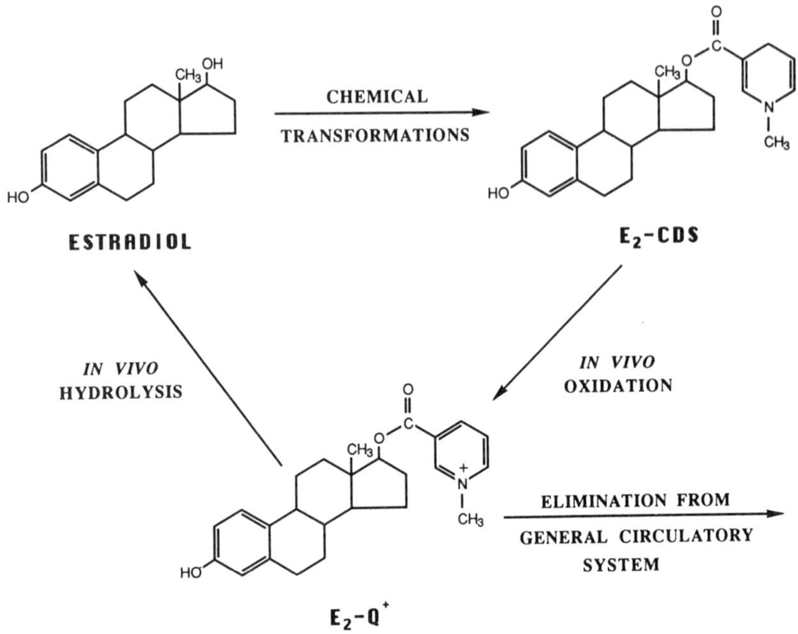

Figure 2 The brain-enhanced delivery of estradiol. Estradiol-CDS (E_2-CDS) is the chemical-delivery system described and the pyridinium form E_2-Q^+ is the charged quaternary salt of the E_2-CDS.

this charged form of the delivery system were elevated and were slowly cleared with a half-life ($t_{1/2}$) of 8–9 days (45).

Following the development of reliable and sensitive assay methods for the simultaneous quantitation of E_2-Q^+ and E_2 (46), we determined the pharmacokinetic deposition of E_2-CDS in a variety of tissues of both male and female rats. After E_2-CDS was administered to male rats (47), brain E_2-Q^+ concentrations increased to 318 ± 14 ng/g tissue (mean ± SEM) on day 1 and declined thereafter with an apparent $t_{1/2}$ of 8–9 days (Fig. 3). By contrast, plasma E_2-Q^+ increased to 6.1 ± 0.3 ng/ml on day 1, then was rapidly cleared with a $t_{1/2}$ of less than 2 days (Fig. 3). The clearance of E_2-Q^+ by the liver was similar to that of plasma (Fig. 3). Brain concentrations of E_2 were increased to 8 ± 0.5 ng/g tissue on day 1 and were cleared with a $t_{1/2}$ identical to that of E_2-Q^+. Plasma and liver E_2 clearance was rapid and similar to that of E_2-Q^+ (Fig. 3).

Dose and time-course evaluation of E_2-CDS were conducted using ovariectomized (OVX) rats (48). OVX rats were treated with a single i.v. injection of

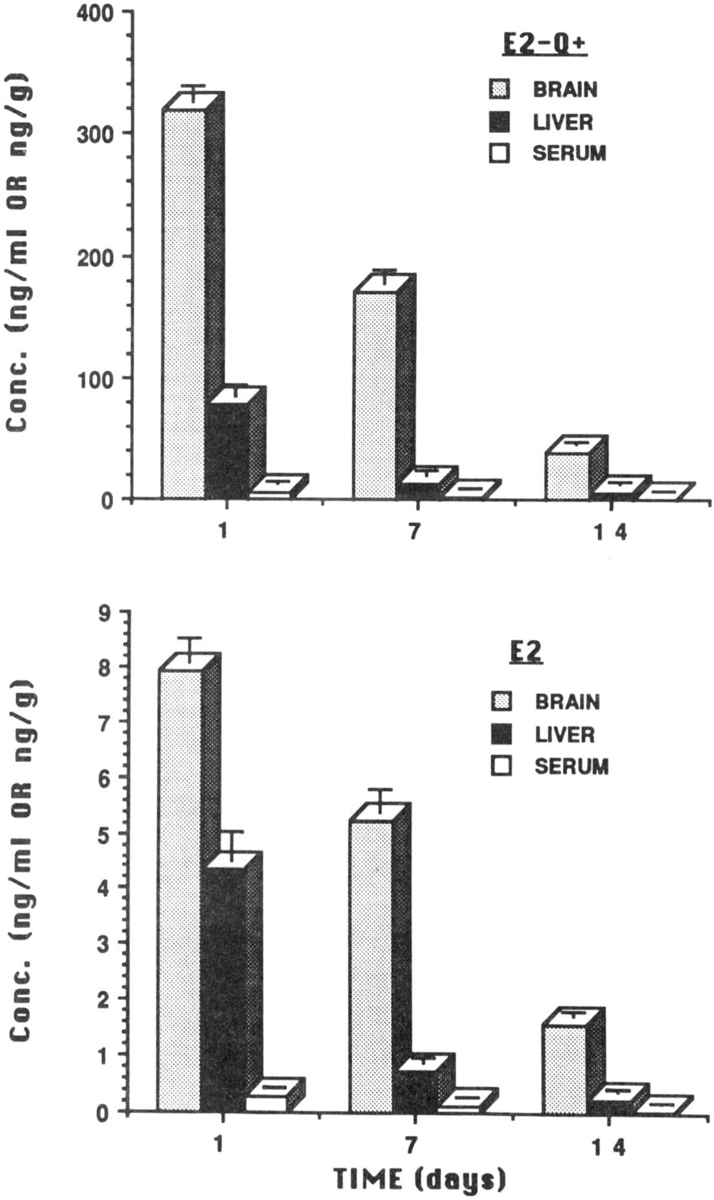

Figure 3 Effects of E_2-CDS on Levels of E_2-Q^+ (upper panel) and E_2 (lower panel) in brain, liver, and serum in the male rat (From Ref. 46.)

0.01, 0.1, or 1.0 mg E_2-CDS/kg body weight and were sampled at 1, 7, 14, 21, or 28 days later for concentrations of E_2-Q^+ and E_2 in whole brain, hypothalamus, plasma, anterior pituitary, kidney, lung, heart, and uterus. In all tissues examined, a dose-dependent increase in E_2-Q^+ and E_2 was observed. The concentration-time profile showed a gradual decline in E_2-Q^+ and E_2 concentrations in the whole brain (Fig. 4) and hypothalamus (data not shown), with an apparent $t_{1/2}$ of 8–9 days. By contrast, E_2-Q^+ and E_2 in plasma (Fig. 5) and other peripheral tissues (data not shown) were rapidly cleared. In comparison to an equimolar dose of E_2, E_2-CDS produced brain E_2 concentrations which were 81–182-fold higher at 1 and 7 days postinjection.

It is reasonable to conclude from these data that E_2-CDS is locked into the brain as the E_2-Q^+ and that E_2 is continuously produced from this depot form of the delivery system. The slow decline in brain E_2 appears to be dependent upon its rate of production from E_2-Q^+ and its rate of elimination from the brain, either by local metabolism or by its redistribution down a concentration gradient into the general circulation. Collectively, these observations are consistent with the proposed biotransformation of E_2-CDS in brain and peripheral tissues.

2. *Pharmacodynamic Studies*

Pharmacodynamic evaluations of the E_2-CDS were conducted to determine if the long brain half-life of E_2-Q^+ and E_2 was reflected in the duration and magnitude of pharmacological responses to the drug. Luteinizing hormone (LH) was evaluated as an indication of the effects of E_2-CDS in view of the primary role of estrogens in the regulation of LH secretion.

Orchidectomized rats were treated with E_2-CDS (3.0 mg/kg body weight), an equimolar dose of E_2, or the vehicle dimethyl sulfoxide (DMSO). Blood samples were obtained at various times thereafter for determination of serum LH and E_2 levels (49). Both E_2 and E_2-CDS decreased LH concentrations by 68–79% compared to DMSO-treated orchidectomized rats (Fig. 6). This effect was maintained from 4–48 hours. In rats treated with E_2, serum LH levels increased progressively to values not different from control levels by 12 days. In contrast, E_2-CDS treated rats continued to exhibit suppressed LH secretion by 82–92% through 12 days post-treatment (last sample time in this study). Serum E_2 concentrations were elevated in both treatment groups through 2 days, then were reduced to the levels of detection of the assay thereafter.

In a subsequent study (49), orchidectomized rats were treated with E_2-CDS, E_2 or DMSO at the doses described above. Animals were sampled 12, 18, or 24 days later. As observed in our first study, LH was suppressed by E_2-CDS by 89%, 88%, and 66% versus DMSO-treated controls at 12, 18, and 24 days post-treatment, respectively. E_2-treated rats showed serum LH levels which were equal to or greater than those of control animals at these three post-treatment times.

Subsequently, we demonstrated that this effect of E_2-CDS is dose-dependent

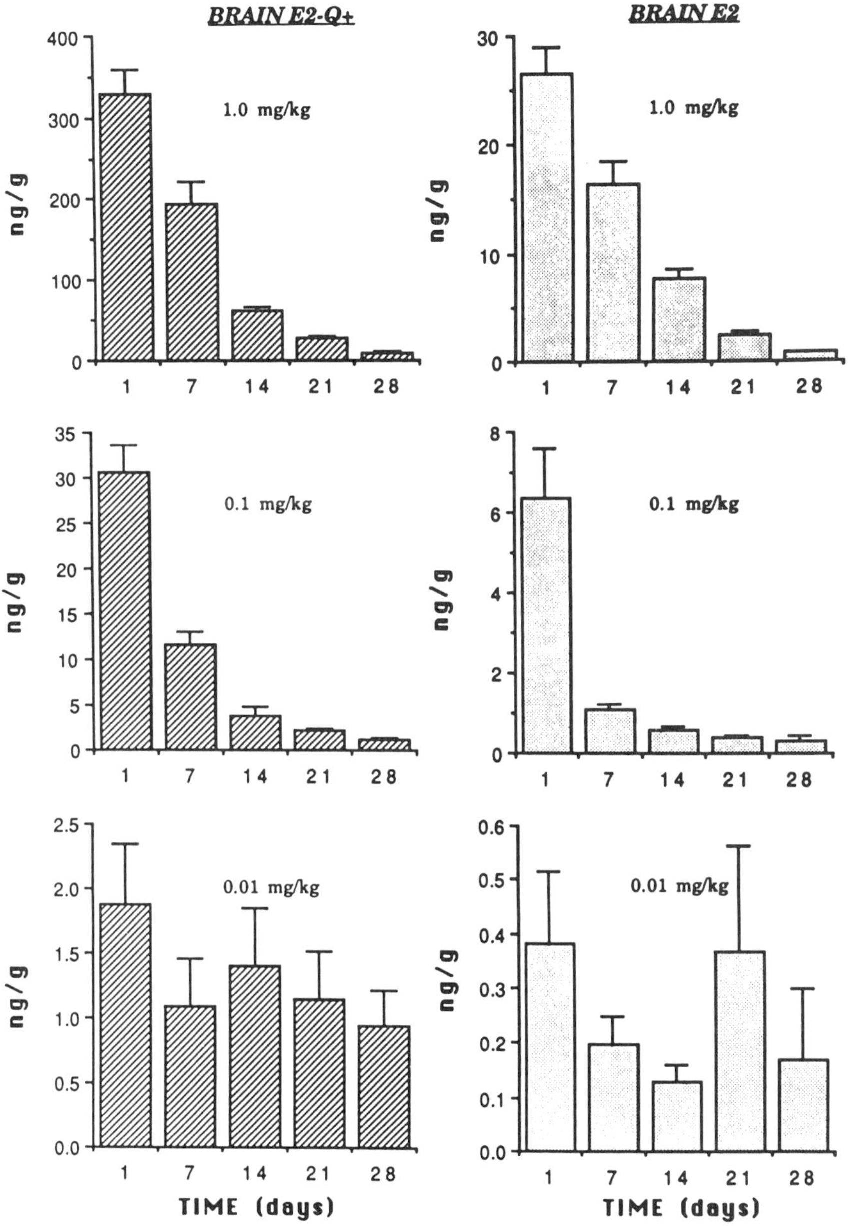

Figure 4 Effects of E_2-CDS on brain concentrations of E_2-Q^+ (left column of panels) and E_2 (right columnof panels) in ovariectomized rats. E_2-CDS was administered at doses of 0.01 (lower panels), 0.1 (middle panels) or 1.0 mg/kg (upper panels). (From Ref. 48.)

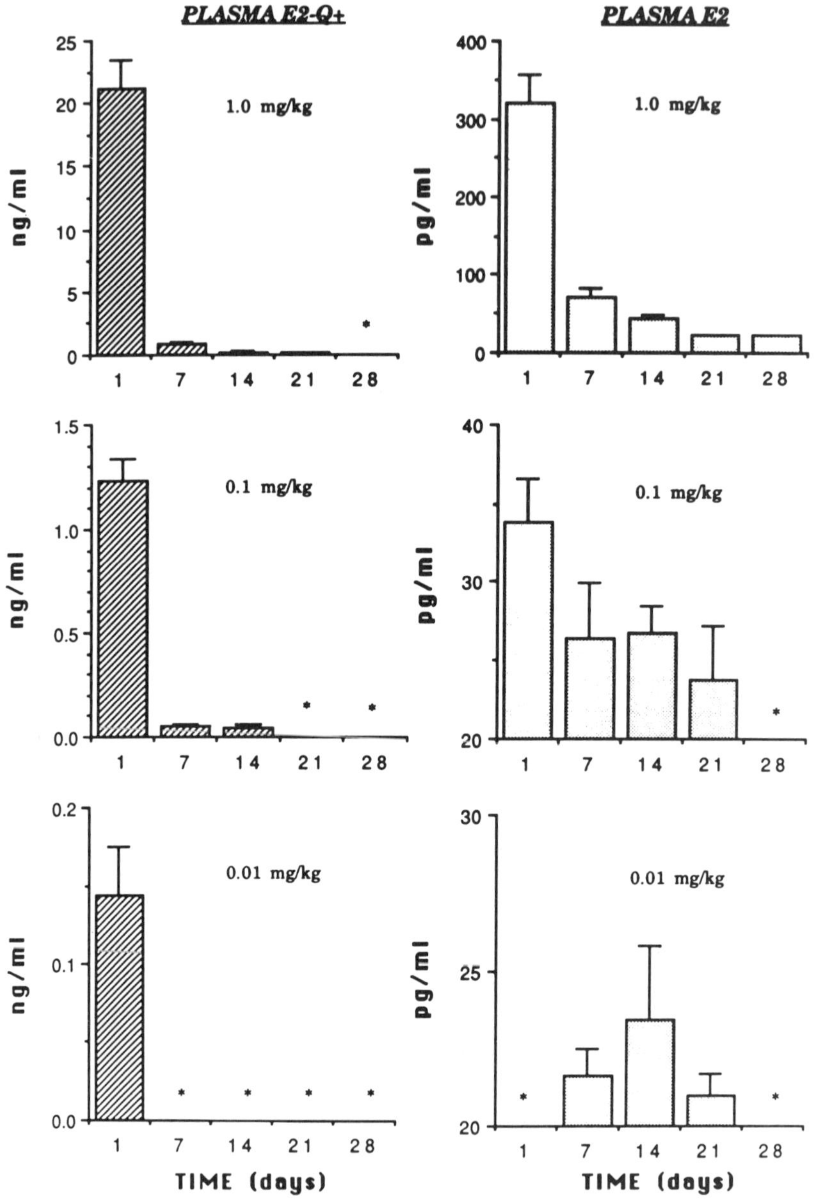

Figure 5 Effects of E_2-CDS on plasma concentrations of E_2-Q^+ (left column of panels) and E_2 (right column of panels) in ovariectomized rats. E_2-CDS was administered at doses of 0.01 (lower panels), 0.1 (middle panels), or 1.0 mg/kg (upper panels). (From Ref. 48.)

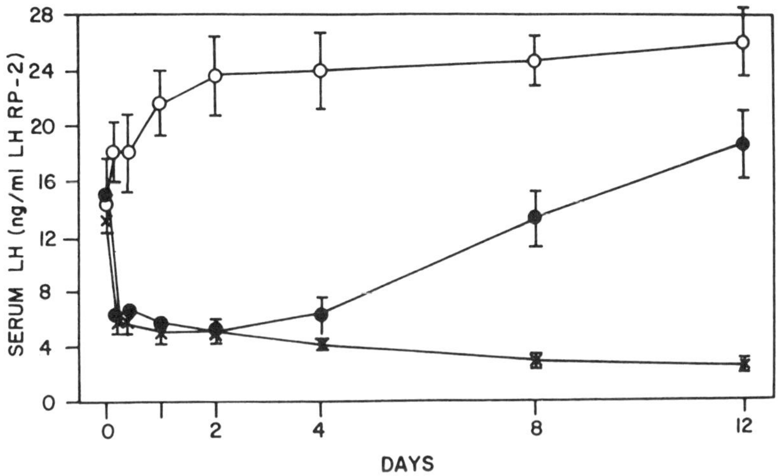

Figure 6 Effects of a single injection of E_2-CDS (x), an equimolar dose of E_2 (●) or the vehicle (○) on serum LH in orchidectomized rats. Mean H SEM are depicted. (From Ref. 49.)

(50,51), is observed at E_2-CDS doses as low as 10 μg/kg (50) and can be achieved without an increase in serum E_2 concentrations (50).

More relevant to the issue of Alzheimer's disease are the behavioral effects of brain-enhanced delivery of E_2. We have evaluated the time-course of two well-described behavioral effects of E_2: stimulation of masculine sexual behavior in castrated male rats (52) and the suppression of food intake in animals (53,54). Castration resulted in a marked diminution in several indicators of male sexual function including the number of mounts and intromissions and a lengthening of the latency to onset of both mounting and intromission behavior. Treatment with a single i.v. injection of E_2-CDS restored sexual behavior to normal for 2 weeks and significantly improved sexual performance (vs. castrated rats) for up to 4 weeks postinjection (52). Similarly, in aged, obese male rats, a dose-dependent reduction in daily food intake was observed which lasted for up to 3 weeks postinjection and resulted in weight reduction for the duration of the 69-day study (53). Collectively, these studies indicate that E_2-CDS results in long behavioral responses following a single dose of E_2-CDS—observations consistent with the long half-life of E_2-Q^+ and E_2 in the brain.

3. *Effects of E_2-CDS on Cholinergic Function*

The rationale for the involvement of estrogens in cognition comes from both animal and clinical studies. Estrogen receptors have been observed in the nuclei of the basal forebrain which are the major loci of cell bodies of cholinergic neurons which innervate the cerebral cortex, limbic system, and hippocampus (55). These brain regions are believed to be involved in the pathology of Alzheimer's disease (56). In rats, cholinergic neurons respond to peripheral administration of estrogen by increasing the activity of choline acetyltransferase, (57) acetylcholine synthesis (58), and high-affinity choline uptake (58). Estrogens may, therefore, serve a modulatory role in the function of cholinergic neurons and may serve as therapeutic agents in the stimulation of brain cholinergic neurons in patients with Alzheimer's disease and other dementia which may be due to a cholinergic deficit.

While preliminary in nature, several clinical studies have indicated that estrogens may be useful in the treatment of dementia, particularly when it is associated with the menopause. Elderly postmenopausal patients were evaluated for psychological function and behavior using the Hospital Adjustment Scale (59,60). Therapy with Premarin ® (conjugated estrogens tablets) did not increase cognition significantly, but it prevented its further decline as compared to a placebo control group (59,60). These studies suggest that chronic estrogen therapy may prevent the progression of loss in cognitive function in postmenopausal patients. In a second study (61), patients diagnosed as "probable Alzheimer's disease" were subjected to a battery of tests to assess cognitive function and depression and were then treated with micronized estradiol for 6 weeks (61). Modest improvements of scores on several tests of cognitive function were observed in one group of patients. In this group, the improvements were related primarily to improvements in attention, orientation, mood, and social interaction. In only one patient was improvement in memory noted.

Other studies have noted improvements in cognitive function which were believed to be secondary to the antidepression actions of estrogen (62). It is well known that emotional status affects memory and learning in both animals and man and that emotional disorders are frequently observed in Alzheimer's patients. Thus, a primary effect of estrogens on mood could result in a secondary improvement in cognition.

E_2-CDS may be potentially useful in the treatment of dementia, since currently there are no effective therapies for dementia and treatment regimens would have to be life-long. As such, peripheral estrogen toxicity would be a persistent problem for chronic peripheral administration of estrogens. The brain-enhanced delivery of estradiol with the E_2-CDS may obviate this potential problem.

Given the aforementioned evidence for an effect of estrogens on cholinergic neuronal function, we evaluated the effects of E_2-CDS on neuronal systems which are known to be dysfunctional in Alzheimer's disease. In an initial study, female rats were ovariectomized (or received sham surgery) and 2 weeks later the OVX rats were treated with the drug vehicle or E_2-CDS (1 mg/kg, i.v.). Five days later, all animals were sacrificed for a determination of high affinity choline uptake in the cerebral cortex, hippocampus, and striatum. Ovariectomy reduced high-affin-

Table 1 Effects of Ovariectomy and E_2-CDS on High-Affinity Choline Uptake in Brain Regions

	Brain region		
	Cortex	Hippocampus	Striatum
Group	(cpm $\times 10^3$/mg protein)		
Intact females and vehicle[a]	176 ± 44	235 ± 33	657 ± 138
OVX[b] and vehicle	100 ± 7	162 ± 2	392 ± 37
OVX and E_2-CDS	181 ± 14	198 ± 21	481 ± 33

[a]Vehicle for all groups was 2-β-hydroxypropylcyclodextrin.
[b]OVX = ovariectomy.

ity choline uptake in all three regions evaluated (Table 1). Treatment with E_2-CDS increased high-affinity choline uptake in the cortex and hippocampus to levels which were not different from intact control values (Table 1). This single-dose study, while preliminary, indicates that E_2-CDS can enhance the activity of cholinergic neurons in an OVX animal model.

V. THE USE OF STEROID DELIVERY SYSTEMS TO DELIVER NEUROACTIVE PEPTIDES TO THE BRAIN

A variety of neuroactive peptides are candidates for memory-enhancing drugs (63) or neurotrophic factors (64). The major pharmaceutical problem limiting their testing and eventual use in the treatment of Alzheimer's disease and other neurodegenerative disorders is the inability of these neuropeptides to cross the BBB.

We have devised a modification of the steroid delivery system to enhance the delivery of neuropeptides to the brain. The first target compound for the proposed delivery technology was leucine-D-ala-encephalin (leu-enk). The N-terminals of leu-enk we attached the dihydropyridine group (dihyotrigonelline) via an amide bond and an alanine spacer. To the C-terminal we attached a cholesterol ester function. This molecular sandwich of the target peptide was administered to rats at a dose of 20 mg/kg by a single i.v. injection. Brain homogenates were analyzed by fast atom bombardment (FAB)-mass spectrometry (MS). Using FAB-MS with the CD_3 analog internal standard, we detected both the "locked in" pyridinium-leu-enk-cholesterol species and the pyridinium-leu-enk complex formed following hydrolysis of the cholesterol ester moeity. Our time-course evaluation of pyridinium-leu-enk revealed a linear decline from peak levels of 35 $\mu g/g$ brain at 15 min to 4 $\mu g/g$ brain at 4 hours postinjection.

These encouraging results with the first neuropeptide evaluated with the modified steroid delivery system suggest that it is possible to deliver to the brain $\mu g/g$ concentrations of a neuroactive peptide using this technology. Further evaluations of this system with memory-enhancing neuropeptides and with trophic factors or smaller active fragment of trophic factors are clearly warranted and are the subject of ongoing research in our laboratory.

ACKNOWLEDGMENTS

The authors wish to thank B. J. Goins and Victoria Redd Patterson for their expert secretarial assistance. Supported in part by NIH grants AG 02021 and HD 22540.

REFERENCES

1. Loftus P. Computer-assisted drug design. In Clark CR., Moos WH (eds): *Drug Discovery Technologies*. Ellis Horwood Ltd, Chichester, England, 1990, pp. 1-21.
2. Lowe MC. Large animal toxicological studies of anticancer drugs. In Hellmann K, Carter SK (eds): *Fundamentals of Cancer Chemotherapy*. McGraw-Hill, New York, 1987, pp. 237-247.
3. Klaussen CD. Principles of Toxicology. In Gilman AG, Goodman LS, Rall TW, Murad F (eds): *The Pharmacological Basis of Therapeutics*, 7th ed. MacMillan, New York, 1985, pp. 1592-1604.
4. Bodor N, Brewster M. Problems of delivery of drugs to the brain. Pharmacol Ther 19: 337-386, 1983.
5. Bianchine JR. Drugs for Parkinson's disease, spasticity and acute muscle spasms. In Gilman AG, Goodman LS, Rall TW, Murad F (eds): *The Pharmacological Basis of Therapeutics*, 7th ed. MacMillan, New York, 1985, pp 473-490.
6. Park GD. Factors affecting pharmacokinetics and pharmacodynamics. In Spector R (ed): *The Scientific Basis of Clinical Pharmacology*. Little Brown and Co., Boston, 1986, pp 113-130.
7. Pardridge WM, Connor JD, Crawford IL. Permeability changes in the blood-brain barriers: causes and consequences. CRC Crit. Rev. Toxic. 1975; 3:150-199.
8. Brightman MW, Reese TS. Junctions between intimately opposed cell membranes in the vertebrate brain. J Cell Biol 40:648-677, 1969.
9. Van Dewis B. Structural aspects of brain barriers, with special reference to the permeability of the cerebral endothelium and choroidal epithelium. Int Rev Cytol 65:117-191, 1980.
10. Oldendorf WH. The blood-brain barrier. Exp Eye Res 25(Suppl):177-190, 1977.
11. Brightman MW. Morphology of blood-brain interfaces. Exp Eye Res 25(Suppl): 1-15, 1977.
12. Broadwell RD, Salomen M. Expanding the definition of the blood-brain barrier to proteins. Proc Natl Acad Sci USA 78:7820-7824, 1981.

13. Hardebo JE, Owman C. Barrier mechanisms for neurotransmitter monoamines and their precursors at the blood-brain barrier. Ann Neurol 8:1–11, 1980.
14. Kaplan GP, Hartman BK, Creveling CR. Immunohistochemical localizationof catechol-o-methyl-transferase in circumventricular organ of the rat: potential variations in the blood brain barrier to native catechols. Brain Res 229:323–335, 1981.
15. Pardridge WM. Transport of nutrients and hormones through the blood-brain barrier. Diabetologia 20:246-254, 1981.
16. Lund-Andersen H. Transport of glucose from blood to brain. Physiol Rev 59:305-352, 1979.
17. Christensen HN. On the development of amino acid transport systems. Proc Soc Exp Biol Med 32:19-28, 1973.
18. Christensen HN. Developments in amino acid transport. Illustrated for the blood-brain barrier. Biochem Pharmacol 28:1989–1992, 1979.
19. Pollay M, Stevens FA. Starvation-induced changes in transport of ketone bodies across the blood-brain barrier. J Neurosci Res 5:163–172, 1980.
20. Cornford EM, Braun LD, Oldenforf WH. Carrier mediated blood-brain barrier transport of choline and certain analogs. J Neurochem 30:299–308, 1978.
21. Braum LD, Cornford EM, Oldenford WH. Newborn rabbit blood-brain barrier is selectively permeable and differs substantially fron the adult. J Neurochem 34:147–152, 1980.
22. Pardridge WM, Meitus LJ. Transport of thyroid and steroid hormones through the blood-brain barrier of new-born rabbits: Primary role of protein-bound hormone. Endocrinology 107:1705–1716, 1980.
23. Barany EH. Bile acids as inhibitors of liver-like anion transport system in the rabbit kidney, urea and choroid plexus. Acta Physiol Scand 92:195–203, 1974.
24. Pappenheimer JP, Heisey SR, Jorday EF. Active transport of diodrast and phenolsulfonphthalein from cerebrospinal fluid to blood. Am J Physiol 200:1–10, 1961.
25. Spector R, Lorenzo AV. The effects of salicylate and probenecid on the cerebrospinal fluid transport of penicillin, amino-salicylic acid and iodide. J Pharmacol Exp Ther 188:55–65, 1974.
26. Schanker LD, Prockop LD, Schov J, et al. Rapid efflux of some quaternary ammonium compounds from cerebrospinal fluid. Life Sci 1:515-521, 1962.
27. Oldendorf WH, Braum L, Hyman S, et al. Blood-brain barrier: Penetration of morphine, codeine, heroin and methadone after carotid injection. Science 178:984–986, 1972.
28. Cruickshank JM, Neil-Dwyer G, Cameron MM, et al. β-ardrenoreceptor-blocking agents and the blood-brain barrier. Clin Sci 59:453s-455s, 1979.
29. Levin VA. Relationship to octanol water partition coefficients and molecular weight to rat brain capillary permeability. J Med Chem 23:682–684, 1980.
30. Sinkula AA, and Yalkowsky SH. Rationale for design of biologically reversible drug derivatives: Prodrugs. J Pharm Sci 64:181–210, 1975.
31. Bodor N. Novel approaches for the design of membrane transport properties of drugs. In Roche EB (ed): *Design of Biopharmaceutical Properties Through Prodrugs and Analogs*. APHA Academy of Pharmaceutical Sciences, Washington DC, 1976, pp 98–135.

32. Connors TA. Possible pro-drugs in cancer chemotherapy. Chem Ind 11:447–451, 1980.
33. Ferres H. Prodrugs of β-lactam antibiotics. Chem Ind 11:436–440, 1980.
34. Bodor N, Farag HH, Brewster ME. Site-specific sustained release of drugs to the brain. Science 214:1370–1372, 1981.
35. Bodor N, Farag H. Improved delivery through biological membranes. XI. A redox chemical drug delivery system and its use for brain specific delivery of phenethylamine. J Med Chem 26:313–318, 1983.
36. Bodor N, Simpkins JW. Brain-specific, sustained release of dopamine with a redox delivery system. Science 221:65–67, 1983.
37. Simpkins JW, Bodor N, Eng A. Direct evidence for brain specific release of dopamine from a redox delivery system. J Pharm Sci 74:1033–1036, 1985.
38. Bodor N, Brewster ME. Improved delivery through biological membranes XV. Sustained brain delivery of Berberine. Eur J Med Chem 18:235–240, 1983.
39. Brewster ME, Bodor N. Improved delivery through biological membranes XVI. Enhancement of the brain-specificity of a dihydropyridine pyridinium salt drug delivery system by controlled infusion. J Parental Sci Tech 37:159–164, 1983.
40. Murakami T, Shek E, Pop E, et al. Improved anticonvulsant activity of phenytoin by a redox brain delivery system: stability in buffers and biological materials. J Pharm Sci 78:732–737, 1989.
41. Anderson W, Simpkins J, Woodard P, et al. Anxiolytic activity of a brain-specific GABA delivery system. Psychopharmacology 92:157–163, 1987.
42. El-Koussi A, Bodor N. Improved delivery through biological membranes XXV. Enhanced and sustained delivery of trifluorothymidine to the brain using a dihydropyridine pyridinium salt type redox delivery system. Drug Des Deliv 1:275–283, 1987.
43. Pop E, Bodor N. Improved delivery through biological membranes XL. Chemical delivery system for some penicillinase-resistant semisynthetic penicillins. J Med Chem 32:1789–1795, 1989.
44. Brewster ME, Robledo-Luiggi C, Miyakeb A, et al. Brain-enhanced delivery of antidementia drugs. In Meyer EM, Simpkins JW, Yamamoto J (eds): *Novel Approaches to the Treatment of Alzheimer's Disease*. Plenum Press, New York, 1989, pp 173–183.
45. Bodor N, McCornack J, Brewster ME. Improved delivery through biological membranes. XXII. Synthesis and distribution of brain-selective estrogen delivery systems. Int J Pharm 35:47–59, 1987.
46. Rahimy MH, Bodor N, Simpkins JW. A rapid, sensitive method for the simultaneous quantitation of estradiol and estradiol conjugates in a variety of tissues: Assay development and evaluation of the distribution of a brain-enhanced estradiol-chemical delivery system. J Steroid Biochem 33:179–187, 1989.
47. Rahimy MH, Simpkins JW, Bodor N. Tissue distribution of a brain-enhanced chemical delivery system for estradiol. Drug Des Deliv 6:29–40, 1990.
48. Rahimy MH, Simpkins JW, Bodor N. Dose and time course evaluation of a redox based estradiol-chemical delivery system for the brain: I. Tissue Distribution. Pharmaceutical Res 7:1061–1067, 1990.
49. Simpkins JW, McCornack J, Estes KS, et al. Sustained brain-specific delivery of

estradiol causes long-term suppression of luteinizing hormone secretion. J Med Chem 29:1809-1812, 1986.
50. Anderson WR, Simpkins JW, Brewster ME, et al. Evidence for suppressionof serum LH without elevation in serum estradiol and prolactin with a brain-enhanced rdox delivery system for estradiol. Life Sci 42:1493-1502, 1988.
51. Rahimy MH, Simpkins JW, Bodor N. Dose and time course evaluation of a redox based estradiol-chemical delivery system for the brain: II. Pharmacodynamic Responses. Pharmaceutical Res 7:1107-1112, 1990.
52. Anderson WR, Simpkins JW, Brewster ME, et al. Evidence for the reestablishment of copulatory behavior in castrated male rats with a brain-enhanced estradiol-chemical delivery system. Pharmacol Biochem Behav 27:265-271, 1987.
53. Simpkins JW, Anderson WR, Dawson R Jr, et al. Chronic weight loss in lean and obese rats with a brain-enhanced chemical delivery system for estradiol. Physiol Behav 44:573-580, 1988.
54. Simpkins JW, Anderson WR, Dawson R Jr., et al. Effects of a brain-enhanced chemical delivery system for estradiol on body weight and food intake in intact and ovariectomized rats. Pharmaceutical Res 6:592-600, 1989.
55. Luine VN, Khylchevskaya RI, McEwen BS. Effects of gonadal steroids on activity of monoamine oxidase and choline acetylase in rat brain. Brain Res 86:293-306, 1975.
56. Coyle JT, Price Dl, Delong MR. Alzheimer's disease: A disorder of cortical cholinergic innervation. Science 219:1184-1190, 1983.
57. Luine VN. Estradiol increases choline acetyltransferase activity in specific basal forebrain nuclei and projection areas in female rats. Exp Neurol 89:484-490, 1985.
58. O'Malley CA, Hautamaki RD, Kelley M, et al. Effects of ovariectomy and estradiol benzoate on high affinity choline uptake, Ach synthesis and release from rat brain cerebral cortical synaptosomes. Brain Res 403:389-392, 1987.
59. Kantor HI, Michael CM, Shore H, et al. Administration of estrogens to older women, a psychometric evaluation. Am J Obstet Gynecol 101:658-661, 1968.
60. Michael CH, Kantor HI, and Shore H. Further psychometric evaluation of older women-the effects of estrogen administration. J Gerontol 25:337-341, 1970.
61. Fillit H, Weinreb H, Cholst I, et al. Observations in a preliminary open trial of estradiol therapy for senile dementia-Alzheimer's type. Psychoneuroendocrinology 11:337-345, 1986.
62. Hackman BW, Galbraith D. Replacement therapy with piperazine oestrone sulfate ("Harmogen") and its effect on memory. Curr Med Res Opin 4:303-306, 1976.
63. DeWied D, van Ree JM. Neuropeptides, mental performance and aging. Life Sci 22: 975-985, 1983.
64. Hefti F. Potential pharmacological use of neurotrophic factors in the treatment of neurodegenerative diseases. In Meyer EM, Simpkins JW, Yamamoto J (eds): *Novel Approaches to the Treatment of Alzheimer's Disease*. Plenum Press, New York, 1989, pp 63-70.

5

Strategies for the Treatment of Alzheimer's Disease: Cholinergic Agonists

Lincoln T. Potter
University of Miami School of Medicine, Miami, Florida

The idea that cholinergic replacement therapy may prove useful for the treatment of memory losses in various forms of Alzheimer's disease (AD) is based on four kinds of information. First, muscarinic antagonists like scopolamine impair cognition, while esterase inhibitors like physostigmine cause small improvements in the performance of memory tasks, in normal humans and laboratory animals (1). Second, experimental cholinergic denervation causes memory deficits in animals, and reinnervation diminishes these effects (2). Third, cholinergic denervation of the cerebral cortex and hippocampus is one of the earliest, most severe, and least variable features of AD (3,4). Postmortem cortical tissue typically shows choline acetyltransferase levels which are one third or less of that found in age-matched controls (5). Fourth, it has been possible to ameliorate the effects of the degenertion of dopaminergic nerves in the brains of persons with Parkinson's disease, by giving the precursor to dopamine, by giving directly acting dopaminergic agonists, and by antagonizing the neural systems which are unbalanced because of decreased levels of dopamine.

I. CHOLINERGIC THERAPEUTIC STRATEGIES

In theory, there are a variety of ways to increase cholinergic activity in the brains of persons with AD. Some focus on the nerves themselves, including attempts to prevent neural degeneration by removal of the (unknown) problem which causes degeneration, attempts to limit degeneration or increase regeneration with specific nerve growth factors, and attempts to cause new innervation by transplantation or with growth factors. Some strategies focus on the ability of the nerves to release acetylcholine; this category includes means to excite cholinergic cell bodies, improvement of choline levels, improvement of intraneuronal acetylcholine levels with esterase inhibitors, and decreased feedback inhibition of release, using appropriate receptor antagonists. Finally, there are potential ways to increase the activation of postsynaptic cells, using esterase inhibitors, exogenous cholinergic agonists, compounds which facilitate desired receptor transduction mechanisms, and antagonists of those muscarinic receptors which are linked to undesired responses.

So far only three of these potential strategies have been explored clinically: the use of choline, esterase inhibitors, and cholinergic agonists. None of these approaches has achieved anywhere near the degree of benefit to AD patients that is achieved easily with drugs like L-dopa for the treatment of Parkinson's disease, and it is appropriate to ask, why not? One real possibility is that in AD, too many nerve cells and kinds of nerve cells have been lost to permit any kind of replacement therapy. It is clear from the major atrophy of AD brains (15–30%) that many cells have degenerated, at least late in the disease, and there is specific evidence for interruptions of noradrenergic, serotonergic, peptidergic, and glutaminergic neurotransmission. On the other hand, a good case can be made that we have not yet adequately demonstrated whether or not cholinergic therapy can work, especially early in the disease process. There is general agreement that the administration of choline and its precursors is not of significant benefit in AD (6). There is, however, little reason to suspect that choline levels are not well maintained in brain tissue, or that choline is a limiting factor for acetylcholine synthesis. More perplexing is the situation with acetylcholinesterase inhibitors. Studies with parenteral physostigmine have indicated that many persons with AD show brief improvement in verbal memory (7), but evidence is accumulating that chronic therapy with oral esterase inhibitors does not yield sustained improvement (8). It is easy to criticize this general approach: enhanced levels of acetylcholine are not at sites of cholinergic denervation; and a general increase in acetylcholine will cause both excitatory and inhibitory effects on the brain (9). Nonetheless, it is disappointing that better results have not been achieved with oral esterase inhibitors early in AD. Finally, five cholinergic agonists have been tested in AD (10,11). Four—pilocarpine, RS-86, arecholine, and oxotremorine—are tertiary amines and unquestionably enter the brain. The fifth, bethanechol, was given intrathecally. While a few persons with AD improved slightly with these agents, the overall results were poor, and oxotremorine, in particular, caused depression. However, none of these agents has a desirable pharmacological profile for causing cerebral excitation; in fact, each would be expected to cause cerebral inhibition (12), for the reasons noted in the following section.

II. INFORMATION WHICH HELPS TO CONSTRAIN THE CHOICE OF A THERAPEUTIC AGENT

Nicotinic acetylcholine receptors account for only a small percent of the total acetylcholine receptors in the brain; the level of nicotinic receptors is decreased by about 50% in AD (12). Anecdotal data suggest that smoking improves mental alertness, but clinical trials of nicotine in AD have not produced significant benefit (13).

The techniques of molecular biology have established the presence of five muscarinic receptors in the brains of humans and animals, now called m1-m5 (14-17,18). Three of these—m1, m3, and m5—are coupled to transduction mechanisms which include an unknown G protein, a phospholipase C, and metabolites of phosphatidylinositides (16,17). In general, the activation of these receptors causes cellular excitation, often by inhibiting potassium fluxes (9). Two receptors—m2 and m4—are coupled to the inhibition of adenylate cyclase (16,17), and their activation typically produces inhibitory effects.

The use of pharmacological antagonists has distinguished three classes of muscarinic receptors, now called M_1, M_2, and M_3 (18). The M_1 type is defined by its high affinity for pirenzepine, the M_2 type by its high affinity for AFDX-116, and the M_3 type by its lower affinity for each of these agents. A number of other antagonists have also proved useful for distinguishing receptors in different tissues (see 16,18,19). The M_1-M_3 classification scheme has proved very useful for pharmacological and physiological work, and is all we have at present for functional studies. However, the m1-m5 and M_1-M_3 schemes overlap. In cloned CHO cells which express m1-m5 receptors separately, pirenzepine shows it s highest affinity for m1 receptors. It shows approximately 5-, 10-, 11-, and 57-fold lower affinity for m4, m5, m3, and m2 receptors, respectively (19). Hence, very low concentrations of ^{3}H-pirenzepine probably label m1 receptors selectively (12). AFDX-116 shows its highest affinity for cloned m2 receptors, and about 2-, 3-, 5-, and 11-fold lower affinity for m4, m3, m1, and m5 receptors, respectively (when the correct value for m2 affinity is used; see 15 as well as the original data in 19). Better selectivity is apparent for AFDX-116 in brain tissues, e.g. as an autoradiographic ligand, ^{3}H-AFDX-116 labels very few sites in the rat caudate nucleus (20), although this region expresses very high levels of mRNA for m1 and m4 receptors (21,22).

The exact numbers and locations of m1-m5 receptors in the brain and other tissues are not known, since the most selective available ligands for muscarinic receptors, ^{3}H-pirenzepine and ^{3}H-AFDX-116, do not distinguish each of these genetically defined receptors accurately. However, the distribution of mRNA for m1-m5 receptors is known with some accuracy (21,22). The most important fact relevant to the treatment of AD is that most of the mRNA in the cerebral cortex and hippocampus is for m1 and m3 receptors. The only other tissue known to have high concentrations of mRNA for m1 receptors is the striatum. However, the blocking effects of pirenzepine in adrenergic ganglia and the ability of the agonist McN-A-343 to activate these ganglia selectively suggests the presence of m1 receptors in ganglia (18). In contrast, mRNA for m3 receptors is widely distributed in glands and smooth muscles as well as the brain (21). Typical locations for the mRNA for the other receptor subtypes include: m2: heart, brainstem and smooth muscles; m4: striatum and cortex, and m5: substantia nigra and globus pallidus (21,22).

Cholinergic agonists act on atropine-sensitive muscarinic receptors in the cortex and hippocampus to cause both excitation and inhibition. In general, excitation is readily blocked by pirenzepine, whereas inhibition is not (9). Inhibition appears to be due to the activation of pirenzepine-resistant receptors on GABAergic, inhibitory, interneurons (9).

Agonists bind to two affinity states of m1 (23,24) and m2 receptors (25), including a guanine nucleotide-sensitive high-affinity state (K_H) and a guanine nucleotide-insensitive low-affinity state (K_L). The K_L/K_H ratio for different agonists correlates closely with the efficacy of the same agonists for producing cortical excitation and phosphoinositide hydolysis (24), or cyclase inhibition (25).

The agonists which have been tested clinically for the treatment of AD—oxotremorine, pilocarpine, arecholine, RS-86, and bethanechol—are all relatively inactive for producing electrophysiological activation of cortical pyramidal cells (9) and phosphoinositide hydrolysis (26), and each shows a low K_L/K_H ratio in binding assays (24). Hence none of these agonists would be expected to have much effect on the predominant m1 and m3 receptors in the cortex. Oxotremorine is known to be an effective agonist at m2 (25) and m4 receptors (27), and to cause cortical inhibition (9). Hence it is not surprising that it causes depression in persons with AD (28).

Blockade of muscarinic receptors in the brain with the M_1-selective antagonist, biperiden (29), causes AD-like symptomatology (30).

Oxotremorine acts on pirenzepine-resistant muscarinic receptors to decrease the release of acetylcholine from nerve terminals (31). Thus there appear to be presynaptic M_2 (m2) receptors on cholinergic nerve terminals which have a role in the feedback regulation of transmitter release.

Comparisons of the affinities of different agonists for the K_H states of m1 (24) and m2 receptors (12,32) indicate that most existing agonists have 10–20-fold higher affinity for inhibitory m2 than excitatory m1 receptors.

A priori, cerebral excitation is more likely to improve memory than is cerebral inhibition. No losses of m1 receptors, compared to controls, are shown by measurements of the numbers of m1 receptors in AD cortex with 1 nM ^{3}H-pirenzepine, and measurements of m1 receptors in the rat hippocampus 1 year after large fimbria/fornix lesions which produce total cholinergic denervation (33). Guanine nucleotide-sensitive high-affinity binding of agonist-m1 receptor-G protein complexes is also near normal in these tissues. Moreover, the ability of agonists to activate phosphoinositide hydrolysis via m1, m3, and m5 receptors remains normal in the denervated tissue (33). It may be concluded that the first steps in the m1 receptor transduction mechanism remain adequate to permit responses to exogenous muscarinic agonists in AD.

Taken together, the evidence above points to one *conclusion*: activation of the cerebral cortex and hippocampus in AD is most likely to be enhanced with selective agonists for m1 and/or m3 receptors. Since m3 receptors are prevalent peripherally whereas m1 receptors are not, the best single choice for further development is an m1 agonist. Aside from producing an increase in cerebral activity, the side effects of an m1 agonist can be expected to be alteration of motor activity, because of the prevalent m1 receptors in the striatum, and tachycardia, because of the presence of m1-like receptors on adrenergic ganglion cells. Tachycardia could be controlled with the peripheral M_1-antagonist, pirenzepine.

The available evidence also offers a plausible explanation for observations that oral esterase inhibition is less effective than parenteral physostigmine for improving memory (6,8). Because acetylcholine shows higher affinity for m2 than m1 receptors, any treatment which tends to maintain a low level of acetylcholine in the brain may cause more cerebral inhibition and blockade of acetylcholine release than cerebral excitation. It is also to be expected that selective activation of excitation, via m1 and m3 receptors, will produce better results than the general activation of m1–m5 receptors throughout the brain.

It has been suggested that an M_2 antagonist might be useful in AD to block feedback inhibition of the release of acetylcholine (34) and to reduce the cerebral inhibition produced by acetylcholine, esterase inhibitors, and nonselective agonists (12). Unfortunately, an M_2 antagonist would have major peripheral side effects on cardiac and smooth muscles.

III. DEVELOPMENT AND TESTING OF NEW AGONISTS

Drug companies can only develop drugs when there is a good test system for screening new drugs. In effect, we have many good agonists and antagonists for the m2 muscarinic receptors which are most prevalent in cardiac and smooth muscles, because of the availability of clearly defined responses in these two tissues to muscarinic agonists. By comparison, until recently there have been few ways to test selective m1 agonists.

For screening new agonists for *efficacy* at m1 receptors, the best available procedure is to examine the ability of the new agent to promote the hydrolysis of ^3H-phosphoinositides in cultured cells which express only these receptors.

Agonist-activated hydrolysis is particularly robust in Chinese hamster ovary cells (35).

For screening new agonists for their *affinity* for the high and low agonist-affinity states of m1 receptors, the best available procedure is to measure competition between the new agent and 1 nM ^{3}H-pirenzepine for muscarinic receptors in the hippocampus (23,24). The ratio of the high and low affinities (K_L/K_H) also offers a quantitative measure of the probable efficacy of the agonist (24).

At present it is difficult to obtain a quantitative idea of the *selectivity* of a new agent for m1 receptors over other receptors. Binding measurements can provide quantitative comparative data, but they are complex to perform for all five m1–m5 receptors. For example, K_H, K_L, and K_L/K_H ratios for m2 receptors can be obtained readily from competition curves between new agents and 0.1 nM ^{3}H-N-methylscopolamine for muscarinic receptors in the brainstem (12). When binding data for m1 and m2 receptors are compared, it is evident that most well-known cholinergic agonists (including all those tested for AD) have higher affinity and efficacy at m2 receptors (Potter, unpublished data). In practice, most drug companies have carried out a wide variety of functional assays. The ability of a new agonist to cause smooth muscle contraction generally correlates with its activity at m2 receptors, whereas activation of glandular secretions is generally mediated via m3 receptors. A more desirable response for an m1-selective agonist for AD is tachycardia, mediated by m1-like receptors on adrenergic gaglion cells.

Ultimately the best single test for a new selective m1 agonist is its ability to cause the excitation of cortical pyramidal cells in a manner which is blocked readily by low concentrations of pirenzepine, without causing increases in interneuron-mediated inhibition (9).

More than a dozen of the world's finest drug companies are engaged in a search for new muscarinic agonists that may improve memory. A number of promising agents have been developed and have reached the stage of animal testing for toxicology. Many more can be expected. There is little doubt but that new drugs can be developed to cause selective muscarinic activation of the cortex and hippocampus.

While the development of a selective m1 agonist can be expected, the critical question remains as to whether such an agent will improve memory or only cause disordered thinking. In the opinion of the author, we will not know the outcome of a large amount of preliminary research on muscarinic agonists until a good m1 agonist is tested clinically for its advantageous and disadvantageous effects on the mental activity of humans. Whatever the outcome, the experience gained from this necessary human experiment will help to define which animal models are useful to predict the efficacy of new drugs that affect memory. If an m1 agonist improves memory, there will be added impetus to examine the activity of m3 agonists, and of combinations of m1 and m3 agonists, despite the higher likelihood of peripheral side effects with m3 agonists.

If an m1 agonist improves memory functions but causes Parkinsonian signs and symptoms, or causes significant downregulation of normal m1 receptor mechanisms, there are a variety of ways to fine-tune the therapeutic strategy. For example, it has been suggested that the use of an esterase-sensitive m1 agonist could overcome both of these problems by targeting the action of an agonist to synapses which have lost acetylcholinesterase (because of cholinergic denervation), and by preventing agonist actions in brain regions which are rich in this enzyme, like the striatum (36).

IV. RESEARCH ISSUES AND FACTORS REQUIRING GREATER EMPHASIS

With respect to the importance of the cholinergic nervous system to the pathogenesis and treatment of AD, the greatest single determinant of progress at present is the (non)availability of highly selective m1-m5 agonists and antagonists. Most of this paper has addressed the reasons for developing and testing only one of the five key agonists and five key antagonists which are necessary to understand the workings of this system. The availability of pirenzepine has been the single most important factor for defining this system so far, but it is far from an ideal ligand. For example, we do not know the exact locations, numbers, functions, life history, or changes in any one of the m1-m5 receptor populations in any brain. We cannot selectively activate or block any of these receptors, and it is still difficult to test new potential drugs for their selective action(s). What is needed most for research work is a selective agonist and antagonist for each receptor, which can be used for functional studies. Imagine, for example, how much information could be gained if we could now activate and block m1 and m3 receptors selectively in the cortex and hippocampus in humans. There is wide agreement among the investigators in this field that receptor-specific antibodies will help define the locations and numbers of m1-m5 receptors. But the development of receptor-specific antibodies has been proceeding slowly, and it is not very likely that these large molecules will diffuse well enough for ideal physiological and pharmacological work, or be useful for clinical studies. A new small snake toxin which shows high selectivity for m1 receptors (37) will help to resolve some issues. But this toxin will not be useful for clinical work and is not reversible for physiological studies. It is very likely that new selective m1 and m3 agonists will be found by the many drug companies which are now seeking a therapeutic agent for AD. It is to be hoped that these companies will also test the thousands of new compounds which have been synthesized, for their ability to selectively block m1-m5 receptors. Antagonists can be tested readily for their selective affinity for these receptors in separate cell lines.

Until we have more selective ligands, it will be extremely difficult to properly evaluate a number of other questions in this field, including the value of different animal models for testing memory, the overlap of effects of different transmitter systems, and the usefulness of combined therapies.

REFERENCES*

1. Bartus RT, Dean RL, Pontecorvo MJ, et al. The cholinergic hypothesis: a historical overview, current perspective and furture directions. Ann NY Acad Sci 444:332–358, 1985.
2. Dunnett SB, Low WC, Iverson SD, et al. Septal transplants restore maze learning in rats with fornix-fimbria lesions. Brain Res 251:335–348, 1982.
3. Francis PT, Palmer Am, Sims NR, et al. Neurochemical studies of early-onset Alzheimer's disease. N Engl J Med 313:7–11, 1985.
4. Coyle JT, Price D, DeLong M. Alzheimer's disease: A disorder of cortical cholinergic innervation. Science 219:1184–1190, 1983.
5. Hansen LA, DeTeresa R, Davies P, et al. Neocortical morphometry, lesion counts, and choline acetyltransferase levels in the age spectrum of Alzheimer's disease. Neurology 38:48–54, 1988.
6. Fovall P, Dysken MY, Davis JM. Treatment of Alzheimer's disease with choline salts. In Reisberg B (ed): *Alzheimer's Disease*, Macmillan, New York, 1983, pp 346–354.
7. Davis KL, Harouturian V. Chapter 3: this volume.
8. Gauthier S, Bouchard R, Lamontagne A, et al. Tetrahydroaminoacridine-lecithin combination treatment in patients with intermediate-stage Alzheimer's disease. N Engl J Med 322:1271–1276, 1990.
9. McCormick DA, Prince DA. Mechanisms of action of acetylcholine in the guinea-pig cerebral cortex in vitro. J Physiol 375:169–194, 1986.
*10. Gray JA, Enz A, Spiegel R. Muscarinic agonists for senile dementia: past experience and future trends. Trends Pharmacol Sci Suppl: 85–88, 1989.
*11. Pomara N, Bagne CA, Stanley M, et al. Prospective strategies for cholinergic interventions in Alzheimer's disease. Prog Neuro-psychopharmacol 10:553–569, 1986.
*12. Potter Lt, Pearce BD, Fisher A. Selection of cholinergic agents which may improve memory. Basic, Clinical and Therapeutic Aspects of Alzheimer's and Parkinson's Diseases, Vol. 2 (Ed. T. Nagatsu), p. 335–340, Plenum Press, New York, 1990.
13. Newhouse PA, Sunderland J, Tariot PN. Intravenous nicotine in Alzheimer's disease: A pilot study. Psychopharmacol 95:171–175, 1988.
14. Fukada K, Kubo T, Maeda A, et al. Selective effector coupling of muscarinic acetylcholine receptor subtypes. Trends Pharmacol Sci Suppl: 4–10, 1989.
15. Bonner TI, Buckley NJ, Young AC, et al. Identification of a family of muscarinic acetylcholine receptor genes. Science 237:527–532, 1987.
16. Bonner TI. New subtypes of muscarinic acetylcholine receptors. Trends Pharmacol Sci Suppl:11–15, 1989.
17. Ashkenazi A, Peralta EG, Winslow JW, et al. Functional diversity of muscarinic receptor subtypes in cellular signal transduction and growth. Trends Pharmacol Sci Suppl:16–22, 1989.

*Recent reviews in the field of cholinergic replacement therapy are marked with an asterisk.

18. Birdsall N and committee. Nomenclature for muscarinic receptor subtypes recommended by symposium. Trends Pharmacol Sci Suppl: VII, 1989.
19. Buckley NJ, Bonner TI, Buckley CM, et al. Antagonist binding properties of five cloned muscarinic receptors expressed in CHO-K1 cells. Mol Pharmacol 35:469-476, 1989.
20. Regenold W, Araujo DM, Quirion R. Quantitative autoradiographic distribution of [^{3}H] AFDX-116 muscarinic M_2 receptor binding sites in rat brain. Synapse 4:115-125, 1989.
21. Buckley NJ, Bonner TI, Brann MR. Localization of a family of muscarinic receptor mRNAs in rat brain. J Neurosci 8:4646-4652, 1988.
22. Weiner DM, Brann MR. Distribution of m1-m5 muscarinic receptor mRNAs in rat brain. Trends Pharmacol Sci Suppl:115, 1989 (Abstract).
23. Potter LT, Ferrendelli CA, Hanchett HE. Two affinity states of M_1 muscarine receptors. Cell Mol Neurobiol 8:181-191, 1988.
24. Potter LT, Ferrendelli CA. Affinities of different cholinergic agonists for the high and low affinity states of hippocampal M_1 muscarine receptors. J Pharmacol 248:974-978, 1989.
25. Ehlert FJ. The relationship between muscarinic receptor occupancy and adenylate cyclase inhibition in the rabbit myocardium. Mol Pharmacol 28:410-421, 1985.
26. Fisher SK, Figueiredo JC, Bartus RT. Differential stimulation of inositol phospholipid turnover in brain by analogs of oxotremorine. J Neurochem 43:1171-1179, 1984.
27. Baumgold J, White T. Pharmacological differences between muscarinic receptors coupled to phosphoinositide turnover and those coupled to adenylate cyclase inhibition. Biochem Pharmacol 38:1605-1615, 1989.
28. Davis KL, Hollander E, Davidson M, et al. Induction of depression with oxotremorine in patients with Alzheimer's disease. Am J Psychiatr 144:468-471, 1987.
29. Syvalahti EKG, Lauren L, Markkanen J, et al. Interactions of psychotropic drugs with brain muscarinic cholinoceptors: Similarities of biperiden with pirenzepine in receptor binding properties. Pharmacol Toxicol 60:66-69, 1987.
30. Kurlan R, Como C. Drug induced Alzheimerism. Arch Neurol 45:356-357, 1988.
31. Hoss W, Messer WS, Monsma FJ, et al. Biochemical and behavioral evidence for muscarinic autoreceptors in the CNS. Brain Res 517:195-201, 1990.
32. Closse A, Bittiger H, Langenegger D, et al. Binding studies with ^{3}H-cis-methyldioxolane in different tissues. NS Arch Pharmacol 335:372-377, 1987.
33. Pearce BD. Experimental basis for cholinergic replacement therapy in Alzheimer's disease. PhD thesis, University of Miami, 1990.
34. Mash DC, Flynn DD, Potter LT. Loss of M_2 muscarine receptors in the cerebral cortex in Alzheimer's disease and after experimental cholinergic denervation. Science 228:1115-1117, 1985.
35. Fraser CM, Wang C-D, Robinson DA, et al. Site-directed mutagenesis of m1 muscarinic acetylcholine receptors: conserved aspartic acids play important roles in receptor functions. Mol Pharmacol 36:840-847, 1989.
36. Potter LT. Muscarine receptors in the cortex and hippocampus in relation to the treatment of Alzheimer's disease. In Cohen S, Sokolovsky M (eds): *International Sympo-*

sium on Muscarinic Cholinergic Mechanisms Freund Publishing Ltd, London, 1987, pp. 294–301.

37. Max SI, Liang J-S, Potter LT. "m1-Toxin": isolation characterization and selectivity for m1 muscarinic receptors. Neurosci Abstr (in press, 1991).

*38. Mayeux R. Therapeutic strategies in Alzheimer's disease. Neurology 40:175–180, 1990.

6

The Use of Molecular Modeling in Alzheimer's Research: Cholinergic Toxins, Amyloid Inhibitors-Diagnostics, and NMDA Agonists and Antagonists

Donald J. Abraham
Medical College of Virginia, Virginia Commonwealth University, Richmond, Virginia

Molecular modeling is a research field that can contribute to new pharmacological approaches by aiding in the design of new medicines and/or diagnostic agents for Alzheimer's disease. Modeling can also provide insights concerning the molecular mechanisms involved in basic neurochemical pathways. Three examples of how we have used or are using molecular modeling in Alzheimer's related research will be illustrated.

I. CHOLINERGIC TOXINS IN THE DEVELOPMENT OF AN ANIMAL MODEL

The hypoactivity of the central cholinergic system has been implicated in several psychiatric disorders, including Alzheimer's disease (1,2). Several years ago, Professor Israel Hanin (when we were both in Pittsburgh) suggested that we design an agent to block high-affinity choline uptake so that an animal model with a cholinergic deficit could be obtained. My first thought was to design the molecules as sterically compatible as possible to the molecular volume of choline. Stereocompatibility between new analogs and agonists or antagonists is a basic principle in drug research that is sometimes overlooked at the early stages of investigation.

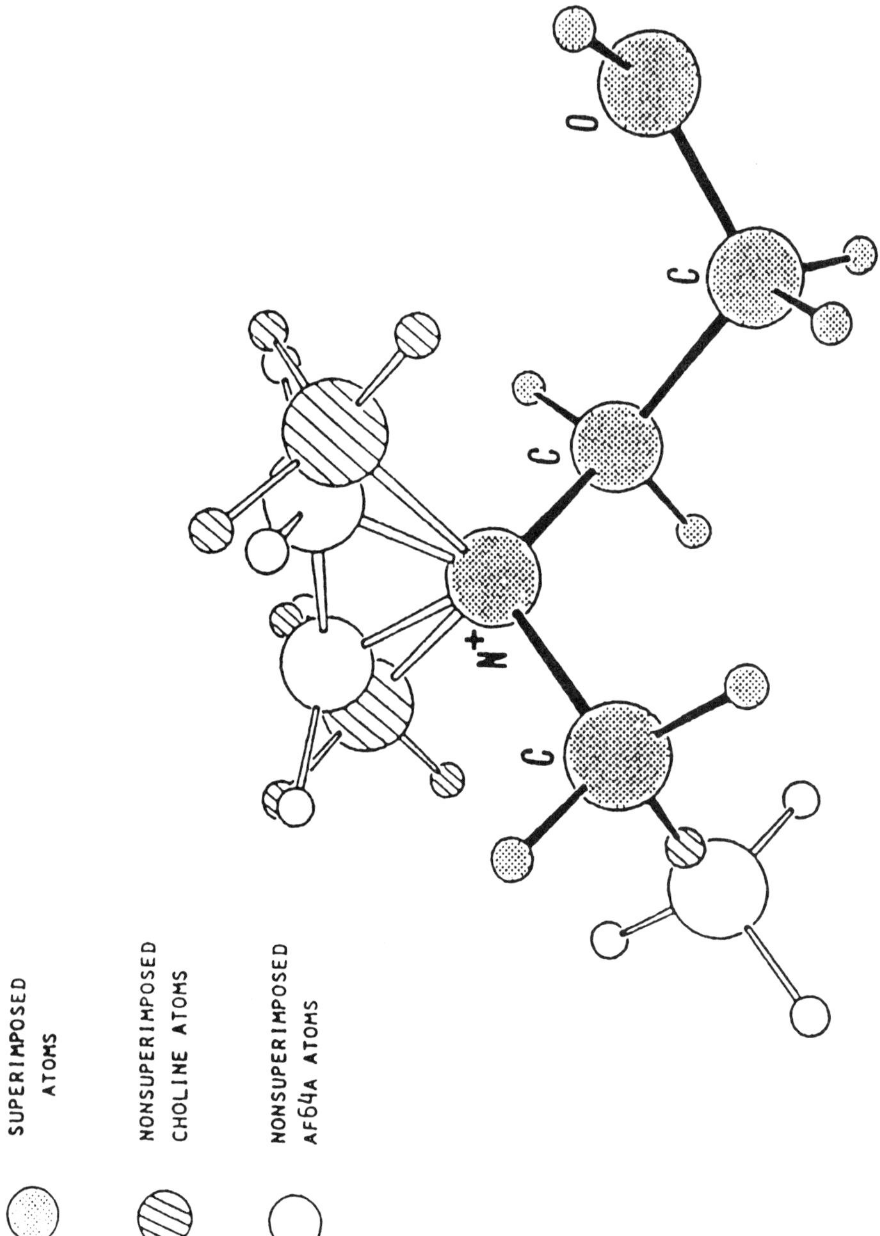
O
C
C
N+
C
SUPERIMPOSED ATOMS
NONSUPERIMPOSED CHOLINE ATOMS
NONSUPERIMPOSED AF64A ATOMS

Figure 1

The next idea was to incorporate a functional group that would bind irreversibly to the high-affinity choline uptake system. Therefore, we started with choline and added a one-arm nitrogen mustard group. The active aziridinium ion intermediate of the ethyl analog of the mustard closely overlaps in steric volume with choline (Fig. 1) (3). The choice of a one-arm mustard was made to reduce the degree of nonspecific reaction observed with two-arm mustards. Abraham Fisher synthesized the one-arm mustard and aziridinium choride and named them AF64 and AF64A, respectively. The aziridinium ion, AF64A, was one of the first activated nitrogen mustard-like molecules to be widely used to attempt to establish a cholinergic deficit in animals (4,5).

The major lesson we learned from this initial work was that a close and effective collaboration between pharmacologists and medicinal chemists with modeling experience produced exciting results almost immediately, although we had no previous experience in this field. Reading the literature and design of the first AF64 compounds were made in 2 weeks. A decade of research on AF64 has followed.

II. MOLECULAR MODELING OF AGENTS OF DIAGNOSE EARLY DEPOSITS OR INHIBIT POLYMERIZATION OF β-AMYLOID FILAMENT PROTEINS

A. Background

β-amyloid protein (BAP) is a 42- or 43-amino acid peptide found in the extracellular neuritic plaques of Alzheimer's patients (6). Kang et al. (7) have sequenced BAP. X-ray diffraction data suggests (8,9) that the fibrils formed by polymerization of BAP are about 8 nm long in the fibril direction and about 4 nm thick, corresponding to approximately four β-pleated sheets. Modeling BAP is possible, since the sequence and some structural information is available. Wischick (10) has proposed that the polymerization process of filament proteins may be similar to the polymerization of sickle hemoglobin (HbS). It was suggested to us by Drs. Zaven Khatchaturian and Claude Wischick that our extensive experience in the design, synthesis, and binding site determination of antisickling agents that hinder the polymerization of HbS might be applicable in discovering agents that interfere with

---

Figure 1 Overlap of AF64A with choline. The overlap of the two molecules demonstrates that the only nonsuperimposed atom is the terminal methyl group of the AF64a ethyl moiety (bottom lower left-open sphere). Two of the methyl groups of choline (hashed spheres) and the methylene atoms of the aziridinium ring (open spheres) are partially overlapped. Seventy-five percent of the structures overlap with similar atom types, i.e., hydrophobic on hydrophobic and polar on polar.

the polymerization of the fibril proteins, such as BAP and the paired helical filament protein (PHF).

B. Mechanistic Understanding of Congo Red Binding

A logical first approach to designing an inhibitor is to search the literature for agents that bind specifically to BAP. It is well known that Congo red stains amyloid proteins, which are thought to play a central role in a variety of disease states (11). The staining is relatively specific (12) and has been employed to demonstrate amyloid in pathological specimens (13) and to gain insights into macromolecular structure (14,15). Our understanding of how Congo red might interact with a β-pleated sheet was first observed through molecular modeling experiments using a single peptide chain folded into two strands of β-pleated sheet. The sulfonic acid oxygen groups of Congo red are separated in energy minimized conformations by 18–21 Å and are in an ideal position to interact with a basic amino acid side chain every seventh residue on one strand of a β-pleated sheet (i.e., the seven α-carbons are separated by 21.9 Å, Fig. 2). The Congo Red aromatic amino groups are separated by 13–14 Å and are in an approximate position to hydrogen bond or form a salt interaction with appropriate polar side chain atoms every fifth residue on the antiparallel β-strand (i.e., the five α-carbons are separated by 14.6 Å; Fig. 2). The polar atoms on Congo red appear to be "tailor-made" to interact with β-pleated sheets when the dye is oriented parallel to the direction of the two peptide chains.

However, it has been suggested that the invariably positive optical character of Congo red–induced birefringence of amyloid implies that the linear dye molecules are arranged parallel on the amyloid, with the long axis of the dye parallel to that of the fibril (16). This would indicate that Congo red binds perpendicular to the direction of the β-pleated strands and not between two antiparallel strands as inferred in Figure 2. We have published another possible mode of binding where Congo red is positioned perpendicular to β-pleated sheets to account for the above observation (17). By either binding mode, it seems clear that the 19–21-Å distance between sulfonic acids on Congo red plays a key role in the interaction with BAP and similar β-pleated sheet fibrils. Structural studies are in progress to elucidate the nature of this interaction.

C. Searching For New Molecules That Bind To BAP

The recent advancement of molecular modeling software has enabled researchers to search large-scale databases for lead compounds once structural features of interest are defined. Aladdin is one such program (18,19). Aladdin searches a database of three-dimensional structures, marks atoms that meet substructure criteria, evaluates geometrical criteria, and prepares a number of files that are input for

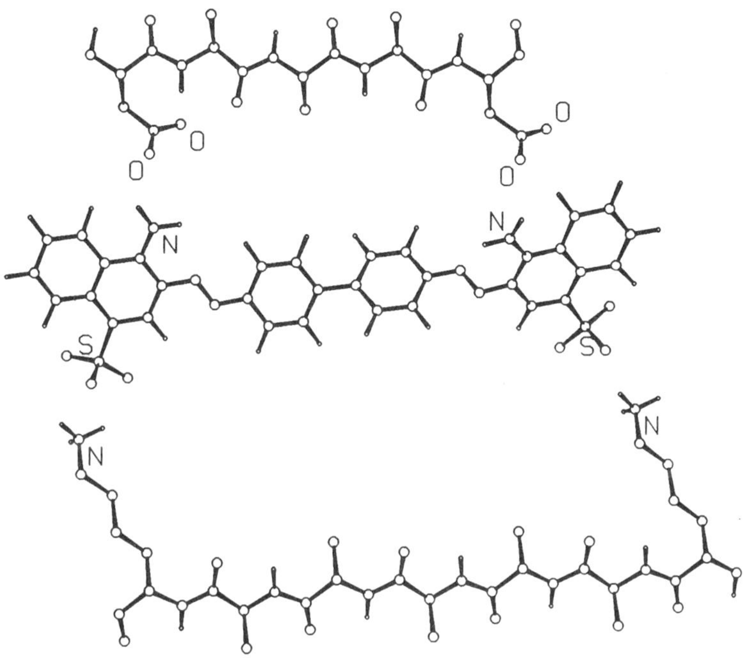

Figure 2 Congo red interaction with a β-pleated sheet. Antiparallel peptides in a β-pleated sheet conformation clearly demonstrate that the sulfonates of Congo red (labeled S) are positioned to interact with suitable basic amino acids, e.g., terminal Lys amino atoms labeled N, every seventh residue. The amino groups of Congo red (labeled N) are positioned to interact with acidic amino acids, e.g., Asp carboxylates labeled O, every fifth residue.

molecular modification, coordinate generation, and molecular graphics. We decided to conduct a 3-D structural search for molecules that might have Congo red binding characteristics.

The most important feature (according to our model for Congo red binding described above and depicted in Fig. 2) is a distance of approximately 19 Å between the two sulfonic acid groups. In the first search, we also added a conjugation constraint extending over a 25-Ådistance. Extensive conjugation gives rise to color in the visible region of the spectrum. Distance and conjugation constraints were used in the database search which targeted disulfonates, dicarboxylates, and mixed functionalities. The Aladdin search (20) of two databases (21) produced a large number of hits.

The Aladdin search suggested structures that we did not conceive as possible analogs that might bind selectively. The new molecules or modified derivatives could have both diagnostic and therapeutic potential in the broad class of diseases which Glenner has termed the β-fibrilloses (1). The interesting ideas to be presented during the panel discussion by Dr. Simpkins (Chapter 4), concerning principles of delivery of agents that cross the blood-brain barrier, must be integrated into the next phase of structure activity studies of active lead compounds.

Finally, it is also conceivable that a 2-D or 3-D NMR solution structure of BAP can be obtained if a suitable solvent can be found to solubilize the peptide. Determining the 3-D structure of BAP and other fibril proteins from brain should be a high priority for basic research in this area.

III. NMDA RECEPTOR MODELING

A. Background

Modeling a receptor complex without secondary, tertiary, or quaternary structural information of the protein components is not very appealing. However, it is possible to model a receptor after a system whose structural details have been elucidated. For example, Efraim Racker has suggested, in a perspective on *Structure, Function, and Assembly of Membrane Proteins* (22): "Data on three-dimensional structures are needed, and physical chemists could help with model designs and experiments that directly demonstrate signal transduction over distances of hundreds of amino acids. Perhaps hemoglobin will serve as a model." Our continuing efforts in designing agents that modify the structure-function of hemoglobin and our past work in the neurosciences provides a background to test Racker's idea by using hemoglobin as a model for the NMDA channel. We selected the NMDA channel to model, since extensive literature exists on the chemistry and pharmacology of this receptor.

Elucidation of the mechanistic operation at the molecular level of the NMDA receptor complex is key to understanding the action of excitatory amino acids and their role in neurochemical pathways. It is known that a voltage-dependent conditional activation of the NMDA-receptor is regulated by magnesium (23,24). The channel conductance and neuronal response consists of short-term membrane conductance associated with long-term biochemical changes. The latter is associated with intracellular calcium concentrations (25). The allosteric facilitation (effector activity) by glycine to a separate site in the receptor complex (26) that prevents desensitization of the receptor (27) is of special mechanistic interest.

B. Hemoglobin Structure and Function

Hemoglobin (Hb) is a tetrameric allosteric protein that binds, transports, and delivers oxygen. Deoxyhemoglobin has a large, central water cavity located between the four subunits (two α and two β) that resembles an open ion channel. A two-fold symmetry axis bisects the molecule through the center of the water channel, so that corresponding amino acid side chains from each subunit that point toward the center of the cavity, also point at each other. For example, the two side chains of Thr 134α1 and 134α2 (the latter designated 534; see Fig. 3 legend for key) reach across the channel and point at each other.

Deoxyhemoglobin is also stabilized by several salt bridges between acidic and basic amino acids. Although the distance is too large in the high-salt deoxy-Hb X-ray crystal structure, one salt bridge is thought to form at physiological conditions between the Arg 141 C-terminal carboxylate ion on one α (α1) subunit and the N-terminal ammonium ion of Val 1 on the other α subunit (α2) (28). Another anion-mediated salt bridge is formed between the guanidinium ion of Arg 141 α1, chloride ion, and the Val 1 α N-terminal amino group (29). The two salt bridges described above occur in pairs due to the two-fold axis and are located near the top of the water channel (i.e., Arg-COO- 141α1 $\leftrightarrow$ Val-NH_3^+ 1α2, and Arg-COO- 141α2 $\leftrightarrow$ Val-NH_3^+ 1α1; and Arg 141α1 $\leftrightarrow$ Cl- $\leftrightarrow$ Val 1α2, and Arg 141α2 $\leftrightarrow$ Cl- $\leftrightarrow$ Val 1α1). Figure 4a depicts these salt bridges and chloride binding sites.

Upon oxygenation, the salt bridges break, the $\alpha 1\beta 1$-subunit pair moves in relation to the $\alpha 2\beta 2$-subunit pair, and the cavity is narrowed and nearly closed at the β-subunit interface (Figure 4a). Hydrogens (termed "Bohr protons") are released from the change in pKA of salt bridge residues. Therefore, R-state hemoglobin is more basic that T-state hemoglobin.

The allosteric equilibrium between the deoxy (T) and the oxy (R) states can be shifted by small molecule effectors or inhibitors that bind in the channel. For example, in humans, the naturally occurring red cell allosteric effector, 2,3-diphosphoglyceric acid (2,3-DPG or DPG), binds at the β-subunit end of the open T-state channel, bridging the molecular two-fold axis (Fig. 5) (30). The negatively charged acid groups of DPG form salt bridges with a pair of histidines and a lysine. DPG has pseudo-two-fold symmetry that matches the two-fold symmetry of the receptor site (Fig. 5).

Another simple allosteric effector, chloride ion (Cl), binds competitively at the DPG site and at the α-subunit opening of the channel in T-state hemoglobin. The latter interaction has been shown (29,31–33) to be located near the Val 1α ammonium ion involved in the Arg 141α salt bridge described above.

Finally, 11 non-naturally occurring allosteric inhibitors (synthetic organic acid molecules) such as the antilipidemic drugs, clofibric acid (clofibrate) and bezafibrate (BZF), have been shown to bind in pairs to "niches" along the Hb central water cavity (Fig. 6a) (34–38). Three of the agents bind to a less defined second site between the α and β subunit interfaces, in the middle of the cavity (Fig. 6b). Most of the interactions between the BZF-like organic acids and the protein are dipolar, microdipolar, or hydrophobic in nature. Stronger interactions between ionized groups of opposite charge and hydrogen bonds are also observed. The acid

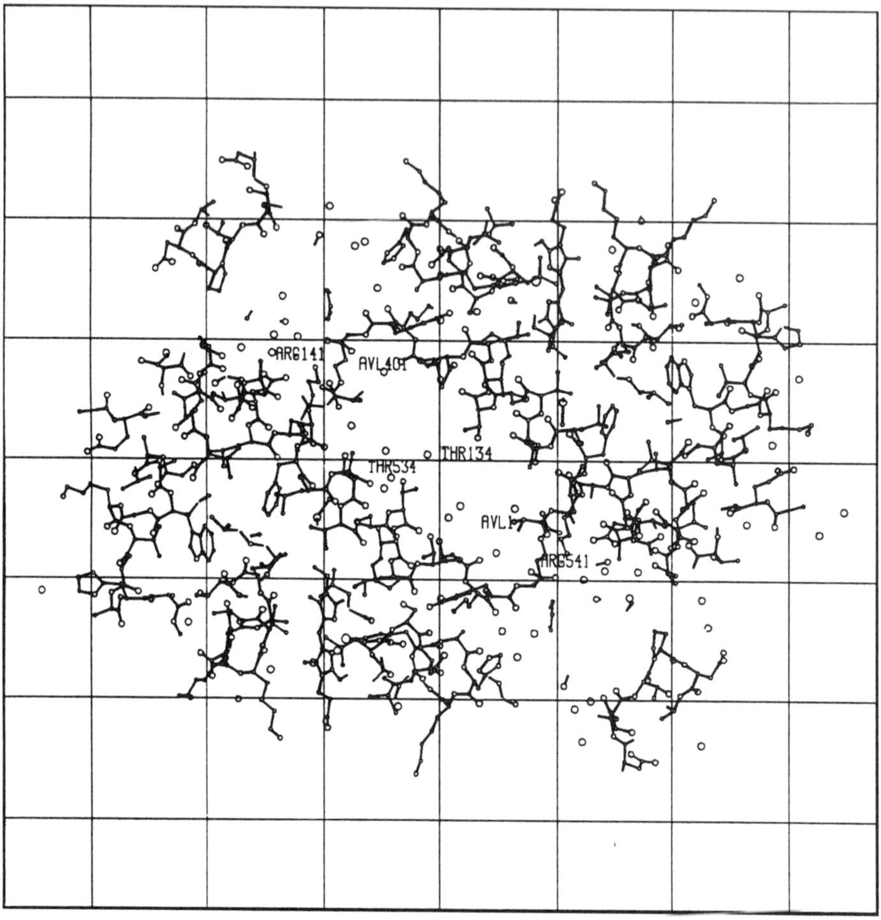

Figure 3 Central H_2O cavity in deoxyhemoglobin. This figure depicts a slice through the top of the hemoglobin α subunits showing the central water cavity. The side chain Thr 534 from the $\alpha 2$ subunit points toward the two-fold axis and the symmetry related $\alpha 1$ Thr 134 side chain. In this figure, all $\alpha 1$ subunit residues are designated with numbers from 1-141 and the $\alpha 2$ subunit residues from 401-541. This nomenclature permits easy identification of residues from all four subunits, where the β-residues are designated from 201-246 for $\beta 1$ and 601-646 for $\beta 2$. The salt bridges depicted in Figure 4a are shown. Arg 141 $\alpha 1$ (labeled Arg 141, upper left corner) is in close proximity to the N-terminal valine ammonium ion of $\alpha 2$ (laveled Avl 401). The symmetry-related pair is at the bottom right corner of the water cavity (Arg 541 = Arg 141 $\alpha 2$ and Avl 1 = Val 1 $\alpha 1$).

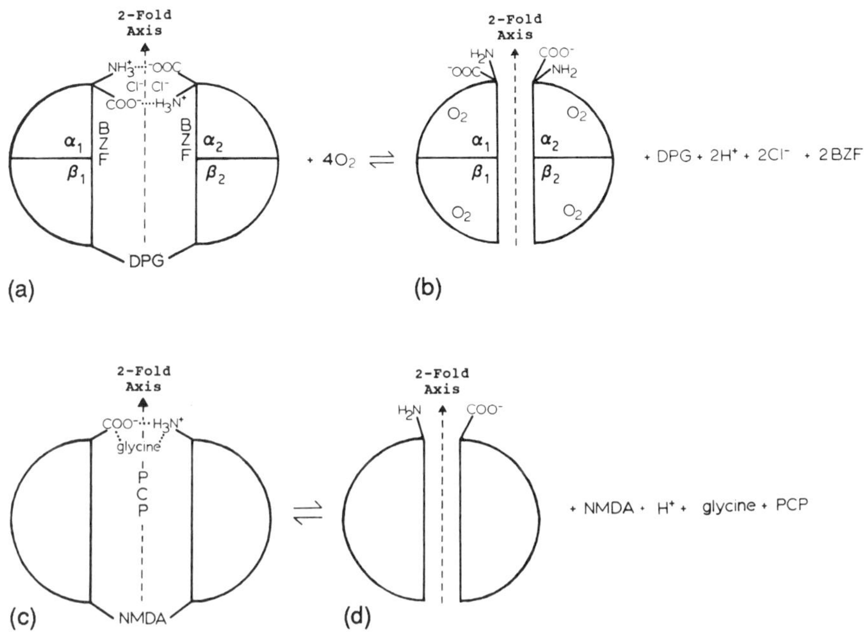

Figure 4 Comparison of the hemoglobin allosteric transition with the proposed allosteric transition of the NMDA receptor.
(a) Deoxyhemoglobin with binding sites of the allosteric modulator DPG, two symmetry-related salt bridges, and two chloride-binding sites bridging the Arg ammonium ion and N-terminal amino group (see text). The symmetry-related binding sites of the antilipidemic drug bezafibrate extend from the top of the α-subunits to the α-β interface in the middle of the channel.
(b) Upon oxygenation, the salt bridges are opened and DPG, chloride, BZF, and protons are released.
(c) The proposed open NMDA channel with bound NMDA, and salt bridge stabilized by glycine. The phencyclidine-binding site, although depicted on the two-fold axis, can be shifted left or right or may exist in pairs similar to BZF in hemoglobin. The number of PCP molecules bound (two or one) would be dependent upon the size of the cavity.
(d) When the cavity is closed, NMDA glycine, PCP, and protons or cations are released (the latter two would be dependent upon changes in pKa of the salt bridge residues between the open and closed channel).

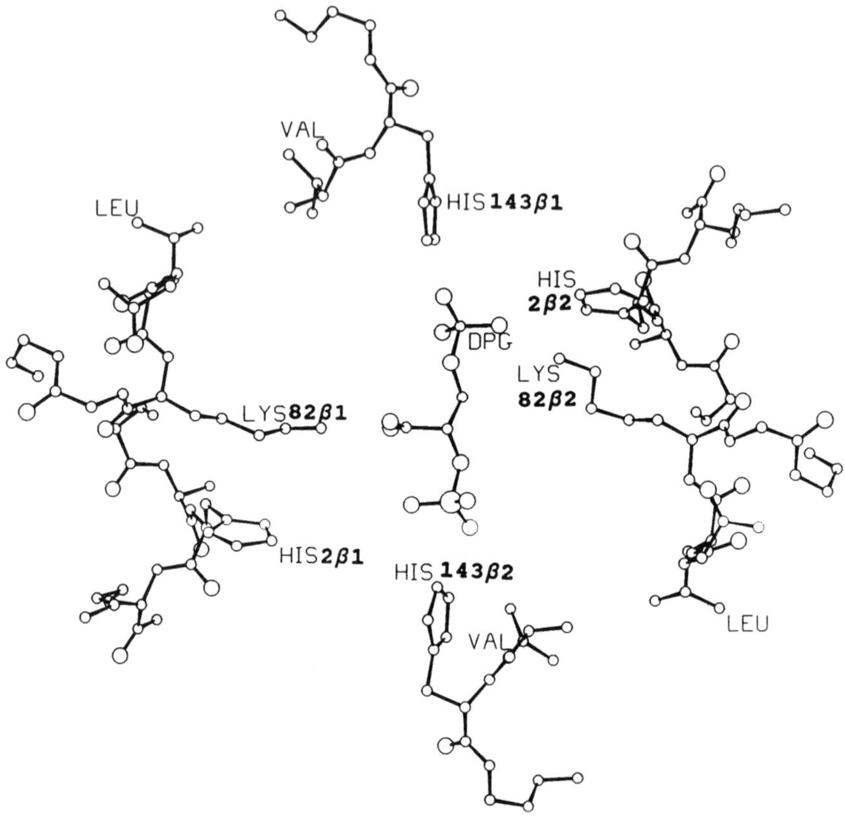

Figure 5 DPG bound to deoxyhemoglobin. 2,3-Diphosphoglyceric acid (DPG) binds across the two-fold axis at the bottom of the β-subunits. The two phosphates form salt interactions with both symmetry-related histidines 2 α1, 2 α2 and 143 α1, 143 α2, while the DPG acid group interacts via another ionic salt bridge with one of the Lys 82 β-residues. DPG therefore binds to the open channel and stabilizes it.

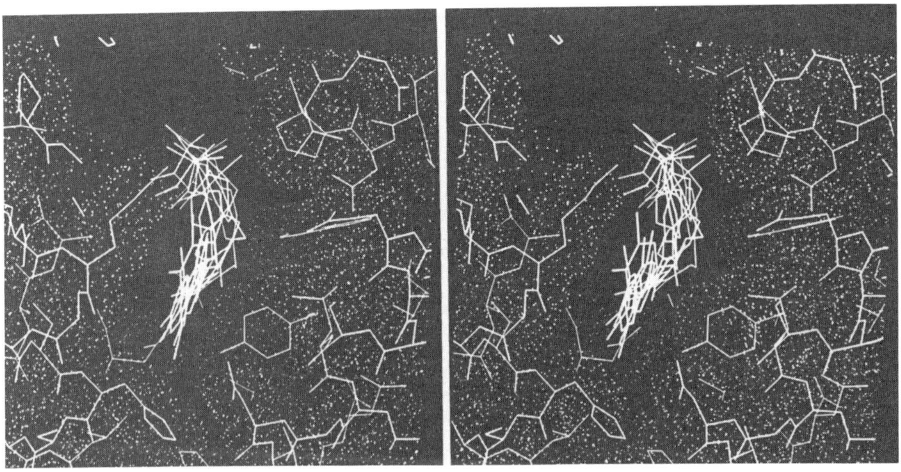

(a)

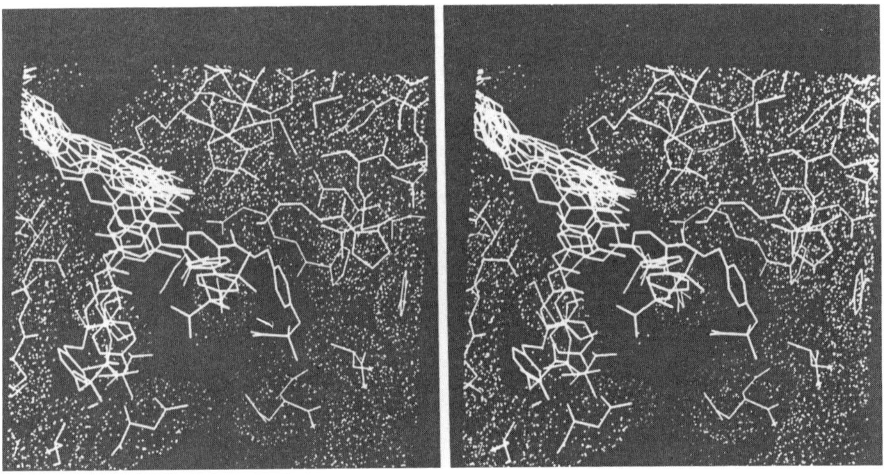

(b)

Figure 6 Central water cavity binding sites of hemoglobin allosteric inhibitors. (a) Stereo pair of six hemoglobin allosteric inhibitor positions superimposed at the major binding niche in the central water cavity. The bound conformations were determined by x-ray crystallographic studies (see ref. 39). Considerable variation in structure and substitution patterns can be made, since the wall of the cavity does not completely surround the inhibitor as would be found for many substrate protein-binding sites. (b) Stereo pair showing a second allosteric inhibitor site for three of the derivatives (see ref. 39 for details). This site (in the center of the photograph) is much less specific than the primary binding site shown in the upper left portion of the figure. There is sufficient nonspecificity at this site so that one of the three bound molecules is able to sit perpendicular to the other two. The major attraction for binding at this site is Arg 104β.

groups of the BZF like compounds interact with the Arg 141α salt bridge and are located near the proposed chloride binding site mentioned above. The allosteric modulation of BZF-like compounds and DPG are additive, since they bind to different sites (Fig. 4a).

C. Hemoglobin as a Model for the NMDA Ion Channel?

Can we use Hb as a model to understand NMDA structure-function, to explain known neurochemical interactions, and to design new agonists and/or antagonists?

Initially we recognized that the structure of N-methyl-D-aspartate (NMDA) has a geometric resemblance to DPG (Fig. 7). The NMDA acid groups can be oriented toward the direction of the DPG phosphates and the NMDA N-methyl group can directed toward the position of the carboxyl group of DPG. NMDA has psuedosymmetry similar to DPG!

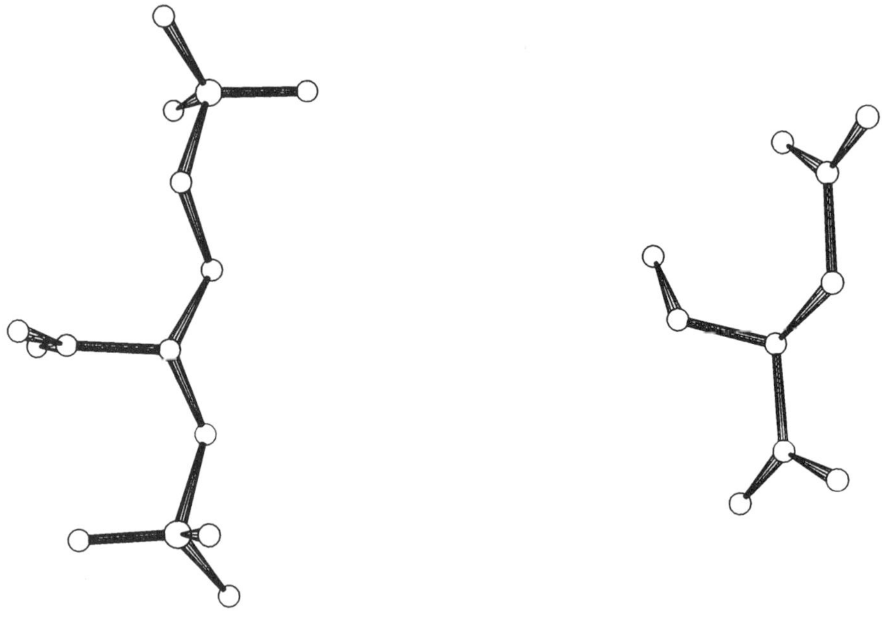

Figure 7 Comparison of the pseudo-two fold symmetry of DPG and NMDA. The similarity in direction of polar residues in both DPG (phosphates and acid groups) and NMDA (acids and amino group) indicates that NMDA could bind across a two-fold axis in a similar manner to DPG.

The similarity of the DPG and NMDA geometries suggests that the NMDA receptor binding site might also be located on a symmetry axis. Therefore, we decided to model the Hb-DPG site to see if it might accommodate NMDA binding. Simple replacement of two symmetry-related Lys residues with Glu in the DPG-binding pocket produced a mutant Hb model with NMDA binding characteristics (Fig. 8). The Glu for Lys substitutions permits NMDA to bridge the two-fold axis between the two β-subunits and interact via three ionic bonds with suitably positioned His and Glu residues in a similar fashion observed for DPG (compare Fig. 5 and 8).

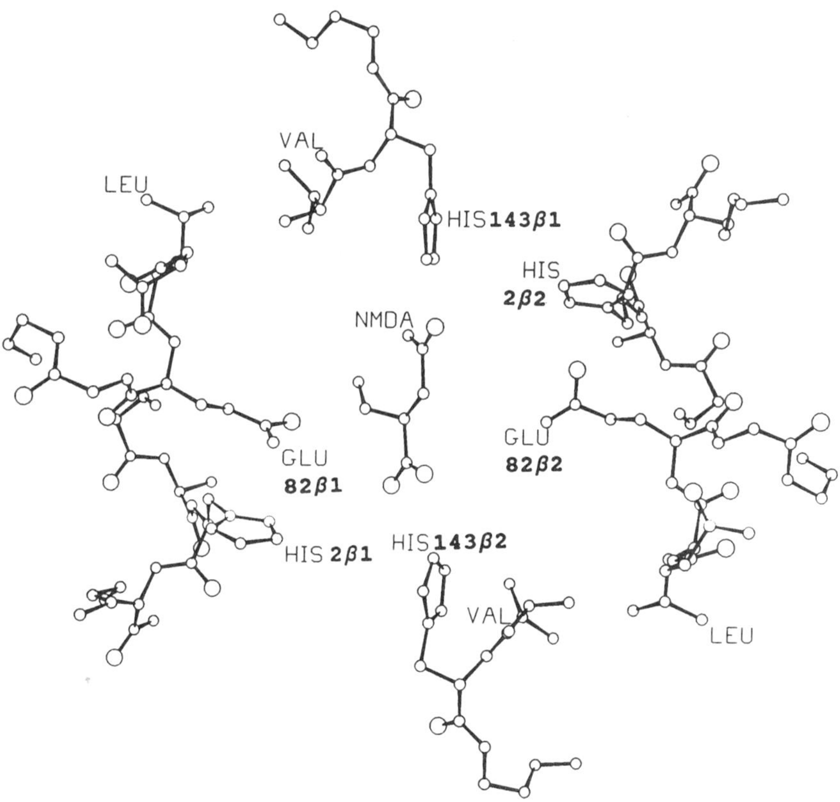

Figure 8 Proposed binding of NMDA to a receptor channel modeled after hemoglobin. By replacing the Lys residue with Glu in the DPG-binding site, a suitable pocket for NMDA is created. In this case the acid groups of NMDA interact with the His residues similar to the DPG phosphate group interactions and the NMDA amino group interacts with the Glu 82β substitution for Lys 82 residue.

The hemoglobin model for the NMDA receptor would indicate that NMDA agonists will contain suitable charge distributions related by an internal psuedo- or real two-fold axis. Molecules that contain a two-fold axis of symmetry with varying steric sizes have been designed to test this hypothesis. If the NMDA cavity is large enough at the NMDA binding site, it is possible for symmetry-related pairs of NMDA or agonists to bind. Such molecules would have symmetry that compliments one half of the two-fold axis.

D. Glycine Activation of the NMDA Receptor: Is It Similar to the Allosteric Effector Stabilization of the Hemoglobin T-State?

Can we incorporate the action of glycine into our proposed model? The co-stabilization of the T-structure in hemoglobin by DPG and BZF-like molecules provides a mechanistic explanation for the co-modulatory effect between NMDA and glycine. DPG- and BZF-like molecules bind at different ends of the channel. Similar binding of glycine and NMDA to different ends or areas of the ion channel would be compatible with the observed effector activity of glycine on NMDA binding (Fig. 4b).

But, how does such a simple molecule as glycine function? If the NMDA open channel is stabilized by salt bridges (as is found in hemoglobin), it can be imagined that glycine (being sterically small) can reinforce a salt bridge, as shown in Figure 9. This would be somewhat analogous to the Hb T-state binding of Cl- to the ammonium ion of the salt bridge between the Val1 α ammonium ion and the Arg 141α C-terminal carboxylate (compare Fig. 4a and 4b). Other small sterically compatible amino acids such as Ala and Ser should function similarly as has been observed (39–41).

Further, a two-fold axis in the NMDA receptor with symmetry-related pairs of salt bridge (as found in hemoglobin) would accommodate a pair of glycine binding sites. Our model would also predict a complimentary binding enhancement of glycine in the presence of NMDA.

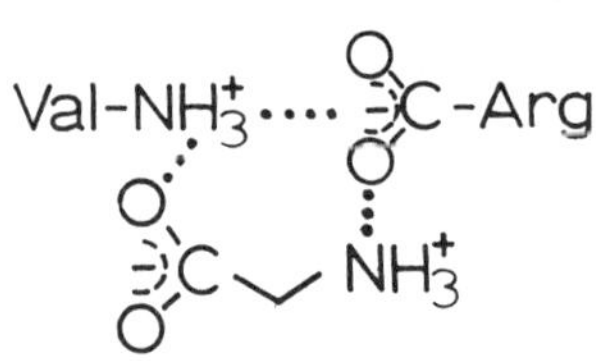

Figure 9 Proposed stabilization of a salt bridge with glycine. A Val-Arg salt bridge interaction illustrates stabilization by further ionic interactions of glycine as shown. Small amino acids, such as Gly, would be more sterically compatible than larger ones that would be obstructed by the residues on the wall of the cavity or the residues around the salt bridge.

E. Phencyclidine (PCP)-Binding Site

Inclusion of antagonist PCP-like binding in this model is also possible. As mentioned earlier, the central cavity of Hb has several surface "niches" that bind a large variety of acid like molecules (Fig. 4b). These "niches" are somewhat nonspecific in stereochemical detail permitting degrees of freedom in making substitutions. A variety of structural classes would be expected for agents that bind along the walls of a water channel, unlike the rigid stereochemical requirements of a substrate binding site. Therefore, we believe that binding of antagonists to "niches" along the NMDA ion channel cavity [similar to that observed in hemoglobin] would explain the observed structural variety of NMDA antagonists.

NMDA antagonists can only block the channel by gaining access to the stabilized open channel. If the cavity is large enough to accommodate pairs of antagonists, the design of new inhibitors would benefit by placement of polar interacting groups to one side of the molecule so they are positioned to interact with the wall of the cavity. If the cavity is narrower at the binding site, then the NMDA antagonist would bind singularly across the symmetry axis. Design of this type of agent would also benefit by having internal symmetry or pseudosymmetry that matches the symmetry of the ion channel. It is also conceivable that the antagonists would be competitive inhibitors of NMDA or glycine if they bind near those sites.

F. Summary of the NMDA-Binding Proposal

The information gained from the binding of allosteric effectors to Hb has permitted us to think about the stereochemical environment of the NMDA-binding site. We propose that the NMDA receptor has inherent symmetry, and that agents that bind to it do so in pairs or singularly dependent upon the size of the cavity at that site. We also propose that binding of more than one effector (NMDA and glycine) at a time can be accommodated, as found in hemoglobin (BZF and DPG), by binding to different areas of the cavity. One would therefore expect a reciprocal allosteric modulator relationship between glycine and NMDA.*

This model for the NMDA receptor, to our knowledge, is the first detailed hypothesis at the structural level that invokes symmetry for the binding site. A recent study demonstrates that NMDA receptors require multiple molecules of agonist for activation (42), which would be in agreement with this model. The concepts presented should permit the design of a number of new agonist and antagonists to test the hypothesis. Figure 4 summarizes and compares the chemical mechanisms

*We have not yet incorporated magnesium-binding sites into our model; however, a salt bridge between symmetry related acids is an obvious binding possibility as well as binding to phosphated amino acids that might be involved in allosteric regulation of the channel. Carboxyl-carboxylate interactions in proteins with associated cations has been observed (see Dayer L, James MNG. *Nature*, 295:79–80, 1982).

governing the allosteric equilibrium for hemoglobin with those similarly proposed for the NMDA receptor.

IV. GENERAL SUMMARY

The criteria of a good model are: 1) that it correlate with the known facts about a system as related to the model; 2) that it be simple in conveying the concept so that complex ideas and mechanisms can readily be grasped; 3) that it be illustrative in a manner that suggests new experiments, and 4) that it be consistent with stereochemical principles. We have attempted to use these guidelines in our work and hope that other neurochemists and pharmacologists might find similar uses for molecular modeling in their studies.

REFERENCES

1. Bowen DJ, Spillane JA, Curzon G, et al. Accelerated ageing or selective neuronal loss as an important cause of dementia? Lancet 1:11, 1979.
2. Davies P. Neurotransmitter-related enzymes in senile dementia of the Alzheimer type. Brain Res. 171:319, 1979.
3. Mistry JS, Abraham DJ, Hanin I. Neurochemistry of aging. 1. Toxins for an animal model of Alzheimer's diseae. J Med Chem 29:376, 1986.
4. Mantione CR, Fisher A, Hanin I. The AF64A-treated mouse: Possible model for central cholinergic hypofunction. Science 213:579, 1981.
5. Fisher A, Mantione CR, Abraham DJ, et al. Long-term central cholinergic hypofunction induced in mice by ethylcholine aziridinium ion (AF64A) in vivo J Pharmacol Exp Ther 222:140, 1982.
6. Glenner GG, Wong CW. Alzheimer's disease: Initial report on the purification and characterization of a novel cerebrovascular amyloid protein. Biochem Biophys Res Commun 122:885–890, 1984.
7. Kang J, Lemaire H-G, Unterbeck A, et al. Nature 325:733–736, 1987.
8. Glenner GG, Wong CW, Quaranta V, et al. The amyloid deposits in Alzheimer's disease: Their nature and pathogenesis. Appl Pathol 2:357–369, 1984.
9. Kirschner DA, Abraham C, Selko DJ. X-ray diffraction from the intraneuronal paired helical filaments and extraneuronal amyloid fibers in Alzheimer's disease indicates cross-beta conformation. Proc Natl Acad Sci USA 83:503–507, 1986.
10. Wischick C. Molecular neuropatholgy of Alzheimer's disease. In Katona CIE (ed): *Dementia Disorders, Advances and Prospects*. Chapman and Hall, London, pp 45–70.
11. Glenner GC. Amyloid deposits and amyloidosis. The beta-fibrilloses. N Eng J Med 302:1283–1333, 1980.
12. Putchtler H, Sweat F, Levin M. On the binding of Congo red by amyloid. J Histochem Cytochem 10:355, 1962.
13. Ladewig P. Double refringence of amyloid Congo red complex in histological section. Nature 156:355, 1945.

14. Glenner GC, Eanes ED, Page DL. The relation of the properties of Congo red-stained amyloid fibrils to the beta-conformation. J Histochem Cytochem 20:821, 1972.
15. Copper JH. Selective amyloid staining as a function of amyloid composition and structure. Lab Invest 31:232, 1974.
16. Romhanyi G. Selective differentiation between amyloid and connective tissue structures based on the collagen specific topo-optical staining with Congo red. Vitchows Arch [Pathol Anat] 354:209, 1971.
17. Klunk WE, Pettegrew JW, Abraham DJ. Quantitative evaluation of Congo red binding to amyloid-like proteins with a beta-pleated sheet conformation. J Histochem Cytochem 1273:1273, 1989.
18. Van Drie JH, Weininger D, Martin YC. Aladdin: An integrated tool for computer-assisted molecular design and pharmacophore recognition from geometric, steric, and substructure searching of three dimensional molecular structures. J Computer-Aided Molecular Design 3:225-251, 1989.
19. Alper J. The microchip microbe hunters Science 247:804-806, 1990.
20. The minimization of Congo red and Aladdin search were conducted by John Shifflett as a research project in a molecular modeling course offered at Virginia Commonwealth University, Spring 1990.
21. Kindly conducted by Dr. Yvonne Martin, Senior Research Fellow, Department 47E, AP9A, Abbott Laboratories, Abbott Park, IL 60064.
22. Racker E. Structure, function, and assembly of membrane proteins. Science 235:959-961, 1987.
23. Novak L, Bregestovski P, Ascher P, et al. Magnesium gates glutamate-activated channels in mouse central neurons. Nature 307:462-465, 1984.
24. Mayer ML, Westbrook G, Guthrie PB. Voltage-dependent block by Mg^{2+} of NMDA responses in spinal chord neurons. Nature 309:261-263, 1984.
25. MacDermott AB, Mayer ML, Westbrook GL, et al. NMDA-receptor activation increases cytoplasmic calcium concentration in cultured spinal chord neurons. Nature 321:519-522, 1986.
26. Johnson JW, Ascher P. Glycine potentiates the NMDA response in cultured mouse brain neurons. Nature 325:529-531, 1987.
27. Mayer ML, Vylicky L Jr, Clements J. Regulation of NMDA receptor desensitization in mouse hippocampal neurons by glycine. Nature 338:425-427, 1989.
28. Fermi G. Three-dimensional Fourier synthesis of human deoxyhaemoglobin at 2.5 Å resolution: refinement of the atomic model. J Mol Biol 97:237-256, 1975.
29. O'Donnell S, Mandaro R, Schuster TM, et al. X-ray diffraction and solution studies of specifically carbamylated human hemoglobin A. J Biol Chem 254:12204-12208, 1979.
30. Arnone A. X-ray diffraction study of binding of 2,3-diphosphoglycerate to human deoxyhaemoglobin. Nature 237:146-149, 1972.
31. Nigen AM, Manning JM, Alben JO. Oxygen-linked binding sites for inorganic anions to hemoglobin. J Biol Chem 255:5525-5529, 1980.
32. Arnone A, O'Donnell S, Schuster T. X-ray diffraction studies of carbamylated human deoxygemoglobin. Fed Proc 35:1604, 1976.

33. Arnone A, Williams DL Jr. Interactions moleculares de l'hemoglobine INSERM (Inst Nat Sante Recher) Collog 70:15–22, 1977.
34. Abraham DJ, Perutz MF, Phillips EV. Physiological and X-ray studies of potential antisickling agents. Proc Natl Acad Sci USA 80:324–328, 1983.
35. Lalezari I, Lalezari P, Poyart C, et al. New effectors of human hemoglobin: Structure and function. Biochemistry 29:1515–1523, 1990.
36. Lalezari I, Rahbar S, Lalezari P, et al. LR16, a compound with potent effects on the oxygen affinity of hemoglobin, on blood cholesterol, and on low density lipoprotein. Proc Natl Acad Sci 85:6117–6121, 1988.
37. Perutz MF, Fermi G, Abraham DJ, et al. Hemoglobin as a receptor of drugs and peptides: X-ray studies of the stereochemistry of binding. J Am Chem Soc 108:1064–1078, 1986.
38. Wireko FC, Kellogg GE, Abraham DJ. Allosteric modifiers of hemoglobin 2. Crystallographically determined binding sites and hydrophobic binding/interaction analysis of novel hemoglobin oxygen effectors. J Med Chem 34:758–767, 1991.
39. Bristow DR, Bowery NG, Woodruff GN. Light microscopic autoradiographic localisation of [^{3}H] glycine and [^{3}H]strychnine binding sites in rat brain. Eur J Pharmacol 126:303–308, 1986.
40. Johnson JW, Ascher P. In Lodge D (ed): *Excitatory Amino Acids in Health and Disease.* John Wiley & Sons, New York, 1988.
41. Snell LD, Morter RS, Johnson KM. Structural requirements for activation of the glycine rceptor that modulates the N-methyl-D-aspartiate operated ion channel. Euro J Pharmacol 156:105–110, 1988.
42. Javitt DC, Frusciante MJ, Zukin SR. Rat brain N-methyl-d-aspartate receptors require multiple molecules of agonists for activation. Mol. Pharmacol. 37:603–607, 1990.

PART III

Neurotrophic Agents—Growth Factors

7

Growth Factors and Neurotrophic Factors in Neurodegenerative Diseases

Franz Hefti, Paul A. Lapchak, and Timothy L. Denton
University of Southern California, Los Angeles, California

Research in the area of growth factors has made rapid progress during recent years and, because of new molecular biological techniques, the number of biochemically characterized and cloned proteins with growth-promoting activity has increased dramatically. Characterization of the regulation of synthesis and release of growth factors, identification of responsive mechanisms and cells, as well as characterization of their biological activities and their physiological role represent vast areas to be investigated. Some of the growth factors stimulate survival and differentiation of neurons and are often referred to as "neurotrophic factors." No generally accepted definition for this term exists, and there are several examples of proteins which promote both differentiation of neurons and proliferation of non-neuronal cells. The historical definition of neurotrophic factors limits this term to proteins which regulate developmental neuronal survival as target-derived, retrogradely acting messengers (1).

Most characterized actions of growth and neurotrophic factors on brain cells relate to developmental processes and suggest that the temporal and local regulation of expression of these proteins plays a key role during the assembly of the nervous system. However, growth factors also appear to be important for adult nervous function by being involved in processes related to plasticity and degeneration/regeneration of nerve cells. Such processes are altered in Alzheimer's disease (AD) and other neurodegenerative diseases, prompting the speculation that growth and neurotrophic factors become involved in the cascades of structural alterations occurring in neurodegenerative diseases. Characterization of neurotrophic mechanisms in the adult and aging brain may help us to understand the pathophysiology of AD and other neurodegenerative diseases. Furthermore, it may be possible to exploit these mechanisms to develop pharmacological manipulations counteracting degenerative events.

The best example of a growth factor studied in the context of neurodegenerative diseases is that of nerve growth factor (NGF) and Alzheimer's disease. NGF is presently being considered for clinical trials in AD because it acts trophically on cholinergic neurons of the adult basal forebrain, which seem to play an important role in memory function and undergo massive degeneration in AD. NGF administration to the brain of animals with experimental lesions of the cholinergic systems prevent the lesion-induced degenerative changes, suggesting that NGF treatment may attenuate the degenerative changes occurring in AD. The rationale for clinical trials with NGF in AD has also been discussed in detail in a recent review (2), and some of the supporting data from animal studies are given at the end of this chapter. The immediately following sections provide a very brief overview of neurotrophic factors, a general exploration of the possibility of utilizing knowledge of neurotrophic factors to further understanding and treatment of neurodegenerative diseases, and examples of recent findings illustrating the basis of these concepts.

I. NEUROTROPHINS

NGF was originally isolated based on its ability to promote survival and neurite outgrowth from responsive sensory neurons (3). Accordingly, the purification of other neurotrophic factors from various sources was approached by using neuronal cell cultures as assay systems. This strategy led to the isolation of ciliary neurotrophic factor (4), Brain-derived neurotrophic factor (BDNF) (5), and previously known proteins now also shown to act on neurons. The isolation and further characterization of BDNF by Barde and collaborators (1) provided the basis for the discovery that NGF is part of a family of proteins, called neurotrophins, which also includes BDNF and neurotrophin-3 (NT-3). BDNF is chemically similar to NGF, and its amino acid and nucleotide sequence shows a high degree of homology with that of NGF (6). The extensive homology between BDNF and NGF led several research groups to use the PCR methodology to search for additional members of a postulated group of NGF-related molecules. So far, this approach has led to the discovery of NT-3, which shares approximately 50% of its amino acids with both NGF and BDNF. Similar to BDNF, NT-3 has been shown to act on subpopulations of sensory neurons and its mRNA is heterogeneously distributed in the brain, suggesting a neurotrophic function for populations of central neurons (7–10). Neurotrophins may also share receptor mechanisms, since a previously characterized low-affinity NGF receptor protein seems to be part of functional high-affinity NGF and BDNF receptors (11).

BDNF promotes survival and fiber growth of neurons from chick sensory ganglia, and injections of BDNF into quail embryos prevent the neuronal death that normally occurs in sensory ganglia (12), clearly indicating a role of BDNF in the development of the peripheral nervous system. However, the function of BDNF in development and function of the brain is of particular interest. BDNF was found to support survival and axonal elongation of rat retinal ganglion cells in culture (13) and to promote the differentiation of basal forebrain cholinergic and GABAergic neurons (14). A function of BDNF in the adult brain is likely, since BDNF has been purified from the brain of adult pigs and since its mRNA seems to be predominately expressed in the brain (6). Levels of BDNF and mRNA in the adult rat brain exceed those of NGF, and BDNF mRNA shows a regionally heterogenous distribution with the highest concentrations occurring in the hippocampus and cerebral cortex (15,16). These findings make it likely that BDNF will be among the most interesting molecules when pharmacological applications to the brain are considered.

II. OTHER GROWTH FACTORS ACTING ON NEURONS

Ciliary neurotrophic factor (CNTF) was purified from chick eye and rat sciatic nerve tissue using chick embryonic ganglion cells as bioassay (4) and has recently been cloned (17,18). Besides acting on ciliary parasympathetic neurons, it supports survival of various chick and rodent sensory and sympathetic ganglia (4). CNTF affects cholinergic neurons in cultures of chick retinal cells (19) but not rat brain cholinergic neurons (20). The highest concentrations of CNTF mRNA were found in the adult sciatic nerve (18), and application of CNTF prevents the degeneration of motor neurons after axotomy in postnatal rats. These observations suggest the possibility that CNTF may become pharmacologically useful to counteract disease-related degenerative changes of motor neurons.

Basic fibroblast growth factor (bFGF) and *acidic fibroblast growth factor* (aFGF) influence neuronal survival and differentiation during development (21,22). While neurons from many brain regions are affected, the proportion of neurons surviving varies among brain regions, suggesting that particular subpopulations of neurons are responsive to FGF (23). Basic FGF promotes survival and differentiation of cholinergic neurons of the rat basal forebrain and of mesencephalic dopaminergic neurons (14,24). The presence of FGF in the adult brain suggests that this factor, in a manner similar to NGF, remains important for maintenance of function of responsive neuronal populations. Pharmacological administration of bFGF to transected neuronal pathways attenuates the loss of neuronal cell bodies. Local administration of bFGF to the proximal nerve stump of a transected sciatic nerve partially prevents the loss of dorsal root ganglion neurons in adult rats (25). In adult rats with fimbrial transections, chronic intraventricular infusions of bFGF attenuate the loss of septal cholinergic neurons, similar to the effects produced by NGF (26). Given the broad spectrum of bFGF responsive neurons, this protein may beneficially influence the recovery of many neuronal systems from injury.

Insulin and the structurally related *insulin-like growth factors I and II* (IGF-I and IGF-II) comprise another family of proteins involved in the regulation of metabolism and cellular growth of many tissues. These three proteins exhibit overlapping specificities for receptors (27). There is abundant evidence for the existence for insulin and IGF receptors in the brain, and the IGFs have been shown to be synthesized in the brain (28). The function of insulin and IGFs in the brain is not clear, despite the many findings showing that they affect various brain cell populations in vitro. Insulin, IGF-I, and IGF-II promote survival and stimulate neurite outgrowth from cultured central and peripheral neurons (29,30). Besides stimulating survival and initial growth of cultured neurons, insulin and the IGFs promote their differentiation and maturation. The neuronal actions of IGFs seem to be relatively nonselective and to involve a majority of neuronal populations (14).

Epidermal growth factor (EGF) is a potent mitogen for several cell types and enhances survival and neurite growth of cultured subneocortical and cerebellar neurons of the neonatal rat brain (31). EGF and EGF receptor immunoreactivity were demonstrated in the rat brain (32). *Transforming growth factor-α* (TGF-α) shows structural homology to EGF, is present in several brain areas, and is synthesized in cell bodies of selected rat forebrain regions (33).

III. RELATIONSHIP OF NEUROTROPHIC FACTORS TO FACTORS OF THE HEMOPOIETIC SYSTEM

Cholinergic neuronal differentiation factor is a factor known to regulate the neurotransmitter phenotype of sympathetic neurons in culture. This factor was purified, partially sequenced, and found to be identical to the leukemia inhibitory factor which regulates growth and differentiation of stem cells and myeloid cells (34). Its actions have been compared to those of interleukins (IL). IL-1 is a potent mitogen for astroglial cells and its synthesis is induced after experimental injury in the brain (35). This protein is able to elevate the expression of NGF in sciatic nerve explants and seems to be responsible for the large increases in NGF synthesis observed after transection of peripheral nerves (36). Injections of IL-1 into the brain elevate NGF mRNA levels in the hippocampus (37). IL-2 promotes the division and maturation of oligodendrocytes and, similar to interleukin-1, has been detected in the vicinity of experimental brain lesions (38). IL-3 and IL-6 were reported to promote survival of cultured postnatal forebrain cholinergic neurons (39,40). These findings suggest a close relationship between neurotrophic and hemopoietic factors and prompt speculations that mechanisms thought to be specific for the immune system may play a role in the CNS as well.

IV. PROTEASES AND PROTEASE INHIBITORS

Several findings point to the possibility of an important role for proteases and protease inhibitors in neuronal growth. Natural and artificial proteases inhibitors stimulate neurite outgrowth from cultured neurons, and it has been speculated that neurite outgrowth and stabilization of axonal terminals at their target cells requires a delicate balance between the activities of proteases and protease inhibitors (41). A glia-derived neurotrophic factor was found to be identical to protease nexin I (41), and this molecule is induced in peripheral nerves after experimental lesions (42). Furthermore, peptide fragments of the amyloid precursor protein have been reported to trophically affect cultured neurons (43), and the secreted part of the molecule (which contains the Kunitz domain) is identical to protease nexin II (44).

V. POSSIBLE INVOLVEMENT OF NEUROTROPHIC FACTORS IN THE PATHOPHYSIOLOGY OF ALZHEIMER'S DISEASE

Neurotrophic and growth factors necessary for the maintenance of structural integrity or the regulation of plasticity of the adult brain may become involved at diverse levels of the pathophysiological processes of neurodegenerative diseases. Synthesis of a growth factor or expression of its receptors might be insufficient, or dysfunction of its transducing mechanism may result in atrophic changes of responsive neurons and enhance their vulnerability to a disease process. Insufficient neurotrophic factor functions could diminish the plastic capabilities of a neuronal system and reduce its functional adaptation to disease-related structural alterations. Alternatively, hyperfunction of growth factor mechanisms may induce synaptic dysfunction or aberrant growth. So far, there is very little evidence in support of any of these speculations; however, only a very few studies have addressed this issue. A single study reported that NGF and mRNA levels remained unchanged in the cortex of Alzheimer brains (45). Given the trophic actions of fragments of the amyloid precursor protein described above and the fact that some forms of this protein act as protease inhibitors, it has been speculated that a dysbalance between peptidases and peptidase inhibitors may be responsible for the aberrant growth often observed around neuritic plaques (46). Clearly, future studies are warranted assessing the status of growth factor mechanisms in AD and other neurodegenerative diseases. If these mechanisms are found to be impaired, application of the corresponding factors as a replacement therapy may stop or attenuate a specific step in the cascade of pathophysiological events.

VI. PHARMACOLOGY OF NEUROTROPHIC FACTORS

Growth factors and neurotrophic factors may become therapeutically useful to stimulate impaired mechanisms or, alternatively, as pharmacological tools to induce hypertrophy of vulnerable neuronal populations. There are several pharmacological strategies which could be pursued to therapeutically exploit neurotrophic factor mechanisms. To be able to reach neuronal populations in the brain, neurotrophic factors will have to be given intracerebrally, since these proteins do not cross the blood-brain barrier. They might be chronically infused into the brain via pumping devices. Such pumps and the intraventricular delivery systems associated with them are at least adequately tolerated in humans (47), but they are not without risk. Stability of the neurotrophic factors during storage in these pump devices may require special preparations.

The demonstration that intraventricular infusion of a neurotrophic factor is clinically effective is likely to stimulate research into alternative methods of administration. It seems possible to develop slow-releasing intracerebral implants. In the case of NGF, existing polymers provide stable release rates over a period of several weeks (48). Combinations of modified neurotrophic factors with polymer matrix materials will offer many possibilities of patent protection and may be an attractive avenue for commercial exploitation. Slow-releasing polymers could be implanted in a simple neurosurgical session and pose less risk than an intraventricular pump.

Grafting of brain tissue replacing degenerated cells is frequently proposed as a potential approach to treat brain dysfunction. Such techniques are not limited to naturally occurring cells but can include genetically modified cells which selectively secrete a desired neurotrophic factor. Rosenberg (49) and Ernfors (50) showed that the implantation of cells producing recombinant NGF evokes trophic actions on NGF responsive cholinergic neurons. It is possible to produce cells which do not proliferate after implantation, are well tolerated by the host, and in which the synthesis of the desired growth factor is under the control of a promoter regulated by drugs. However, such cells may release a multitude of other active molecules making it difficult to limit their specificity.

Rather than administering entire trophic factor molecules, it may be possible to use active fragments or molecules mimicking the active sites of neurotrophic factors. So far, very little is known about the possibility of producing active fragments of NGF or other neurotrophic factors. Longo (51) reported the production of peptide fragments which inhibit biological actions of NGF. Fragments of EGF, bFGF, IGF-I, and IGF-II appear to retain activity (52–55). A synthetic peptide analog of TGF-α was shown to specifically inhibit EGF and TGF-α growth stimulatory actions on a responsive cell line (56). While effective concentrations of the active peptides were often much higher than those of the native proteins, these reports demonstrate the feasibility of the approach which attempts to reduce trophic factors to smaller molecules exerting the same actions on the specific receptors.

Studies with peptide fragments and modified peptides will provide a basis for molecular modeling studies attempting to replace peptides with nonpeptide effectors. Theoretical feasibility of this approach is illustrated by the example of endorphins and morphine, which both act on the same receptors. While this approach has the potential to lead to trophic factor agonists which can be administered systemically, it has to be pointed out that the systemic administration of such an active molecule may substantially elevate the possibility of undesired side effects. Effects on neurons of the peripheral nervous system may lead to autonomous disturbances.

Another approach to influence neurotrophic actions may be to search for ways to specifically manipulate the synthesis of endogenous neurotrophic factors. At the present time, very little is known about the regulation of synthesis of NGF or other neurotrophic factors, and the mechanisms controlling the selective expression of their genes are poorly understood. IL-1 elevates expression of NGF in sciatic nerve and hippocampus (35,36). Retinoic acid has recently been reported to increase the number of receptors for NGF in neuroblastoma cells (57) and to elevate the levels of NGF and its mRNA in L cells (58). Morphological and biochemical differentiation of human neuroblastoma cells is affected by retinoic acid (59,60). Thyroid hormones are essential for the normal development of the brain, and these hormones have been reported to influence axonal regeneration in adult animals (61) and may act by altering growth factor mechanisms.

Given the manifold systems affected by neurotrophic factors, one has to direct awareness to the possibility that pharmacological use of growth factors and trophic agents may be detrimental to neuronal function, contrary to the beneficial role implied by the term "trophic." Such detrimental actions have to be considered and ruled out before clinically using trophic molecules. Neurotrophic agents may, by promoting the function of selective neuronal systems, alter the balance among various systems within neuronal networks. Trophic agents may induce the formation of aberrant synaptic connections which may disrupt normal signal flow. They may induce the expression of abnormal proteins by both neuronal and non-neuronal cells and stimulate pathological proliferation of non-neuronal cells.

VII. PHARMACOLOGICAL ACTIONS OF RECOMBINANT HUMAN NERVE GROWTH FACTOR ON LESIONED CENTRAL CHOLINERGIC NEURONS

The decline of cholinergic function and cholinergic markers observed in the human AD hippocampus (62,63) are mimicked by a partial lesion of the septohippocampal pathway in the adult rat brain (64). In this model, a knife-cut transection of the fimbria—the axonal pathway which provides the majority of cholinergic innervation to the hippocampus from cholinergic septal cell bodies—results in decreases of choline acetyltransferase (ChAT) activity and acetylcholinersterase (AChE) activity in the hippocampal formation; the most pronounced decreases are observed toward the temporal pole of the hippocampus (64,65). The decreases of ChAT activity are paralleled by reductions in the ability of hippocampal slices to synthesize [^{3}H]acetylcholine (ACh) from the precursor molecule [^{3}H]choline in vitro possibly due to reduced uptake of precursor into cholinergic terminals (65). Spontaneous and evoked [^{3}H]ACh release from hippocampal slices is also reduced substantially by the transection of cholinergic axons. Previous results from our group have shown that chronic treatment with NGF increases ChAT activity and AChE staining in the hippocampus following partial fimbrial lesions (64). More recent studies summarized here determined whether chronic recombinant human nerve growth factor (rhNGF) treatment alters synthesis and release of [^{3}H]acetylcholine (ACh) from the precursor molecule [^{3}H]choline in vitro.

Adult rats received partial fimbrial transections and were treated with rhNGF during 3 weeks. Every second day, the treated animals received an intracerebroventricular injection of 1 μg of rhNGF. Three weeks following partial fimbrial lesions, animals were taken for analysis of [^{3}H]ACh synthesis and release in hippocampal slices using techniques described in detail elsewhere (65). In lesioned control animals, [^{3}H]ACh synthesis was reduced by 52% on the lesioned side. In rats that received chronic rhNGF treatment, [^{3}H]ACh was increased to 78% of control values, representing a 26% increase in the ability of hippocampal slices to synthesize [^{3}H]ACh (Fig. 1). Chronic rhNGF treatment did not alter [^{3}H]ACh synthesis by hippocampal slices contralateral to the fimbrial transection. Partial fimbrial lesions reduced spontaneous and evoked [^{3}H]ACh release from hippocampal slices by 64% and 39%, respectively, compared to control values. However, following chronic rhNGF treatment, spontaneous [^{3}H]ACh release approached normal control levels and evoked [^{3}H]ACh release was increased to 73% of control levels (Fig. 1).

Additional experiments defined the exact treatment regimen required to observe rhNGF-induced increases of presynaptic cholinergic function in hippocampal slices. Animals were lesioned and then treated with rhNGF for various periods, as shown in Figure 2. Single injections of rhNGF at the time of lesion produced a slight decrease in the ability of hippocampal slices to synthesize [^{3}H]ACh measured 3 weeks postlesion. However, both 3 and 9 weeks of continuous rhNGF treatment initiated on the day of lesion resulted in a significant enhancement of [^{3}H]ACh synthesis (45% and 118%, respectively), as determined from hippocampal slices. The rhNGF-induced increase in the capacity of hippocampal slices to synthesize [^{3}H]ACh was long-lasting and persisted for 3 weeks following the termination of chronic 3-week rhNGF administration (3 weeks followed by 3 weeks without treatment). rhNGF treatment was ineffective at increasing measures of [^{3}H]ACh synthesis if treatment was started 3 or 9 weeks

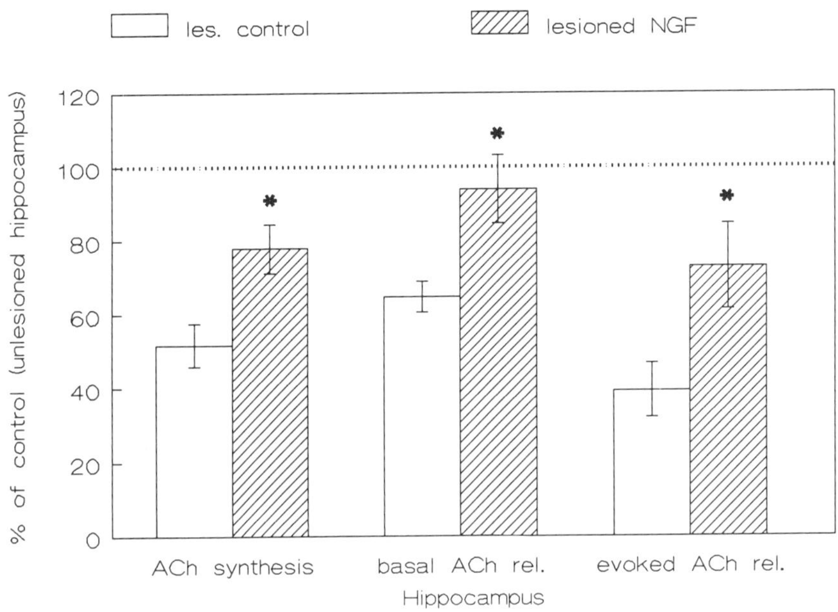

Figure 1 Effect of chronic rhNGF treatment on the synthesis and release of [^{3}H]ACh from hippocampal slices following partial fimbrial lesions. Partial fimbrial lesions reduced synthesis as well as basal and evoked release of [^{3}H]ACh release of hippocampal slices of the lesioned side (open bars = lesioned side of untreated control animals). Chronic rhNGF treatment increases these parameters (hatched bars). The values in NGF-treated rats are significantly different from those of lesioned control animals (*$p < 0.05$).

following partial fimbrial lesions (3 week delay 3 week and 9 week delay 3 week, respectively).

These studies indicate that chronic treatment with rhNGF produces long-lasting increases in the capacity of hippocampal neurons surviving partial fimbrial lesions to synthesize, store, and release ACh. Furthermore, this study suggests that treatment with rhNGF is required during the period of ongoing degenerative processes in order to produce increases in cholinergic parameters. The results of the present study are of relevance, considering the proposed clinical trials to treat AD patients with rhNGF (66). In AD, brain nerve growth factor (NGF) receptors are co-localized with ChAT in remaining cholinergic cell bodies which are present in the nucleus basalis (67,68), suggesting the possibility that basal forebrain cholinergic neurons may be responsive to exogenously applied growth factor. The slow degeneration of cholinergic neurons of the septohippocampal pathway which is observed in AD is comparable to that of the rapid degeneration which

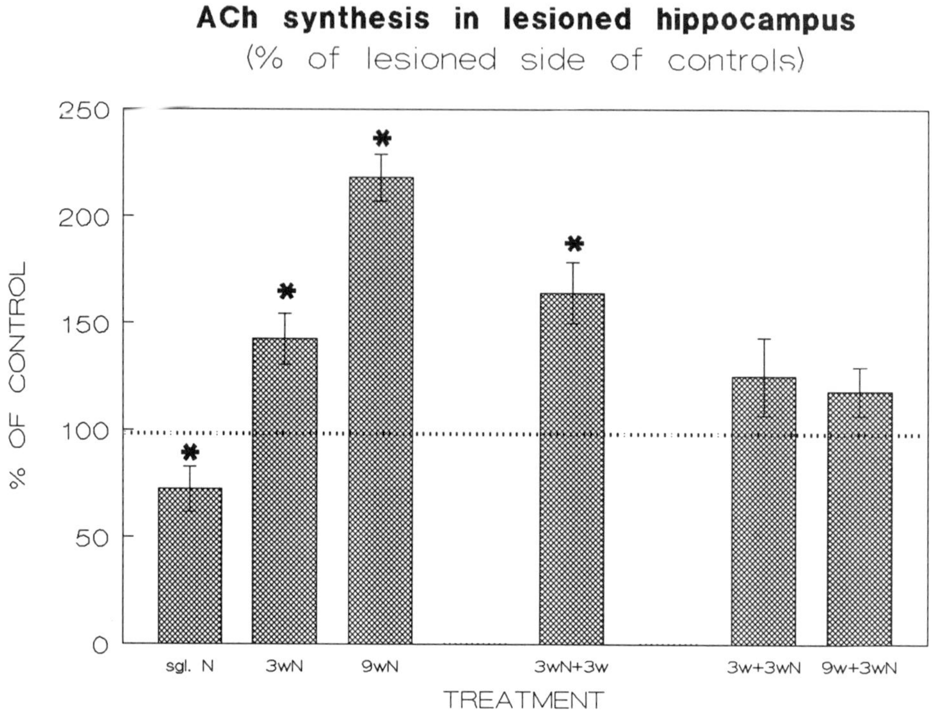

Figure 2 Effect of various rhNGF administration regimens on the capacity of hippocampal slices to synthesize [^{3}H]ACh from [^{3}H]choline following partial fimbrial lesions. Values are shown as % of control (rhNGF values/control animal values). Thus, a valuc of 100% indicates no effect of drug treatment compared to the respective control. sgl.N = single rhNGF injection immediately after fimbrial transection, animals sacrificed 3 weeks later; 3wN = rhNGF treatment during 3 weeks; 9wN = rhNGF treatment during 9 weeks; 3wN + 3w = 3 weeks of rhNGF treatment followed by 3 weeks without treatment: 3w + 3wN = 3 weeks without treatment followed by 3 weeks of rhNGF treatment; 9w + 3wN = 9 weeks without treatment followed by 3 weeks of rhNGF treatment. * Significantly different from lesioned animals treated with a control protein ($p < 0.05$).

occurs in the rat following the transection of fimbrial axons. Therefore, it is possible that the chronic treatment of AD patients with rhNGF would increase the functional capacity of septohippocampal cholinergic neurons, thus attenuating the decline of cognitive processes.

VIII. CONCLUSIONS

A growing body of findings suggests that growth factors and neurotrophic factors are involved in the regulation of survival and plasticity of the adult nervous system. Administration of neurotrophic factors can attenuate age-related and experimentally induced degeneration and behavioral deficits in animals; this suggests that they, or molecules derived from them, may be useful in the treatment of diseases involving structural disintegration of nervous tissue. NGF may be beneficial in Alzheimer's disease, which is associated with a loss of the NGF-responsive population of cholinergic neurons in the basal forebrain. Available information suggests that other, more recently discovered neurotrophic factors have a different and, probably, broader spectrum of action than NGF. Various pharmacological strategies to utilize neurotrophic molecules exist for the development of effective therapy of neurodegenerative diseases.

ACKNOWLEDGMENTS

The authors were supported by grants from NIH, NSF, AFAR, and the National Parkinson Foundation.

REFERENCES

1. Barde YA. Trophic factors and neuronal survival. Neuron 2: 1525–1534, 1989.
2. Hefti F, Schneider LS. Rationale for the planned clinical trials with nerve growth factor in Alzheimer's disease. Psychiatr Dev 4:297–315, 1989.
3. Levi-Montalcini R. Developmental neurobiology and the natural history of nerve growth factor. Ann Rev Neurosci 5:341–362, 1982.
4. Barbin G, Selak I, Manthorpe M, et al. Use of central neuronal cultures for the detection of neurotrophic agents. Neuroscience 12:33–43, 1984.
5. Barde YA, Davies AM, Johnson JE, et al. Brain-derived neurotrophic factor. Prog Brain Res 71:185–189, 1987.
6. Leibrock J, Lottspeich F, Hohn A, et al. Molecular cloning and expression of brain-derived neurotrophic factor. Nature 341:149–152, 1989.
7. Ernfors P, Ibanex CF, Ebendal T, et al. Molecular cloning and neurotrophic activities of a protein with structural similarities to nerve growth factor: Developmental and topographical expression in the brain. Proc Natl Acad Sci USA 87:5454–5458, 1990.
8. Hohn A, Leibrock J, Bailey K, et al. Identification and characterization of a novel member of the nerve growth factor/brain-derived neurotrophic factor family. Nature 344:339–341, 1990.

9. Maisonpierre PC, Belluscio L, Squinto S, et al. Neurotrophin-3: A neurotrophic factor related to NGF and BDNF. Science 247:1446–1451, 1990.
10. Rosenthal A, Goeddel DV, Nguyen T, et al. Primary structure and biological activity of a novel human neurotrophic factor. Neuron 4:767–773, 1990.
11. Rodriguez-Tebar A, Dechant G, Barde YA. Binding of brain-derived neurotrophic factor to the nerve growth factor receptor. Neuron 4:487–492, 1990.
12. Hofer MM, Barde YA. Brain-derived neurotrophic factor prevents neuronal death in vivo. Nature 331:261–262, 1988.
13. Thanos S, Bahr M, Barde YA, et al. Survival and axonal elongation of adult rat retinal ganglion cells. In vitro effects of lesioned sciatic nerve and brain derived neurotrophic factor. Euro J Neurosci 1:19–26, 1989.
14. Knusel B, Michel PP, Schwaber J, et al. Selective and nonselective stimulation of central cholinergic and dopaminergic development in vitro by nerve growth factor, basic fibroblast growth factor, epidermal growth factor, insulin and the insulin-like growth factors I and II. J of Neurosci 10:558–570, 1990.
15. Hofer M, Pagliusi SR, Hohn A, et al. Regional distribution of brain-derived neurotrophic factor mRNA in the adult mouse brain. EMBO J 9:2459–2464, 1990.
16. Phillips H, Winslow J, Nikolics K. Distribution of BDNF mRNA in the rat brain. Science 250:290–294, 1990.
17. Lin LFH, Mismer D, Lile JD, et al. Purification, cloning, and expression of ciliary neurotrophic factor (CNTF). Science 246:1023–1025, 1989.
18. Stockli KA, Lottspeich F, Sendtner M, et al. Molecular cloning, expression and regional distribution of rat ciliary neurotrophic factor. Nature 342:920–923, 1989.
19. Hofmann HD. Ciliary neuronotrophic factor stimulates choline acetyltransferase activity in cultured chicken retina neurons. J Neurochem 51:109–113, 1988.
20. Knusel B, Hefti F. Development of cholinergic pedunculopontine neurons in vitro: Comparison with cholinergic septal cells and response to nerve growth factor, ciliary neuronotrophic factor, and retinoic acid. J Neurosci Res 21:365–375, 1988.
21. Morrison RS, Sharma A, DeVellis J, et al. Basic fibroblast growth factor supports the survival of cerebral cortical neurons in primary culture. Proc Natl Acad Sci USA 83:7537–7541, 1986.
22. Walicke P, Cowan WM, Ueno N, et al. Fibroblast growth factor promotes survival of dissociated hippocampal neurons and enhances neurite extension. Proc Natl Acad Sci USA 83:3012–3016, 1986.
23. Walicke PA. Basic and acidic fibroblast growth factors have trophic effects on neurons from multiple CNS regions. J Neurosci 8:2618–2627, 1988.
24. Grothe C, Otto D, Unsicker K. Basic fibroblast growth factor promotes in vitro survival and cholinergic development of rat septal neurons: Comparison with the effects of nerve growth factor. Neuroscience 31:649–661, 1989.
25. Otto D, Unsicker K, Grothe C. Pharmacological effects of nerve growth factor and fibroblast growth factor applied to the transectioned sciatic nerve on neuron death in adult rat dorsal root ganglia. Neurosci Lett 83:156–160, 1987.
26. Anderson KJ, Dam D, Lee S, et al. Basic fibroblast growth factor prevents death of lesioned cholinergic neurons in vivo. Nature 443:360–362, 1988.

27. Rechler MM, Nissley SP. The nature and regulation of the receptors for insulin-like growth factors. Ann Rev Physiol 47:425-442, 1985.
28. Sara VR, Carlsson-Skwirut C. The role of the insulin-like growth factors in the regulation of brain development. Prog Brain Res 73:87-99, 1988.
29. Aizenman Y, Weischsel ME Jr, De Vellis J. Changes in insulin and transferrin requirements of pure brain neuronal cultures during embryonic development. Proc Natl Acad Sci USA 83:2263-2266, 1986.
30. Recio-Pinto E, Rechler MM, Ishii DN. Effects of insulin, insulin-like growth factor-II, and nerve growth factor on neurite formation and survival in cultured sympathetic and sensory neurons. J Neurosci 6:1211-1219, 1986.
31. Morrison RS, Keating RF, Moskal JR. Basic fibroblast growth factor and epidermal growth factor exert differential trophic effects on CNS neurons. J Neurosci Res 21:71-79, 1988.
32. Fallon JH, Seroogy KB, Morrison RS, et al. Epidermal growth factor immunoreactive material in the central nervous system: Location and development. Science 224:1107-1109, 1984.
33. Derynck R. Transforming growth factor alpha. Cell 54:593-595, 1988.
34. Yamamori T, Fukada K, Aebersold R, et al. The cholinergic neuronal differentiation factor from heart cells is identical to leukemia inhibitory factor. Science 246:1412-1416, 1989.
35. Nieto-Sampedro M, Berman MA. Interleukin-1-like activity in rat brain: Sources, target, and effect of injury. J Neurosci res 17:214-219, 1987.
36. Lindholm D, Heumann R, Meyer M, et al. Interleukin I regulates synthesis of nerve growth factor in non-neuronal cells of rat sciatic nerve. Nature 330:658-659, 1987.
37. Spranger M, Lindholm D, Bandtlow C, et al. Regulation of nerve growth factor (NGF) synthesis in the rat central nervous system: Comparision bertween the effects of interleukin-1 and various growth factors in astrocyte cultures and in vivo. Euro J Neurosci 2:69-76, 1990.
38. Nieto-Sampedro M, Chandy KG. Interleukin-2-like activity in injured rat brain. Neurochem Res 12:723-727, 1987.
39. Hama T, Miyamoto M, Tsukui H, et al. Interleukin-6 as a neurotrophic factor for promoting the survival of cultured basal forebrain cholinergic neurons from postnatal rats. Neurosci Lett 104:340-344, 1989.
40. Kamegai M, Miijima K, Kunishita T, et al. Interleukin 3 as a trophic factor for central cholinergic neurons in vitro and vivo. Neuron 2:420-436, 1990.
41. Monard D. Role of protease inhibition in cellular migration and neuritic growth. Biochem Pharmacol 36:1389-1392, 1987.
42. Meier R, Spreyer P, Ortmann R, et al. Inductionof glia-derived nexin after lesion of a peripheral nerve. Nature 342:548-550, 1989.
43. Zurn, A.D., Nick, H. and Monard, D. A glia-derived nexin promotes neurite outgrowth in cultured chick sympathetic neurons. Dev. Neurosci. 10:17-24, 1988.
44. Oltersdorf T, Fritz LC, Schenk DB, et al. The secreted form of the Alzheimer's amyloid precursor protein with the Kunitz domain is protease nexin-II. Nature 341:144-147, 1989.
45. Goedert M, Fine A, Hunt Sp, et al. Nerve growth factor mRNA in peripheral and cen-

tral rat tissues and in the human central nervous system: Lesion effects in the rat brain and levels in Alzheimer's disease. Mol Brain Res 1:85–92, 1986.
46. Whitson JS, Glabe CG, Shintani E, et al. Beta-amuyloid protein promotes neuritic branching in hippocampal cultures. Neurosci Lett 110:319–324, 1990.
47. Harbaugh RE. Intracerebroventricular cholinergic drug administration in Alzheimer's disease: Preliminary results of a double-blind study. J Neural Transm Suppl 24:271–277, 1987.
48. Powell EM, Sobarzo MR, Saltzman WM. Controlled release of nerve growth factor from a polymeric implant. Brain Res 515:309–311, 1990.
49. Rosenberg M, Friedmann T, Robertson RC, et al. Grafting genetically modified cells to the damaged brain: Restorative effects of NGF expression. Science 242:1275-1278, 1988.
50. Ernfors P, Ebendal T, Olson L, et al. A cell line producing recombinant nerve growth factor evokes growth responses in intrinsic and grafted central cholinergic neurons. Proc Natl Acad Sci 86:4756–4760, 1989.
51. Longo FM, Vu TH, Mobley WC. In vitro biological effect of nerve growth factor inhibited by synthetic NGF peptides. Soc Neuroscience Abst 15:17, 1989.
52. Baird A, Schubert D, Ling N, et al. Receptor-and heparin-binding domains of basic fibroblast growth factor. Proc Natl Acad Sci USA 85:2324–2328, 1988.
53. Ballard FJ, Francis GL, Ross M, et al. Natural and synthetic forms of insulin-like growth factor-1 (IGF-1) and the potent derivative, destripeptide IGF-1: Biological activities and receptor binding. Biochem Biophys Res Commun 149:398–404, 1987.
54. Komiriya A, Hortsch M, Meyers C, et al. Biologically active synthetic fragments of epidermal growth factor: Localization of a major receptor-binding region. Proc Natl Acad Sci 81:1351–1355, 1984.
55. Konishi Y, Knotts CE, Bullock LD, et al. Fragments of bovine insulin-like growth factors I and II stimulate proliferation of rat L6 myoblast cells. Biochemistry 28: 8872–8877, 1989.
56. Eppstein DA, Marsh YV, Schryver BB, et al. Inhibition of epidermal growth factor/ transforming growth factor-alpha-stimulated cell growth by a synthetic peptide. J Cell Physiol 141:420–430, 1989.
57. Haskell BE, Stach RW, Werrbach-Perez K, et al. Effect of retinoic acid on nerve growth factor receptors. Cell Tissue Res 247:67–73, 1987.
58. Wion D, Houlgatte R, Barbot N, et al. Retinoic acid increases the expression of NGF gene in mouse L cells. Biochem Biophys Res Comm 149:510–514, 1987.
59. Thiele CJ, Reynolds CP, Israel MA. Decreased expression of N-myc precedes retinoic-acid induced morphological differentiation of human neuroblastoma. Nature 313:404–406, 1985.
60. Casper D, Davies P. Stimulation of choline acetyltransferase activity by retinoic acid and sodium butyrate in a cultured human neuroblastoma Brain Res 478:74–84, 1989.
61. Grave GD. *Thyroid Hormones and Brain Development.* Raven Press, New York, 1977.
62. Davies P, Maloney AJF. Selective loss of central cholinergic neurons in Alzheimer's disease. Lancet 2:1403–1406, 1977.

63. Whitehouse PJ, Price DL, Struble RG, et al. Alzheimer's disease and senile dementia: Loss of neurons in the basal forebrain. Science 215:1237-1239, 1982.
64. Hefti F, Dravid A, Hartikka J. Chronic intraventricular injections of nerve growth factor elevate hippocampal choline acetyltransferase activity in adult rats with partial septo-hippocampal lesions. Brain Res 293:305-311, 1984.
65. Lapchak PA, Hefti F. Effect of recombinant human nerve growth factor on presynaptic cholinergic function in rat hippocampal slices following partial septo-hippocampal lesions: measures of [^{3}H]acetylcholine synthesis, [^{3}H]acetylcholine release and choline acetyltransferase activity. Neuroscience, 1991 (in press).
66. Phelps CH, Gage FH, Growdon JH, et al. Potential use of nerve growth factor to treat Alzheimer's disease. Neurobiol Aging 10:205-207, 1989.
67. Hefti F, Mash DC. Localization of nerve growth factor receptors in the normal human brain and in Alzheimer's disease. Neurobiol Aging 10:75-87, 1989.
68. Kordower JH, Gash DM, Bothwell M, et al. Nerve growth factor receptor and choline acetyltransferase remain colocalized in the nucleus basalis (Ch4) of Alzheimer's patients. Neurobiol Aging 10:67-74, 1989.

8

Functional Effects of Chronic Nerve Growth Factor Infusions on Adult and Aged Basal Forebrain Cholinergic Neurons

Karen S. Chen, Mark H. Tuszynski, and Fred H. Gage
University of California, San Diego, La Jolla, California

Gerald A. Higgins
National Institute on Aging, National Institutes of Health, Bethesda, Maryland

As the percentage of elderly people in the population increases, the number of individuals afflicted with various neurodegenerative diseases also continues to increase. The most prevalent form of dementia is Alzheimer's disease (AD), which accounts for at least 50% of the diagnosed dementias (1). AD is characterized by intellectual deterioration, as well as neuropathological changes which include cortical atrophy, neuronal loss, neurofibrillary tangles, neuritic plaques (see 2, 3 for review) and synaptic loss (4,5). Various neurotransmitter systems including the noradrenergic (6-9), serotonergic (10-12), and somatostatinergic (13,14) systems have been shown to undergo alterations in AD, but the most consistent changes have been observed in the basal forebrain cholinergic system (15-25). Furthermore, of the neurotransmitter deficits known to be present in AD, cholinergic deficits have correlated most highly with the degree of cognitive impairment (26-29). Thus several therapeutic strategies have focused upon ameliorating cholinergic dysfunction in AD.

It is therefore of some interest that nerve growth factor (NGF) has been shown to have a neurotrophic effect upon basal forebrain cholinergic neurons. The highest concentrations of NGF and its messenger RNA are found in the hippocampus and neocortex, the target regions for these cholinergic neurons (30-32). NGF injected into the target areas is transported retrogradely by basal forebrain cholinergic cells (33,34), and administration of NGF increases choline acetyltransferase

(ChAT) activity in basal forebrain neurons (35–39). NGF receptors have been localized on cholinergic neurons in the medial septum, vertical limb of the diagonal band, and the nucleus basalis of Meynert (NMB) (40–45). NGF effects on cholinergic neurons may begin as early as the period of neuronal development, when increases in ChAT immunoreactivity in the medial septum are just preceded and paralleled by increases in levels of NGF expression in the hippocampus (46–49). This chapter reviews some of the effects of chronic infusions of NGF on cholinergic neurons in the adult and aged mammalian brain with an attempt to examine the specificity of these functional responses.

I. NGF AND ITS RECEPTOR

NGF can induce the expression of its own receptor. Normally, cholinergic neurons of the adult striatum do not possess demonstrable levels of low-affinity NGF receptor (NGF-R). During development, however, NGF-Rs are presented transiently on striatal cholinergic interneurons (36,39,50) and then decline postnatally. In the adult peripheral nervous system (PNS), damage to peripheral nerves will induce the reexpression of NGF-Rs on Schwann cells within the denervated distal portion of the nerve (51). To determine whether damage in the central nervous system (CNS) may similarly result in reexpression of NGF-Rs, the adult rat neostriatum was lesioned by chronic infusions of a vehicle solution (52). Cannulae connected to osmotic minipumps were implanted into the striatum, and vehicle was infused for 2 weeks. Striatal damage following infusion of vehicle resulted in the appearance of NGF-R-immunoreactivity on many cholinergic interneurons. NGF was also infused into the striatum to determine whether the presence of NGF results in effects beyond those observed after damage alone. NGF infusions dramatically increased the size and staining intensity of ChAT-immunoreactive striatal cholinergic neurons, in addition to causing the appearance of NGF-R-immunoreactivity (Fig. 1). Further, NGF infusions increased mRNA levels for NGF-R, demonstrated by in situ hybridization, compared to normal control animals. Interestingly, infusion of anti-NGF serum partially inhibited the increase in NGF-R-immunoreactivity. Thus, NGF treatment is necessary for the induction of NGF-R gene expression and to increase the size of cholinergic neurons in the striatum, but lesion-induced damage alone can increase NGF-R protein levels through nontranscriptional mechanisms, possibly by "unmasking" NGF-Rs already present on the cell.

To determine whether NGF can induce NGF-R gene expression in basal forebrain cholinergic neurons that already normally express NGF-R protein in the adult animal, NGF was chronically infused into the lateral ventricles of adult rats (53). NGF infusion produced hypertrophy of cholinergic neurons compared to vehicle infusion (shown in an earlier study (54)) and increased NGF-R mRNA and ChAT mRNA per cell. Chronic NGF infusions, but not vehicle infusions, also in-

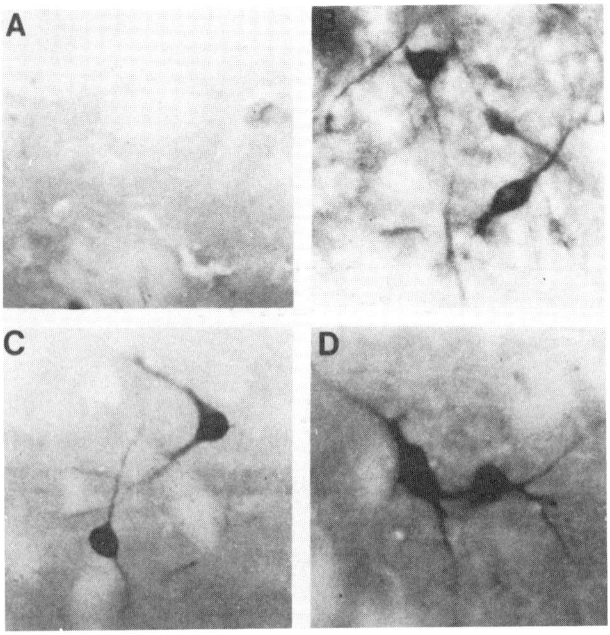

Figure 1 Photomicrograph of the adult neostriatum (A) Stained with antibody for NGF-R (no staining was observed even at dilutions of 1:1) (B) Stained with antibody for NGF-R following infusions of vehicle alone. (C) Stained with antibody for ChAT. (D) Stained with antibody for ChAT following infusions of NGF.

duced the expression of NGF-R mRNA as shown by in situ hybridization within the medial septum, diagonal band, and NBM basal forebrain neurons. These cells had not previously exhibited detectable levels of NGF-R mRNA. Therefore, NGF can induce the expression of its own receptor and produce cholinergic neuronal hypertrophy through induction of NGF-R gene expression within the basal forebrain. While information continues to accumulate on the mechanisms of NGF action, the studies discussed here reveal that considerable gaps in our knowledge remain concerning the intracellular effects of NGF on its target neurons. More is known on the systemic effects of NGF, as will be reviewed in the following sections.

II. NGF AND FIMBRIA-FORNIX LESIONS

A preliminary study in 1979 (33) suggested that the cholinergic neuronal subpopulation in the CNS might exhibit NGF responsiveness; specific effects of NGF in the adult CNS were subsequently investigated. Two model systems have typically been used to examine the effects of NGF upon cholinergic neurons in the CNS, including lesions of the medial septohippocampal projection (fimbria-fornix transections) and natural atrophy of basal forebrain cholinergic neurons during aging. In the rat, neurons of the medial septum and vertical limb of the diagonal band project dorsally to the hippocampus, mainly through the fimbria-fornix fiber bundle pathway. This projection provides the hippocampus with 90% of its cholinergic input (55–57); approximately 50% of the neurons that send their axons through the fimbria-fornix are cholinergic (58,59). Complete transection of the fimbria-fornix in adult rats results in rapid retrograde degeneration of many cholinergic and noncholinergic septal/diagonal band neurons that send axonal projections via the fimbria-fornix, and in complete cholinergic denervation of the dorsal hippocampus (35,60–62). Retrograde degeneration of 70–90% of medial septal cholinergic cells has been demonstrated by the use of several markers, including retrogradely transported fluorescent dyes and Nissl stains (63,64), acetylcholinesterase (AChE) or ChAT expression (63,65), and NGF-R expression (64,66,67). While one recent study suggested that the cells may be in a dysfunctional state rather than dead following fimbria-fornix transection (68), other studies report that many of the cells actually die after a period of prolonged degeneration (64,67,69,70).

The discovery that chronic intraventricular infusions of NGF into adult rats following fimbria-fornix lesions can prevent retrograde degeneration of axotomized basal forebrain cholinergic cells represented a significant step in potentially preventing naturally occurring neuronal degeneration (62,71–73). Prevention of retrograde degeneration in 90–100% of septal/diagonal band neurons can be achieved by infusions of NGF into the ventricular system at the time of fimbria-fornix lesions. Further, NGF can induce sprouting of axotomized cholinergic fibers, as evidenced by cholinergic neuritic sprouting into the dorsolateral quadrant of the septum 2 weeks following fimbria-fornix lesions (70). These findings led to the "neurotrophic hypotheses" that axotomy-induced degeneration of septal/diagonal band neurons may be a result of deprivation from a critical supply of NGF normally provided by postsynaptic neurons and/or glial cells located within the hippocampal formation (37,42,74–78).

These studies demonstrated the ability of NGF to prevent CNS basal forebrain cholinergic neuron degeneration in the adult rat, but it remained to be determined whether NGF was also biologically active on basal forebrain cholinergic neurons in the primate. To address this question, we adapted the fimbria-fornix transection model to the nonhuman primate, *macacas fascicularis* (79). Eight young primates underwent unilateral fornix transections, thereby interrupting the septohippocampal projection. Four animals received intracerebroventricular infusions of mouse 2.5S NGF, and four animals received infusions of a control solution of artificial cerebrospinal fluid. In all animals, as expected, a severe reduction in the number

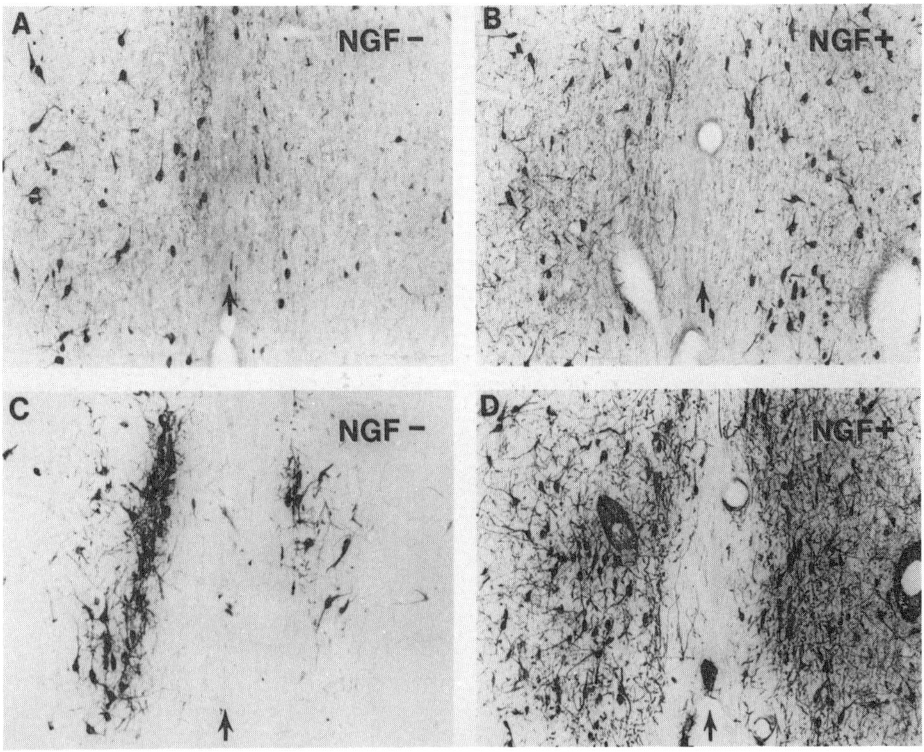

Figure 2 Photomicrograph of the medial septum of an adult primate stained with antibodies for ChAT (A, B) and NGF-R (C, D) following infusions of vehicle alone (A, C) or NGF (B, D). Animals underwent a lesion of the right fornix 1 month prior to sacrifice.

of cholinergic fibers in the hippocampus was found. In the medial septal region, control animals that did not receive NGF infusions showed persistent labeling of only 45 ± 5% of ChAT-labeled neurons (±SEM) on the lesioned side of the medial septum compared to the contralateral, unlesioned side of the same animal (Fig. 2). In contrast, NGF-treated animals showed persistent labeling of 80±6% of cholinergic neurons. Similarly, labeling for NGF-R-immunoreactive neurons showed that only 41±4% of medial septal neurons remained labeled in control animals, while NGF-treated animals showed a persistence of 70±5% of NGF-R-immunoreactive neurons. Thus, NGF is also able to prevent lesion-induced cholinergic neuron degeneration in the CNS of adult primates.

III. NGF AND AGING

Basal forebrain cholinergic cells have been shown to atrophy during aging (23,27). Shrinkage, and in some cases loss, of cholinergic cells correlates with decreased cognitive ability both in rats (54) and in humans (26–28). RNA blotting and protein data suggest a reduction in NGF levels in the hippocampus of aged rats compared to the levels in young adult rats (80).

Behaviorally, aged rats as a group are significantly impaired compared to young rats on the Morris water maze task, a test of spatial learning and memory (54,81–83). In this task, the rats must swim to a hidden platform submerged below the surface of a pool of water, using spatial cues in the environment to remember the location of the platform. Although aged animals as a group are impaired as compared to young rats, only a subgroup (one fourth to one third) of aged rats demonstrates a marked impairment on this task. There is a significant correlation between forebrain AChE-positive cell loss and/or atrophy and degree of cognitive impairment (54,81).

We attempted to determine whether age-related behavioral deficits observed on the water maze task and morphological changes in basal forebrain cholinergic neurons could be ameliorated by chronically infusing NGF into the lateral ventricles of cognitively impaired, aged rats (54). A group of aged and young adult rats was tested in the Morris water maze for 2 weeks to determine which animals were initially impaired (Fig. 3). The impaired aged animals were equally divided into a group that would receive NGF infusions and a group that would receive vehicle infusions. During the second and fourth weeks following the beginning of the infusions, all of the rats (unimpaired aged, NGF-treated aged, vehicle-treated aged, and young rats) were retested on the water maze task. The performance of both groups of impaired aged rats did not improve, compared to unimpaired aged rats, on the first retest during the second week of infusion. By the second retest on the fourth week of infusion, aged rats that received NGF showed a significant improvement in retention of the platform location in the water maze relative to vehicle-infused rats, due primarily to improved retention of information acquired during the first retest. Additionally, there was a significant increase in the size of cholinergic neruons in the basal forebrain region ipsilateral to the infusion site in NGF-treated aged rats compared to vehicle-treated aged rats. Therefore, NGF can improve some of the behavioral and morphological alterations associated with aging.

IV. NGF AND AMYLOID PROTEIN PRECURSOR mRNA

One of several genes whose expression may be regulated by NGF is the amyloid protein precursor (APP) which encodes the amyloid β/A4 protein. The β/A4 protein is a major constituent of neuritic plaques and cerebrovascular amyloid depos-

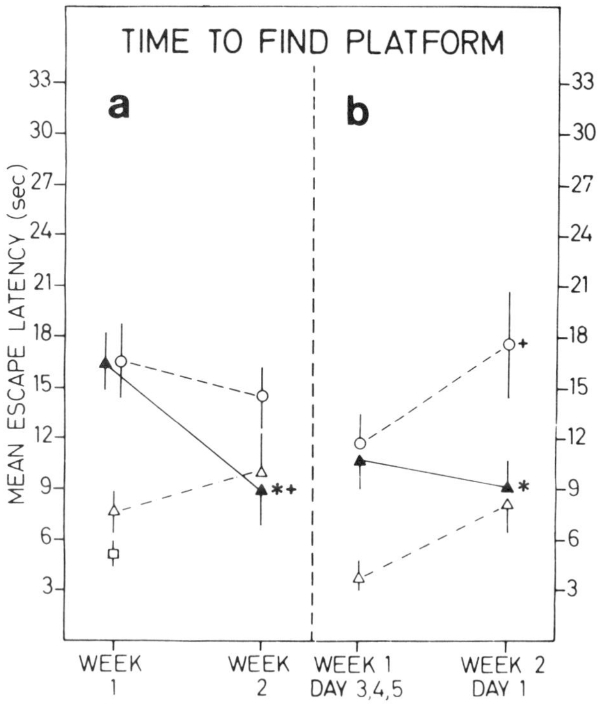

Figure 3 Performance of three groups of aged rats on the water maze test (Δ = aged, nonimpaired; o = aged, impaired; ▲ = NGF-treated, aged, impaired) in test weeks 1 and 2, expressed as escape latency, and one group of young rats (□ = young). (a) Mean performance (± SEM) over all trials. (b) Memory retention expressed as the difference between the mean performance in the last 3 days of test week 1 and the first test day of test week 2. * = Significant difference from aged impaired. $p < 0.025$ on a one-way ANOVA; + in panel a denotes significantly improved performance on test week 2, $p < 0.025$; + in panel b = significantly impaired performance on week 2, day 1, $p < 0.025$.

its in AD brains (84,85). Increased APP levels have been observed in the basal forebrain and hippocampal regions in the brains of patients with AD (86,87). It has been postulated that formation of neuritic plaques might result from increased amyloid expression. Thus it is important to understand the regulation of the APP gene.

Amyloid protein has also been demonstrated to enhance neuronal survival of developing hippocampal pyramidal neurons in culture (88). Therefore, Whitson et al. (88) hypothesized that the physiological product of APP normally performs a trophic function but, when processed aberrantly, is precipitated as amyloid in an inactive form, which may lead to the death of cells dependent upon it for trophic support. This is yet another example of the role that APP might have in neuronal degeneration in AD.

There are four different forms of APP. Three forms contain an insertion homologous to the Kunitz domain of serine protease inhibitors (KPI): APP-751, APP-770, and APP-related 563 (the latter does not encode the β/A4 protein). The fourth form, APP-695, does not contain the KPI insert (89,90). The presence of multiple forms of APP has prompted efforts to understand how differential APP gene expression may be etiologically relevant to amyloid deposition in AD. Overexpression of one form of APP mRNA may be preferentially associated with neuritic plaque formation and cerebrovascular amyloidosis. A recent study showed different anatomical distributions of APP-695 and APP-751/770 mRNAs in normal adult human brain and alterations in the distribution of the mRNAs of these forms in AD frontal cortex (91). Palmert et al. (92) suggested that selective elevation of the noninserted APP-695 form may be responsible for the observed total increase in APP mRNA in the NBM of AD patients. In contrast, Johnson et al. (93,94) showed decreased levels of APP-695 message in the cortex and hippocampus of the brains of AD patients, which was not simply the result of the loss of APP-695 neurons (95). Additionally, Tanaka et al. (96) observed increased levels of APP-770 mRNA in the brains of AD patients compared to the brains of age-matched controls. Thus, currently, evidence of alterations in the levels of the different forms of APP in AD is contradictory, and the final role the different APP forms may play is a field of active investigation.

Studies of APP gene expression in animals may prove useful in elucidating this issue. APP gene expression has been examined in the basal forebrain of aged and adult rats that have been behaviorally tested in the water maze (97). Increased levels of APP-751 mRNA relative to APP-695 mRNA have been observed in the medial septum, diagonal band, and NBM regions of aged rats with spatial memory deficits compared to nonimpaired aged rats and young rats (Fig. 4). Therefore, not only does atrophy of cholinergic neurons in the basal forebrain region of aged rats correlate with behavioral deficits in learning and memory tasks (described above), but alterations in the ratio of APP mRNAs may also correlate with neuronal atrophy in the subpopulation of behaviorally impaired aged rats. Presently, it appears that an increase in the ratio of KPI-containing to non-KPI-containing APP mRNA correlates with cognitive impairment in aged rodents.

We attempted to evaluate NGF effects on the different forms of APP expression by chronically infusing NGF into the lateral ventricles of young adult rats (98). Two-week NGF infusion produced increases in the ratio of APP-695 mRNA to APP-751 mRNA in the basal forebrain region, as well as increases in NGF-R mRNA hybridization, NGF-R-immunoreactivity, and ChAT mRNA hydridization. Hypertrophy of ChAT-positive neurons also resulted from NGF treatment. NGF injection into developing rodent basal forebrain was also able to increase

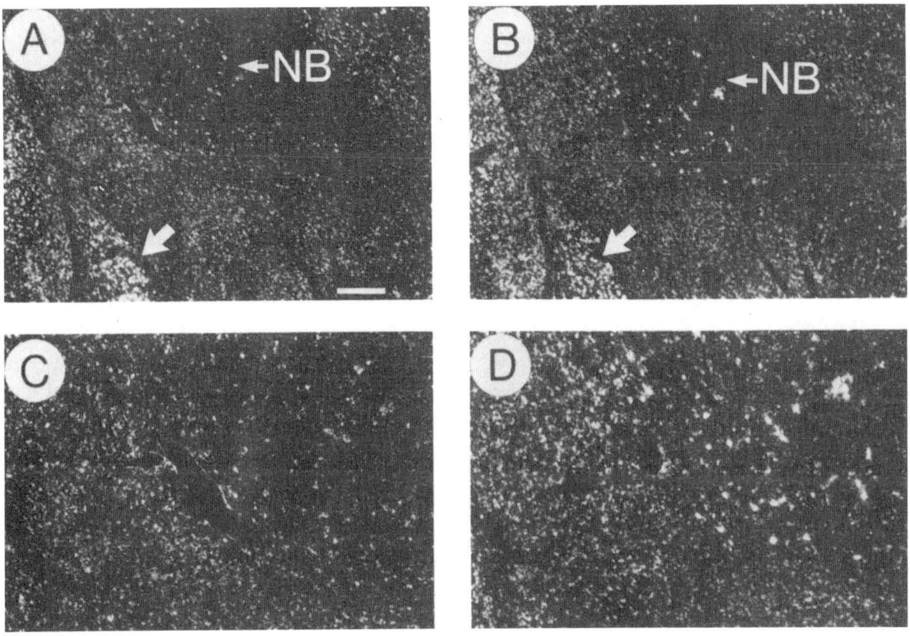

Figure 4 Dark-field photomicrograph of the nucleus basalis (NB) region showing in situ hybridization using a rat ^{35}S-labeled oligonucleotide probe in an aged, unimpaired animal (A, C) and an aged, impaired animal (B, D). (C, D) High-power views of A and B. Large arrows indicate the lateral nucleus of the amygdala, which appears to contain similar levels of APP and mRNA in both animals.

total APP mRNA levels (Higgins GA, unpublished observation). Additionally, the postnatal peak of APP-695 expression corresponds to the period of greatest NGF sensitivity within the basal forebrain. Thus it appears NGF can regulate APP gene expression, with the 695 form of the protein being potentially the most responsive to NGF.

We are currently testing the hypothesis that administration of NGF into behaviorally impaired aged rats may be able to reverse the APP-751/APP-695 mRNA ratio through induction of the NGF-responsive form of APP mRNA (i.e., APP-695). We will also examine the capacity of aged basal forebrain neurons to induce NGF receptor and ChAT expression in response to NGF infusion to determine whether defects in induction underlie age-related morphological changes in the basal forebrain region of these rats.

V. RECOMBINANT HUMAN β-NGF

Evidence from fimbria-fornix lesion studies and studies on aged animals strongly support the hypothesis that NGF has an ameliorative effect upon degenerating basal forebrain cholinergic neurons. Since cholinergic neuronal degeneration is a prominent component of neuronal loss in AD, as noted above, the use of NGF as a therapeutic approach in AD has been suggested. A recent meeting sponsored by the National Institute on Aging (99) sought to assess the potential utility of neurotrophic factor therapy in AD and recommended that several prerequisites be met before NGF trials are initiated in AD patients. One was "a critical need for a reliable source of well-characterized human NGF with known activity in sufficient quantity for a comprehensive program of research."

Previous experiments have demonstrated that continuous intracerebral infusions of the 2.5S form of *mouse* β-NGF can reverse some of the degenerative changes resulting from compromise of the basal forebrain cholinergic system. Recently, a baculovirus expression vector was constructed containing the coding sequence for *human* prepro β-NGF; upon infection of insect cells with the recombinant virus mature human β-NGF (rhNGF) was released into the culture fluid (100). We then chronically infused this rhNGF into the lateral ventricles of rats with fimbria-fornix lesions in order to determine whether rhNGF exerts biological effects and to compare the efficacy of rhNGF to mouse NGF (mNGF) in vivo (100). Two differing doses of mNGF and rhNGF were examined: 0.36 μg/d and 0.72 μg/d. Control animals lacking NGF infusions showed a persistence of only 43% of cells labeled for ChAT after unilateral fimbria-fornix lesions. In contrast, rats receiving the lower dose of mNGF showed a persistence of 97% of medial septal cholinergic neurons, while rats receiving the higher dose of mNGF showed persistence of 100% of cholinergic neurons. Animals receiving the low dose of rhNGF showed a persistence of 79% of medial septal cholinergic neurons, whereas animals receiving the higher dose showed a persistence of 92% of cholinergic neurons. Thus, similar to the previous results obtained with intraven-tricular infusions of mNGF, rhNGF was able to prevent the retrograde degeneration of septal/diagonal band neurons following transection, and mNGF was slightly more biologically active in rats than rhNGF—a result that is not unexpected, given that the sequence homology between mouse and rat NGF is closer than that between human and rat NGF. We are currently conducting trials of rhNGF in our primate model of cholinergic degeneration. Preliminary results indicate that rhNGF is biologically active in the primate as well.

To examine the effects of rhNGF on aged animals, rhNGF was chronically infused into the lateral ventricles of aged rats that exhibited an impairment on a pretest in the water maze compared to both young rats and aged unimpaired rats (101). During the second and fourth weeks of infusion, the rats were retested on the water maze task. As was the case with mNGF, the performance of the impaired

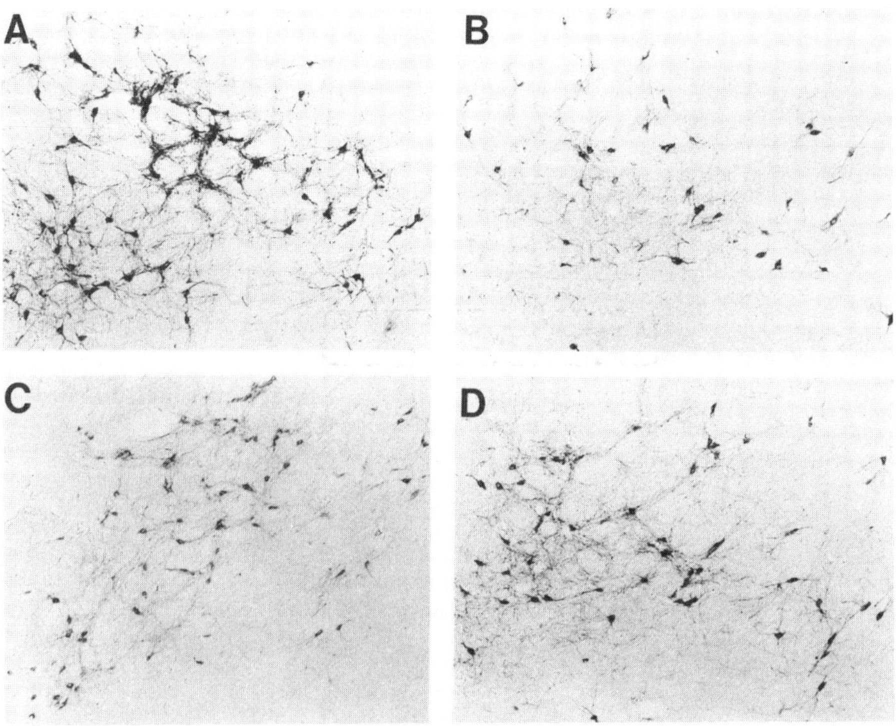

Figure 5 Photomicrograph of the nucleus basalis region stained with antibodies for NGF-R in (a) an aged, impaired animal that received infusions of rhNGF; (b) an aged, impaired animal that received infusions of vehicle alone; (c) an aged, unimpaired animal; and (d) a young animal.

aged rats in both groups was not improved on the first retest, but by the second retest NGF-infused aged rats showed a significant improvement in retention of the platform location in the water maze relative to vehicle-infused, impaired aged rats. This improvement was due primarily to improved retention of information acquired during the first retest. Histologically, there was a loss of NGF receptor-positive cells in the basal forebrain region of both behaviorally impaired aged groups (rhNGF-treated and vehicle-treated groups) compared to the unimpaired aged and young groups (Fig. 5). Chronic infusions of rhNGF increased the size of the NGF receptor-positive neurons relative to the vehicle-treated group, as well as the unimpaired aged and young groups. However, NGF infusions did not affect the number of NGF-R-positive neurons. The NGF effects on cell size were most evident on the side of the brain ipsilateral to the rhNGF infusion. These findings demonstrate that *human* recombinant β-NGF, like *mouse* β-NGF, has morphological effects upon neurons in the aged basal forebrain, and an ameliorative effect upon retention deficits exhibited by aged rats on the water maze.

VI. GRAFTING OF GENETICALLY MODIFIED CELLS

Grafting cells to the CNS has been used as a therapeutic approach to selectively replace cells lost as a result of damage or disease. Recently, techniques that attempt to directly correct genetic deficits have begun to be developed. This strategy of treating human genetic disease in vivo through the replacement of damaged or deficient genes with functional genes has been called gene therapy (102). Gene therapy involves either the modification of the expression of a mutant gene or the introduction of new genetic information into defective cells in vivo. We have recently proposed a combination of gene transfer via efficient viral vectors into cultured cells followed by intracerebral grafting of the genetically modified cells as an effective approach to restore function in the damaged or diseased CNS (103). In particular, we have harvested and cultured primary or immortalized skin fibroblasts, infected the cells with the transgene using retroviruses, selected the cells expressing the gene at high levels, and then grafted these cells into the brain.

To assess the potential therapeutic efficacy of this approach, we grafted genetically modified fibroblasts into adult rats following unilateral fimbria-fornix transections (104). A retroviral vector was constructed from Moloney murine leukemia virus to contain the fragment of mouse NGF cDNA that encodes the precursor to NGF that is secreted. Either retrovirus-infected (NGF-secreting) or control-uninfected fibroblasts were injected into the fimbria-fornix lesion cavity and lateral ventricle ipsilateral to the cavity. After 2 weeks, staining for fibronectin, a fibroblast-specific marker, revealed robust survival of the grafts in both groups of animals (Fig. 6). However, there was a significantly greater number of medial septal cholinergic neurons labeled for both ChAT and NGF-R, as well as a greater sprouting response of AChE-positive fibers in the dorsal lateral quadrant of the septum, in animals that received grafts of NGF-secreting fibroblasts compared to animals that received non-NGF-secreting fibroblasts. Therefore, intracerebral grafting of genetically modified cells may provide a useful tool for delivering biologically active NGF to the brain.

VII. FUTURE DIRECTIONS

Animal models of some of the morphological alterations and behavioral deficits associated with AD have yielded many insights into the relationships among the basal forebrain cholinergic system, amyloid protein precursor, and NGF. There is

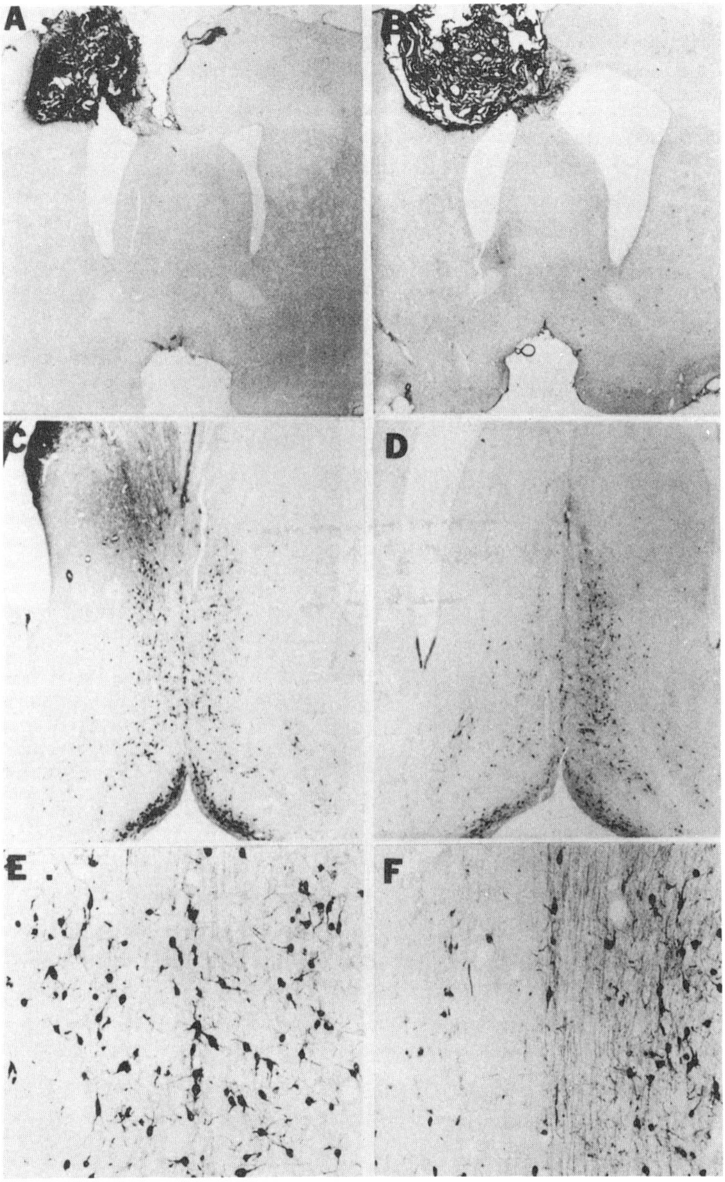

Figure 6 Photomicrograph of fibroblasts grafted into the fimbria-fornix cavity on the left side in the medial septal region stained with antibodies for fibronectin (A, B) and ChAT (C, D). Animal with graft of retrovirus-infected cells (A, C) and graft of control cells (B, D). (E, F) High-power views of C and D.

considerable evidence that chronic infusions of NGF can save cholinergic neurons in the basal forebrain region, a region that is involved in learning and memory and is particularly affected in AD. Additionally, NGF infusions can affect the various forms of APP which may be associated with amyloid deposition and are differentially affected during aging. Thus administration of NGF to AD patients may partially reverse some of the morphological alterations and ameliorate some of the functional deficits. Some additional issues need to be addressed:

1. *Does the chronic administration of NGF have any toxic or undesirable systemic side effects?* As stated earlier, NGF can affect APP mRNA levels. Whether such alterations are related to the pathological changes associated with AD remains to be determined. For example, the carboxyl terminus of the APP molecule has been shown to have a potent neurotoxic effect on NGF-primed PC12 cells and rat hippocampal neurons (105), which could contribute to the widespread cell death in AD. Also, amyloid protein may have trophic and tropic properties and may promote aberrant neuritic sprouting in the brain (88). In fact, NGF itself has been shown to promote aberrant sympathetic neuritic sprouting (106). Additionally, a recent report showed that NGF induces not only expression of APP genes but also genes for the prion protein which may be involved in the etiology of AD (107).

2. *What is the minimum dose of NGF which can affect cholinergic neurons?* Extensive dose response studies in experimental animals, including nonhuman primates, should be performed to determine the optimal dose of NGF that can save cholinergic neurons. This may also decrease the possibility of undesirable side effects of NGF treatment.

3. *What is the duration of NGF treatment necessary to permanently support cholinergic cells?* Is permanent NGF treatment necessary to retain improvements that result from NGF infusions, or can short-term NGF infusions provide permanent protection to the cells? Studies that examine the effects of discontinuing NGF administration after a period of time should be performed.

4. *Where should NGF be delivered into the brain?* Most animal studies have examined the effects of intraventricular NGF administration on medial septal neurons. However, a more widely distributed population of cholinergic neurons is affected in AD. Thus the extent the NGF penetrates and diffuses into brain parenchyma, as well as the optimal site for administration, need to be determined.

5. *How can NGF be most effectively delivered into the brain?* If long-term NGF treatment is found to be necessary, a delivery system that ensures the stability of the NGF protein for prolonged periods of time or employs a replenishable source of NGF must be developed. Chronic infusions via intracerebral cannulae may result in infection and damage to CNS tissue. Studies using recombinant human β-NGF and grafts of genetically manipulated fibroblasts that secrete NGF demonstrate the efficacy of alternatives to chronic mouse NGF infusions.

VIII. SUMMARY

There is substantial evidence for a relationship among NGF, the cholinergic system, cognitive function, and APP. The role that NGF may play in preventing progression of AD remains an enigma.

ACKNOWLEDGMENTS

This research was supported by NIA AGO 03553A, 6088, 8514.

REFERENCES

1. Katzman R. The prevalence and malignancy of Alzheimer's disease. Arch Neurol 33:217–218, 1976.
2. Price DL. New perspectives on Alzheimer's Disease. Annu Rev Neurosci 9:489–512, 1986.
3. Katzman R. Alzheimer's disease. N Engl J Med 314:964–973, 1986.
4. Hamos JE, DeGennaro LJ, Drachman DA. Synaptic loss in Alzheimer's disease and other dementias. Neurology 39:355, 1989.
5. Masliah E, Terry RD, DeTeresa R, et al. Immuno-histochemical quantification of the synapse related protein synaptophysin in Alzheimer's disease. Neurosci Lett 103:234–239, 1989.
6. Adolfsson R, Gottfries CG, Oreland L, et al. Reduced levels of catecholamines in the brain and increased activity of monoamine oxidase in platelets in Alzheimer's disease. In Katzman R, Terry RD, Bick KL (eds): *Alzheimer's Disease: Senile Dementia and Related Disorders (Aging).* Raven Press, New York, pp. 441–451, 1978.
7. Cross AJ, Crow TJ, Perry EK, et al. Reduced dopamine-β-hydroxylase activity in Alzheimer's disease. Br Med J 282:93–94, 1981.
8. Winblad B, Adolfsson R, Carlsson A, et al. Biogenic amines in brains of patients with Alzheimer disease. In Corkin S, Davis KL, Growdon JH, et al. (eds): *Alzheimer's Disease: A Report of Progress in Research (Aging).* Raven Press, New York, pp. 25–33, 1982.
9. Yates CM, Simpson J, Gordon A, et al. Catecholamines and cholinergic enzymes in pre-senile and senile Alzheimer-type demetia and Down's syndrome. Brain Res 280:119–126, 1983.
10. Ishii T. Distribution of Alzheimer's neurofibrillary changes in the brain stem and hypothalamus of senile dementia. Acta Neuropathol 6:181–187, 1966.
11. Curcio CA, Kemper T. Nucleus raphe dorsalis in dementia of the Alzheimer type: Neurofibrillary changes and neuron packing density. J Neuropath Exp Neurol 43:359–368, 1984.
12. Yamamoto T, Hirano A. Nucleus raphe dorsalis in Alzheimer's disease: Neurofibrillary tangles and loss of large neurons. Ann Neurol 17:573–577, 1985.
13. Davies P, Katzman R, Terry RD. Reduced somatostatin-like immunoreactivity in cerebral cortex from cases of Alzheimer disease and Alzheimer senile dementia. Nature 288:279–280, 1980.

14. Rossor MN, Emson PC, Mountjoy CQ, et al. Reduced amounts of immunoreactive somatostatin in the temporal cortex in senile dementia of Alzheimer type. Neurosci Lett 20:373–377, 1980.
15. Perry EK, Perry RH, Blessed G, et al. Necropsy evidence of central cholinergic deficits in senile dementia. Lancet 2:143, 1977.
16. Arendt T, Taubert G, Bigl V, et al. Amyloid deposition in the nucleus basalis of Meynert complex: A topographic marker for degenerating cell clusters in Alzheimer's disease. Acta Neuropathol (Berl) 75:226–232, 1988.
17. Arendt T, Bigl V, Tennstedt A, et al. Correlation between cortical plaque count and neuronal loss in the nucleus basalis in Alzheimer's disease. Neurosci Lett 48:81–85, 1984.
18. Arendt T, Bigl V, Tennstedt A, et al. Neuronal loss in different parts of the nucleus basalis is related to neuritic plaque formation in cortical target areas in Alzheimer's disease. Neurosci 14:1–14, 1985.
19. Bowen DM, Smith CB, White P, et al. Neurotransmitter-related enzymes and indices of hypoxia in senile dementia and other abiotrophies. Brain 99:459–496, 1976.
20. Etienne P, Robitaille Y, Wood P, et al. Nucleus basalis neuronal loss, neuritic plaques and choline acetyltransferas activity in advanced Alzheimer's disease. Neurosci 19: 1279–1291, 1986.
21. Nagai T, McGeer PL, Peng JH, et al. Choline acetyltransferase immunohistochemistry in brains of Alzheimer's disease patients and controls. Neurosci Lett 36:195–199, 1983.
22. Whitehouse PJ, Price DJ, Clark A, et al. Alzheimer's disease: Evidence for selective loss of cholinergic neurons in the nucleus basalis. Ann Neurol 10:122–126, 1981.
23. Whitehouse PJ, Price DL, Struble RG, et al. Alzheimer's disease and senile dementia: Loss of neurons in the basal forebrain. Science 215:1237–1239, 1982.
24. Davies P, Maloney AJF. Selective loss of central cholinergic neurons in Alzheimer's disease. Lancet 2:1403, 1976.
25. White P, Goodhardt MJ, Keet JK, et al. Neocortical cholinergic neurons in elderly people. Lancet 1:668–671, 1977.
26. Perry Ek, Tomlinson BE, Blessed G, et al. Correlation of cholinergic abnormalities with senile plaques and mental test scores in senile dementia. Br Med J 2:1457–1459, 1978.
27. Bartus RT, Dean RL, Beer B, et al. The cholinergic hypothesis of geriatric memory dysfunction. Science 217:408–417, 1982.
28. Coyle JT, Price PH, DeLong MR. Alzheimer's disease: A disorder of cortical cholinergic innervation. Science 219:1184–1189, 1983.
29. Collerton D. Cholinergic function and intellectual decline in Alzheimer's disease. Neuroscience 19:1–28, 1986.
30. Korsching S, Auburger G, Heumann R, et al. Levels of nerve growth factor and its mRNA in the central nervous system of the rat correlate with cholinergic innervation. EMBO J 4:1289–1293, 1985.
31. Shelton DL, Reichardt LF. Studies on the expression of beta NGF gene in the central nervous system: Level and regional distribution of NGF mRNA suggest that NGF

functions as a trophic factor for several neuronal populations. Proc Natl Acad Sci USA 83:2714-2718, 1986.
32. Ayer-LeLievre C, Olson L, Ebendahl T, et al. Expression of the beta-nerve growth factor gene in hippocampal neurons. Science 240:1339-1341, 1988.
33. Schwab ME, Otten U, Agid Y, et al. Nerve growth factor (NGF) in the rat CNS: Absence of specific retrograde axonal transport and tyrosine hydroxylase induction in locus coeruleus and substantia nigra. Brain Res 168:473-483, 1979.
34. Seiler M, Schwab ME. Specific retrograde transport of nerve growth factor (NGF) from cortex to nucleus basalis in the rat. Brain Res 300:33-39, 1984.
35. Hefti F, Dravid A, Hartikka JJ. Chronic intraventricular injections of nerve growth factor elevate hippocampal choline acetyltransferase activity in adult rats with partial septohippocampal lesions. J Brain Res 293:305-311, 1984.
36. Mobley WC, Rutkowski JL, Tennekoon GI, et al. Choline acetyltransferase activity in striatum of neonatal rats increased by nerve growth factor. Science 229:284-287, 1985.
37. Gnahn H, Hefti F, Heumann R, et al. NGF-mediated increase in choline acetyltransferase (ChAT) in the neonatal rat forebrain; evidence for physiological role of NGF in the brain? Dev Brain Res 9:45-52, 1983.
38. Mobley WC, Rutkowski JL, Tennekoon GI, et al. Nerve growth factor increases choline acetyltransferase activity in developing basal forebrain neurons. Mol Brain Res 1:53-62, 1986.
39. Johnston MV, Rutkowski JL, Wainer BH, et al. NGF effects on developing forebrain cholinergic neurons are regionally specific. Neurochem Res 12:985-994, 1987.
40. Batchelor PE, Armstrong DM, Blaker SM, et al. Nerve growth factor receptor and choline acetyltransferase colocalization in neurons within the rat forebrain: Response to fimbria-fornix transection. J Comp Neurol 284:187-204, 1989.
41. Richardson PM, Verge Isse VMK, Riopelle RJ. Distribution of neuronal receptors for nerve growth factor in the rat. J Neurosci 6:2312-2321, 1986.
42. Taniuchi M, Johnson EM. Characterization of the binding properties and retrograde axonal transport of monoclonal antibody directed against the rat nerve growth factor receptor. J Cell Biol 101:1100-1106, 1985.
43. Hefti F, Hartikka J, Knusel B. Function of neurotrophic factors in the adult and aging brain and their possible use in the treatment of neurodegenerative diseases. Neurobiol Aging 10:515-533, 1989.
44. Schatteman GC, Gibbs L, Lanahan AA, et al. Expression of NGF receptor in the developing and adult primate central nervous system. J Neurosci 8:860-873, 1988.
45. Kordower JH, Bartus RT, Bothwell M, et al. Nerve growth factor receptor immunoreactivity in the non-human primate (Cebus apella): distribution, morphology, and colocalization with cholinergic enzymes. J Comp Neurol 277:465-486, 1988.
46. Armstrong DM, Bruce G, Hersh LB, et al. Development of cholinergic neurons in the septal/diagonal band complex of the rat. Dev Brain Res 36:249-256, 1987.
47. Auburger GR, Heumann R, Hellweg S, et al. Developmental changes of nerve growth factor and its mRNA inthe rat hippocampus: comparison with choline acetyltransferase. Dev Biol 120:322-328, 1987.

48. Large TH, Bodary SC, Clegg Do, et al. Nerve growth factor gene expression in the developing rat brain. Science 234:352–355, 1986.
49. Whittmor Sr, Ebendal T, Larkfors L, et al. Developmental and regional expression of B nerve growth factor messenger RNA and protein in the rat central nervous system. Proc Natl Acad Sci USA 83:817–821, 1986.
50. Martinez HJ, Dreyfus CF, Jonakait GM, et al. Nerve growth factor promotes cholinergic development in brain striatal cultures. Proc Natl Acad Sci USA 82:7777–7781, 1985.
51. Taniuchi M, Clark HB, Johnson EM Jr. Induction of nerve growth factor receptor in Schwann cells after axotomy. Proc Natl Acad Sci USA 83:4094–4098, 1986.
52. Gage FH, Batchelor P, Chen KS, et al. NGF receptor reexpression and NGF mediated cholinergic neuronal hypertrophy in the damaged adult neostriatum. Neuron 2:1177–1184, 1989.
53. Higgins GA, Koh S, Chen KS, et al. NGF induction of NGF receptor gene expression and cholinergic neuronal hypertrophy within the basal forebrain of the adult rat. Neuron 3:247–256, 1989.
54. Fischer W, Wictorin K, Bjorklund A, et al. Amelioration of cholinergic neuron atrophy and spatial memory impairment in aged rats by nerve growth factor. Nature 329:65–68, 1987.
55. Gage FH, Bjorklund A, Stenevi U. Functional correlates of compensatory sprouting by biogenic amine and cholinergic afferents in the hippocampal formation. Brain Res 268:27–37, 1983.
56. Gage FH, Bjorklund A. Compensatory collateral sprouting of aminergic systems in the hippocampal formation following partial deafferentation. In Isaacson RL, Pribram KH (eds): *The Hippocampus.* Plenum Publishing Corp, New York, 1986.
57. Milner TA, Amaral DG. Evidence for a ventral septal projection to the hippocampal formation of the rat. Exp Brain Res 55:579–585, 1984.
58. Amaral DG, Kurz J. An analysis of the origins of the cholinergic and noncholinergic septal projections to the hippocampal formation of the rat. J Comp Neurol 240:37–59, 1985.
59. Wainer BH, Levey AI, Rye DB, et al. Cholinergic and non-cholinergic septohippocampal pathways. Neurosci Lett 54:45–52, 1985.
60. Grady S, Reeves T, Steward O. Time course of retrograde degeneration of the cells of origin of the septohippocampal pathway after fimbria-fornix transections. Dev Brain Res 9:45–52, 1984.
61. Kromer LF, Bjorklund A, Stenevi U. Intracephalic embryonic neural implants in the adult rat brain. I. Growth and mature organization of brain stem, cerebellar, and hippocampal implants. J Comp Neurol 218:433–459, 1983.
62. Hefti F. Nerve growth factor (NGF) promotes survival of septal cholinergic neurons after fimbrial transection. J Neurosci 6:2155–2162, 1986.
63. Gage FH, Wictorin K, Fischer W, et al. Life and death of cholinergic neurons: In the septal and diagonal band region following complete fimbria-fornix transection. Neurosci 19:241–255, 1986.
64. Tuszynski MH, Armstrong DM, Gage FH. Basal forebrain cell loss following fimbria/fornix transection. Brain Res 508:241–248, 1989.

65. Armstrong DM, Terry RD, DeTeresa RM, et al. Response of septal cholinergic neurons to axotomy. J Comp Neurol 264:421-436, 1987.
66. Springer JE, Koh S, Tayrien MW, et al. Basal forebrain magnocellular neurons stain for nerve growth factor receptor: Correlation with cholinergic cell bodies and effects of axotomy. J Neurosci Res 17:111-118, 1987.
67. Montero CN, Hefti F. Rescue of lesioned septal cholinergic neurons by nerve growth factor: Specificity and requirement for chronic treatment. J Neurosci 8:2986-2999, 1988.
68. Hagg T, Manthorpe M, Vahlsing HL, et al. Delayed treatment with nerve growth factor reverses the apparent loss of cholinergic neurons after acute brain damage. Exp Neurol 101:303-312, 1988.
69. Arimatsu Y, Miyamoto M, Tsukui H, et al. Nerve growth factor enhances survival of identified projection neurons in the rat septal and diagonal band regions in vitro. Soc Neurosci Abstr 14:1114, 1988.
70. O'Brien TS, Svendsen CN, Isacson O, et al. Loss of True blue labelling from the medial septum following transection of the fimbria-fornix: Evidence for the death of cholinergic and noncholinergic neurons. Brain Res 508:249-256, 1990.
71. Gage FH, Armstrong Dm, Williams LR, et al. Morphological response of axotomized septal neurons to nerve growth factor. J Comp Neurol 269:147-155, 1988.
72. Kromer LF. Nerve growth factor treatment after brain injury prevents neuronal death. Science 235:214-216, 1987.
73. Williams LR, Varon S, Peterson Gm, et al. Continuous infusion of nerve growth factor prevents basal forebrain neuronal death after fimbria-fornix transection. Proc Natl Acad Sci USA 83:9231-9235, 1986.
74. Gage FH, Bjorklund A, Stenevi U. Denervation releases a neuronal survival factor in adult rat hippocampus. Nature 308:637-639, 1984.
75. Bjorklund A, Stenevi U. In vivo evidence of a hippocampal adrenergic neurotrophic factor specifically released on septal deafferentation. Brain Res 229:403-428, 1981.
76. Collins F, Crutcher KA. Neurotrophic activity in the adult rat hippocampal formation: Regional distribution and increase after septal lesion. J Neurosci 5:2809-2814, 1985.
77. Gage FH, Bjorklund A. Cholinergic septal grafts into the hippocampal formation improve spatial learning and memory in aged rats by an atropine-sensitive mechanism. J Neurosci 6:2837-2847, 1986.
78. Boyd FT, Clarke DW, Raizada MK. Insulin inhibits specific norepinephrine uptake in neuronal cultures from rat brain. Brain Res 398:1-5, 1986.
79. Tuszynski MH, U HS, Amaral DG, et al. Nerve growth factor infusion in primate brain reduces lesion-induced cholinergic neuronal degeneration. J Neurosci 10:3604-3614, 1990.
80. Larkfors L, Ebendal T, Whittemore SR, et al. Decreased level of nerve growth factor (NGF) and its messenger RNA in the aged rat brain. Mol Brain Res 3:55-60, 1987.
81. Fischer W, Gage FH, Bjorklund A. Degenerative changes in forebrain cholinergic nuclei correlate with cognitive impairments in aged rats. Europ J Neurosci 1:34-45, 1989.
82. Gage FH, Dunnett SB, Bjorklund A. Spatial learning and motor deficits in aged rats. Neurobiol Aging 5:43-48, 1984.

83. Gage FH, Kelly PAT, Bjorklund A. Regional changes in brain glucose metabolism reflect cognitive impairments in aged rats. J Neurosci 4:2856–2865, 1984.
84. Glenner GG, Wong CW. Alzheimer's disease-initial report of the purification and characterization of a novel cerebrovascular amyloid protein. Biochem Biophys Res Comm 120:885–890, 1984.
85. Masters CL, Simms G, Weinman NA, et al. Amyloid plaque core protein in Alzheimer-disease and Down syndrome. Proc Natl Acad Sci USA 82:4245–4249, 1985.
86. Cohen ML, Golde TE, Usiak MF, et al. In situ hybridization of nucleus basalis neurons shows increased beta-amyloid mRNA in Alzheimer's disease. Proc Natl Acad Sci USA 85:1227–1231, 1988.
87. Higgins GA, Lewis DA, Goldaber D, et al. Differential regulation of amyloid-B-protein mRNA expression within hippocampal neuronal subpopulations in Alzheimer disease. PNAS 85:1297–1301, 1988.
88. Whitson JS, Selkoe DJ, Cotman CW. Amyloid β protein enhances the survival of hippocampal neurons in vitro. Science 243:1488–1490, 1989.
89. Kitaguchi N, Takahashi Y, Tokushima Y, et al. Novel precursor of Alzheimer's disease amyloid protein shows protease inhibitory activity. Nature 331:530–532, 1988.
90. Ponte P, Gonzalez-DeWhitt P, Schilling J, et al. New A4 amyloid mRNA contains a domain homologous to serine proteinase inhibitors. Nature 331:525–527, 1988.
91. Neve RL, Finch EA, Dawes LR. Expression of the Alzheimer amyloid precursor gene transcripts in the human brain. Neuron 1:669–677, 1988.
92. Palmert MR, Golde TE, Cohen ML, et al. Amyloid protein precursor messenger RNAs: Differential expression in Alzheimer's disease. Science 241:1080–1083, 1988.
93. Johnson SA, Pasinetti FM, May PC, et al. Selective reduction of mRNA for the β-amyloid precursor protein that lacks a Kunitz-type protease inhibitor motif in cortex from Alzheimer brains. Exp Neurol 102:264–268, 1988.
94. Johnson SA, Rogers J, Finch CE. APP-695 transcript prevalence is selectively reduced during Alzheimer's disease in cortex and hippocampus but not in cerebellum. Neurobiol Aging 10:267–272, 1989.
95. Johnson SA, Finch CE. Alzheimer's disease does not alter the proportion of hippocampal neurons with APP-695 or APP-751 mRNA. Soc Neurosci Abstr 15:1379, 1989.
96. Tanaka S, Nakamura S, Ueda K, et al. Three types of amyloid protein precursor mRNA in human brain: their differential expression in Alzheimer's disease. Biochem Biophys Res Commun 157:472–479, 1988.
97. Higgins GA, Oyler GA, Neve RL, et al. Altered levels of amyloid protein precursor transcripts in the basal forebrain of behaviorally impaired aged rats. Proc Natl Acad Sci USA 87:3032–3036, 1990.
98. Higgins GA, Neve RL, Chen KS, et al. Nerve growth factor (NGF) regulation of amyloid gene expression in aged rat forebrain. Soc Neurosci Abst 15:1378, 1989.
99. Phelps CH, Gage FH, Growdon H, et al. Potential use of nerve growth factor to treat Alzheimer's disease. Neurobiol Aging 10:205–207, 1989.
100. Barnett J, Baecker P, Routledge-Ward C, et al. Human beta nerve growth factor ob-

tained from a baculovirus expression system has potent in vitro and in vivo neurotrophic activity. Exp Neurol 110: 11-24, 1990.
101. Chen KS, Barnett J, Chan H, et al. Chronic intraventricular infusions of recombinant human β-NGF into the aged rat: A behavioral and morphological study. Soc Neurosci Abstr 16:479, 1990.
102. Friedmann T. Progress toward human gene therapy. Science 244:1275-1281, 1989.
103. Gage FH, Wolff JA, Rosenberg MB, et al. Grafting genetically modified cells to the brain: Possibilities for the future. Neurosci 23:795-807, 1987.
104. Rosenberg MB, Friedmann T, Robertson RC, et al. Grafting genetically modified cells to the damaged brain: restorative effects of NGF expression. Science 242: 1575-1578, 1988.
105. Yankner BA, Dawes LR, Fisher S, et al. Neurotoxicity of a fragment of the amyloid precursor associated with Alzheimer's disease. Science 245:417-420, 1990.
106. Isaacson LG, Saffran BN, Crutcher KA. Intracerebral NGF infusion induces hyperinnervation of cerebral blood vessels. Neurobiol Aging 11:51-55, 1990.
107. Mobley WC, Neve RL, Prusiner SB, et al. Nerve growth factor induces gene expression for prion- and Alzheimer's beta-amyloid proteins. Proc Natl Acad Sci USA 85:9811-9815, 1988.

9

The Potential Use of Neurotrophic Factors in the Treatment of Alzheimer's Disease

Lars Olson
Karolinska Institute, Stockholm, Sweden

Barry J. Hoffer
University of Colorado, Denver, Colorado

The problem of dementia in the western world is of mounting medical concern. In fact, medical progress in treating other somatic illnesses, leading to a longer average life expectancy, has automatically increased the number of people suffering from various degrees of mental disorders of the presenile/senile dementia type. Memory impairments come first in Alzheimer's disease (AD). Intellectual disturbances, including dysphasia, dysgnosia, and dyspraxia follow. Recent studies (1) suggest that the prevalence of Alzheimer's disease may be higher than previously reported, encompassing 3% of the population aged 65-74, 18.7% of those aged 75-84, and 47.2% of those over 85 years of age. Unless progress in the understanding and treatment of dementias of the Alzheimer type is rapidly effected, it will become a health problem of enormous proportions.

The clinical diagnosis of Alzheimer's disease is based on a history of symptoms and neurological examination (2). In addition, positron emission tomography (PET) scans reveal decreased glucose utilization, particularly in temporal and parietal areas. Unequivocal diagnosis, however, rests upon finding the characteristic neuropathological changes at autopsy. The classical description of tangles and plaques by Alois Alzheimer (3-5) still stands as a relatively complete description of the neurodegenerative changes seen in the cortices at the light microscopical level. Temporal and parietal lobes are severely affected, while motor and sensory cortex areas, including the occipital cortices, are less affected. The hippocampus is severely affected. Modern cellular and molecular neurobiological techniques have added information about the nature of amyloid deposition and the relative involvement of various transmitter-specific neuronal systems. Several reviews on current research topics related to the epidemiology, pathology, genetics, neurotransmitter disturbances, and molecular biology of amyloid and biological markers of Alzheimer's disease have recently been published (6–8). While a number of different fiber systems projecting both to and from cortex cerebri and hippocampus have been demonstrated to be affected in AD, the most remarkable and consistent finding appears to be degeneration of the long, ascending, unmyelinated cholinergic fiber tracts from the basal forebrain to cortex cerebri and hippocampus. Thus there is marked loss of cholinergic nerve cell bodies in nucleus basalis of Meynert and in certain other associated groups of cholinergic neurons and a corresponding loss of cortical cholinergic nerve terminals as assessed by markers such as choline acetylase (ChAT) levels. Similar severe cholinergic deficits, as evidenced by decreases in ChAT activity, have been shown in senile dementia of Lewy body type (9).

I. ANIMAL MODELS OF ALZHEIMER'S DISEASE

The etiology of Alzheimer's disease, including the familial forms, remains unknown. It appears not to exist in rodents; its existence in any animals, including nonhumans, is unclear. Extensive animal experimentation has revealed the importance of the cholinergic projections to the cortices for memory and cognitive functions (10). Animal models of Alzheimer's disease are therefore often based on cholinergic lesions. Such lesions include mechanical transections of the cholinergic projections from the medial septal nuclei and the diagonal band via the fimbria-fornix to the hippocampus, as well as neurotoxin (e.g., ibotenic acid)-induced lesions of the cholinergic cell bodies such as those in nucleus basalis projecting to cortex cerebri (11,12).

II. THE NGF FAMILY OF GROWTH FACTORS

In situ hybridization has shown that nerve growth factor (NGF) mRNA is present in neurons rather than glial cells in the normal adult rodent brain (13). This evidence was derived from the localization of a hybridization signal over nerve cell cytoplasm rather than glial cells in normal hippocampal tissue, and from the results of neurotoxic lesion experiments with kainic acid and colchicine. Thus neuronal death was correlated with loss of hybridization signal, in spite of concomitant glial proliferation (13). These experiments therefore suggested that NGF can function as a direct neuron-to-neuron trophic signal in the central nervous system.

Recently, NGF (14,15) was shown to have structurally similar "relatives," forming a family of factors currently including three members (see ref. 16). This new development began with the landmark report of Leibrock and colleagues (17) showing that brain-derived neurotrophic factor (BDNF) has a remarkably high sequence homology to NGF, sharing some 50% of the amino acid residues. Soon afterwards, five different groups almost simultaneously reported a third member in the NGF family, variously called hippocampal-derived neurotrophic factor (HDNF) (18), neurotrophin-3 (19,20), neuronotrophin-3 (21) or NGF-2 (22). In the following, we shall use HDNF to denote this third factor.

Recently, using oligonucleotide probes, it has been demonstrated that BDNF and HDNF mRNA are also expressed by neurons rather than glial cells in the nonlesioned adult brain (23,24). The specificity of the labeling was ascertained in several ways, including 1) the demonstration of identical patterns of labeling using different probes to the same factor; 2) the fact that other probes applied to consecutive sections in the same experiments (such as probes for the NGF receptor) generate different, reproducible, and previously defined labeling; and 3) the fact that only certain restricted sets of neurons are labeled with any given growth factor probe. Moreover, using high-stringency conditions, mRNA for the three different growth factors have at least partially nonoverlapping distributions in the brain. Finally, regional studies using northern blot analyses of mRNA levels are in general agreement with the detailed results provided by in situ hybridization data. The fact that neurons in the brain express mRNA for NGF, BDNF, and HDNF suggests that they synthesize the corresponding proteins and may release them locally to attract and maintain specific sets of synaptic inputs.

A. NGF, BDNF, and HDNF Are All Made by Neurons in the Hippocampal Formation

There is a remarkable concentration of neurons expressing mRNA for the NGF family members in the hippocampal formation of the adult rodent brain. While all three factors, to a varying degree, are also found elsewhere in the CNS, the fact they are so abundant in the hippocampal formation makes it tempting to speculate that their presence is related to a high degree of plasticity in this brain area, perhaps related to such phenomena as long-term potentiation, kindling, memory formation, and information processing. Indeed, recent studies indicate that mRNA levels for the NGF family of growth factors change rapidly in response to experimentally induced seizures (25) and to mechanical as well as neurotoxin-induced insults to the hippocampal formation (26). The uniqueness of the adult hippocampus as a source of growth factors is further emphasized by the presence of basic fibroblast growth factor mRNA hybridizing neurons in this region (27).

Neurons expressing NGF mRNA are found scattered along the entire hippocampal pyramidal cell layer in the rat brain. Labeled cells are also found outside the pyramidal layer, particularly in stratum oriens. particularly strongly labeled neurons are found in the hilar region of the dentate gyrus, especially close to the inner border of the dentate granular cell layer. The dentate granular neurons themselves express moderate amounts of NGF mRNA (24).

BDNF mRNA-containing neurons are more numerous than NGF-expressing neurons in the pyramidal layer. Many pyramidal neurons all the way from medial CA1 to the hilar region express BDNF, although the strongest labeled neurons are found in CA2, CA3, and the hilar region of the dentate gyrus. The dentate neurons express moderate levels of BDNF mRNA (23,24). A similar pattern of labeling with BDNF oligonucleotide probes is found in the pig hippocampus (23).

The pattern of HDNF-expressing neurons in the hippocampal formation is clearly different from that of the other two NGF family members. Labeled neurons are seen in medial CA1 and, very characteristically, in all of CA2. In addition, lateral parts of CA1 contain scattered HDNF-expressing neurons. Dentate granule cells also express HDNF (18,24).

B. BDNF in Cortex Cerebri and Claustrum

BDNF-hybridizing neurons are found throughout the *cerebral cortex* of both pig (23) and rat (23,24), including pyramidal cells in both the inner and the outer pyramidal cell layer. Neurons expressing BDNF are particularly abundant in *temporal, perirhinal, cingulate,* and *piriform* cortex. Scattered BDNF-expressing neurons are also found in the *amygdaloid* area (24).

Strongly BDNF-hybridizing cells are furthermore found in *claustrum* of both pig (23) and rat (23,24). In this area, a majority of the neurons appeared labeled, suggesting that BDNF expression might be related to the presumed role of claustrum in sensory input processing (28,29).

III. TREATMENT STRATEGIES BASED ON NEUROTROPHIC FACTORS

Unlike the case of Parkinson's disease, in which the neurodegeneration is highly localized, the loss of cholinergic nerve terminals in Alzheimer's disease is very widespread, affecting huge areas of cortex and the hippocampal formation. This fact would appear to make a therapy based on grafting fetal cholinergic neurons less attractive, although such therapy is feasible. Aspects of neuronal grafting and Alzheimer's disease have recently been summarized (30). A better strategy may be to attempt to stop the progressive degenerative changes and, if possible, to reverse them by treatment with specific neurotrophic agents. As will be detailed below, there is now strong evidence to suggest that many cholinergic neurons in the brain are sensitive to and depend upon continuous access to NGF. Therefore, whether a disturbed NGF production or utilization of NGF is involved in the disease process or not, treatment with exogenous NGF as a pharmacological agent might rescue cholinergic neurons in diseased condition, and indeed cause the sprouting of new fibers into denervated areas. Additionally, other neurotrophic factors, such as the new members of the NGF family or the FGFs that may act on neuronal systems which regress in Alzheimer's disease, might be similarly used. For instance, BDNF has recently been shown to increase survival and induce differentiation of fetal septal cholinergic neurons in culture (31). If trophic effects of BDNF on cholinergic neurons are maintained in adult neurons, a combination treatment with NGF and BDNF might prove advantageous.

A. Strategies to Increase Brain Levels of Neurotrophic Factors

There are several ways in which the intracerebral levels of a neurotrophic factor might be increased. These possibilities can be exemplified for NGF as follows.

1. *Administration of Purified NGF*

Several techniques have been used to deliver NGF acutely and chronically to the central nervous system, both intraventricularly and intraparenchymally. Indwelling cannulas or dialysis fibers reaching sterotaxically defined targets and connected to subcutaneous osmotic pumps permit constant infusion over weeks or months. This duration of NGF administration may be needed to obtain significant fiber growth responses.

2. *Transplantation of Cells That Make NGF*

Cells That Naturally Make NGF. Male mouse *submandibular gland* tissue is an extremely rich source of the factor. Such tissue, however, does not give good long-term survival after grafting. Moreover, the cells of the striated ducts secrete many other factors which may not be wanted. *Schwann cells* synthesize NGF, particularly after having been deprived of their nerves. Therefore, minces of peripheral nerves, rich in Schwann cells, or cultures of Schwann cells could be transplanted alone or cografted with NGF-sensitive neurons.

Genetically Modified Cells. Cell lines can be genetically modified to secrete large amounts of NGF (32). Thus a mouse fibroblast cell line was established (11) that secretes biologically active NGF. The cells can be grafted to the brain and exert effects on NGF-sensitive intrinsic as well as grafted neurons (32,33).

3. *Regulation of Endogenous Trophic Factor Production*

Recent studies using dispersed cultures of fetal hippocampus (34) suggest that factors that cause or mediate inflammatory responses, such as lipopolysaccharide, interleukin-1, and prostaglandins can upregulate NGF mRNA and protein levels. In vitro, glial cells also make NGF, particularly when grown at low density. Addition of serum to astroglial cultures is another potent upregulator of NGF in these cells. It thus appears that in the normal adult CNS, NGF is made primarily by neurons which are target cells for NGF-dependent nerve fibers. However, glial cells, particularly astrocytes, also make NGF after injury or in disease states accompanied by extravasated blood, inflammatory processes, and other reactive changes. It is possible that other trophic factors undergo similar upregulation. Thus, it may be possible to augment endogenous levels of NGF in the CNS.

IV. FUNCTIONAL CONSIDERATIONS

It is becoming increasingly clear that NGF is an important trophic factor in the central nervous system. The regional presence of NGF and its receptor, demonstrated at both the mRNA and protein level, as well as experimental data with NGF applications in vitro and in vivo, suggests that several neuronal systems, including the cholinergic projections from septum and the basal forebrain to hippocampus and cortex cerebri, are sensitive to, and probably dependent upon NGF (see ref. 16). By analogy, it may be assumed that BDNF and HDNF might play similar trophic roles for specific sets of CNS neurons. In support of such an assumption are the in vitro data showing that BDNF and HDNF also affect ganglia in differential ways, making it possible to distinguish NGF, BDNF, and HDNF from one another (16) (see also ref. 18).

V. A RATIONALE FOR CLINICAL TRIALS WITH NGF IN PATIENTS WITH ALZHEIMER'S DISEASE

Trials of new treatment strategies in patients are always associated with risks. Such trials must be based on substantial animal research data. The potential hazards of morbidity and mortality associated with any new treatment must also be considered in the context of the available conventional treatments and of the prognosis of the disease under consideration. In the case of Alzheimer's disease, we argue that it is reasonable to initiate small, carefully controlled clinical trials with NGF infusion. The reasoning leading to this conclusion is based on the work cited above and below and can be summarized as follows:

1. Patients with Alzheimer's disease lose cholinergic innervation of cortex and hippocampus.
2. Lesions of cholinergic pathways to the cortices in rodents lead to cognitive deficits reminiscent of some of the symptoms seen in Alzheimer's disease patients.
3. In rodents, NGF can rescue axotomized cholinergic neurons and counteract the functional effects of cholinergic losses.
4. Remaining cholinergic neurons in nucleus basalis of Meynert in Alzheimer's disease patients express normal or supranormal levels of the 75kD NGF-R mRNA (35).

5. Infusion of purified mouse β-NGF (4 mg over 3 weeks) into the putamen of a patient with Parkinson's disease, to support adrenal medullary autografts (37), has not led to immunization against NGF. There have not been any measurable negative effects in this patient. Long-term improvement in parkinsonian symptoms has been observed.
6. Alzheimer's disease is a progressive and devastating disease, leading to disintegration of mental functions.
7. There is no presently available treatment that can retard the progression of Alzheimer's disease.

In developing this rationale, we have reasoned that mouse salivary β-NGF is an acceptable substitute for human NGF. Mouse β-NGF can be purified in adequate amounts at reasonable costs. It is very similar to human NGF, differing approximately as much as swine insulin differs from human insulin. When human recombinant NGF, now undergoing preliminary trials in animals, becomes available in pure and biologically active form in adequate quantities, it is obviously to be preferred. However, infusion of species-specific NGF is no guarantee against problems of immunization. For instance, mice can be effectively immunized using mouse NGF, provided that effective immunization protocols are followed (37). Moreover, there are no known differences in biological activity between human and mouse NGF as tested in either rodent or human NGF-sensitive systems.

In addition to the general surgical risks involved with chronic infusion into the CNS, there are possible specific risks associated with NGF, such as growth-stimulating effects on other neuronal systems or in other areas of the CNS counteracting the desired effects as well as other "nontrophic" effects of an acute or chronic nature, such as actions on electrical activity of neurons (cf. ref. 38).

We have concluded, however, based on the above reasoning, that the possible benefits outweigh the risks. If promising, initial results could be used as a basis for more extended trials with NGF, and perhaps other neurotrophic factors, as a way to counteract Alzheimer's disease and other types of neurodegenerative diseases.

ACKNOWLEDGMENTS

Supported by the Swedish Medical Research Council, the Swedish Natural Environment Protection Board, Karolinska Institutets Fonder, and USPHS grants AG-04418 and NS-09199.

REFERENCES

1. Evand D, Funkenstein H, Albert M, et al. Prevalence of Alzheimer's disease in a community population of older persons. Higher than previously reported. JAMA 262: 2551–2556, 1989.
2. McKhann G, Drachman D, Folstein M, et al. Clinical diagnosis of Alzheimer's dis-

ease: Report of the NINCDS-ADRDA work group under the auspices of Department of Health and Human Services Task Force on Alzheimer's disease. Neurology 34: 939–944, 1984.

3. Alzheimer A. Über einen eigenartigen schweren Krankheitsprozess der Hirnrinde. Zentralbl Nervenkh 25:1134, 1906.
4. Alzheimer A. Über einen eigenartigen schweren Krankenheitsprozess der Hirnrinde. Zentralbl Nervernkh 30:177, 1907.
5. Alzheimer A. Über eine eigenartige Erkrankung der Hirnrinde. Allg Z Psychiatr 64:146, 1907.
6. Boller F, Katzman R, Rasco A, et al. *Biological Markers of Alzheimer's Disease. Research and Perspectives in Alzheimer's Disease.* Fondation IPSEN. Springer Verlag, Berlin-Hiedelberg, 1989.
7. Petit H, Leys D, Christen Y. *Imaging, Cerebral Topography and Alzheimer's Disease. Research and Perspectives in Alzheimer's Disease.* Fondation IPSEN. Springer Verlag, Berlin-Heidelberg, 1990.
8. Wurtman R, Corkin S, Growdfon J, et al. *Alzheimer's Disease.* Advances in Neurology. Raven Press, New York, 1990.
9. Perry E, Kerwin J, Perry R, et al. Cerebral cholinergic activity is related to the incidence of visual hallucinations in senile dementia of the Lewy body type. Dementia 1:2–4, 1990.
10. Gage F, Chen K, Buzsaki G, et al. Experimental approaches to age-related cognitive impairments. Neurobiol Aging 9:645–655, 1988.
11. Ernfors P, Ebendal T, Olson L, Mouton P, et al. A cell line producing recombinant nerve growth factor evokes growth responses in intrinsic and grafted central cholinergic neurons. Proc Natl Acad Sci USA 86:4756–4760, 1989.
12. Tyszynski M, Armstrong D, Gage G. Basal forebrain cell loss following fimbria/fornix transection. Brain Res 508:241–248, 1990.
13. Ayer-LeLievre C, Olson L, Ebendal T, et al. Expression of the β-nerve growth factor gene in hippocampal neurons. Science 240:1339–1341, 1988.
14. Levi-Montalcini R. The nerve growth factor: its mode of action on sensory and sympathetic nerve cells. Harvey Lect 60:217–259, 1966.
15. Levi-Montalcini R. The nerve growth factor: Thirty-five years later. Science 237: 1154–1162, 1987.
16. Ebendal T, Söderström S, Hallböök F, et al. Human nerve growth factor: Biological and immunological activities, and clinical possibilities in neurodegenerative disease. In *Plasticity and Regeneration in the Nervous System.* Plenum Press, New York, Timiras P, Privat A (eds): 1991 (in press).
17. Leibrock J, Lottspeich F, Hohn A, et al. Molecular cloning and expression of brain-derived neurotrophic factor. Nature 341:149–152, 1989.
18. Ernfors P, Ibanez CF, Ebendal T, et al. Molecular cloning and neurotrophic activities of a protein with structural similarities to β-nerve growth factor: Developmental and topographical expression in the brain. Proc Natl Acad Sci USA, 1990 87:5454–5458.
19. Hohn A, Leibrock J, Bailey K, et al. Identification and characterization of a novel member of the nerve growth factor/brain-derived neurotrophic factor family. Nature 344:339–341, 1990.

20. Maisonpierre PC, Belluscio L, Squinto S, et al. Neurotrophin-3: A neurotrophic factor related to NGF and BDNF. Science 247:1446–1451, 1990.
21. Rosenthal A, Goeddel DV, Nguyen T, et al. Primary structure and biological activity of a novel human neurotrophic factor. Neuron 4:767–773, 1990.
22. Kaisho Y, Yoshimura K, Nakahama K. Cloning and expression of a cDNA encoding a novel human neurotrophic factor. FEBS Letters 266:187–191, 1990.
23. Wetmore C, Ernfors P, Persson H, et al. Localization of brain-derived neurotrophic factor mRNA to neurons in the brain by in situ hybridization. Exp Neurol 109:141–152, 1990.
24. Ernfors P, Wetmore C, Olson L, et al. Identification of cells in rat brain and peripheral tissues expressing mRNA for the members of the nerve growth factor family. Neuron 1990 5:511–526.
25. Gall CM, Isackson PJ. Limbic seizures increase neuronal production of messenger RNA for nerve growth factor. Science 245:758–761, 1989.
26. Ballarín M, Ernfors P, Lindefors N, et al. Rapid induction of mRNA for brain-derived neurotrophic factor after intrahippocampal injection of kainic acid. Exp Neurol 114 1991 (in press).
27. Walicke P, Cowan W, Ueno N, et al. Fibroblast growth factor promotes survival of dissociated hippocampal neurons and enhances neurite extension. Proc Natl Acad Sci USA 83:3012–3016, 1986.
28. Witter M, Room H, Groenewegen H, et al. Reciprocal connections of the insular and piriform claustrum with limbic cortex: An anatomical study in the cat. Neuroscience 24:519–539, 1988.
29. Sherk H, Levay S. Visual claustrum: Topography and receptive field properties in the cat. Science 212:87–89, 1989.
30. Gage F, Privat A, Cristen Y. *Neuronal Grafting in Alzheimer's Disease. Research Perspectives in Alzheimer's Disease*. Fondation IPSEN. Springer Verlag, Berlin-Heidelberg, 1989.
31. Alderson R, Alterman A, Barde Y-A, et al. Brain-derived neurotrophic factor increases survival and differentiated functions of rat septal cholinergic neurons in culture. Neuron 5:297–306, 1990.
32. Rosenberg MB, Friedmann T, Robertson RC, et al. Grafting genetically modified cells to the damaged brain: Restorative effects of NGF expression. Science 242:1575–1578, 1988.
33. Strömberg I, Wetmore CJ, Ebendal T, et al. Rescue of basal forebrain cholinergic neurons after implantation of genetically modified cells producing recombinant NGF. J Neurosci Res 25:405–411, 1990.
34. Friedman WJ, Lärkfors L, Ayer-LeLievre C, et al. Regulation of β-nerve growth factor expression by inflammatory mediators in hippocampal cultures. J Neurosci Res 1990.
35. Ernfors P, Lindefors N, Chan-Palay V, et al. Cholinergic neurons of nucleus basalis express elevated levels of nerve growth factor receptor mRNA in senile dementia of the Alzheimer type. Proc Natl Acad Sci USA 1990 (in press).
36. Olson L, Backlund E, Ebendal T, et al. Intraputaminal infusion of nerve growth factor

to support adrenal medullary autografts in Parkinson's disease: One-year follow-up of first clinical trial. Arch Neurol 1991 48:373–381.

37. Korsching S, Thoenen H. Nerve growth factor in sympathetic ganglia and corresponding target organs of the rat: Correlation with density of sympathetic innervation. Proc Natl Acad Sci USA 80:3513–3516, 1983.
38. Palmer M, Wuerthele S, Hoffer B. Physical and physiological characteristics of micropressure ejection of drugs from multibarreled pipettes. Neuropharmacology 19: 931–938, 1980.

PART IV

Anti-Inflammatory Drugs

10

Human Antibodies to Alzheimer's Disease and Normal Neural Elements

Felicia Gaskin
University of Virginia School of Medicine, Charlottesville, Virginia

The hypothesis discussed in this chapter is that there is a specific immune response in Alzheimer's disease (AD). The response is identifiable, albeit weak. This immune response may contribute to the pathogenesis of AD. It is also compatible with recent documentation of low-grade chronic inflammation in AD brain with HLA-DR positive microglia, T-cells, increased cytokines, complement components of the classical pathway, and scattered Ig staining. All of these are described in Chapter 11.

Evidence obtained in our laboratory and those of other investigators shows that there are autoantibodies against neural elements in AD patients and that specific anti-AD brain antibodies are present. Two types of evidence are present.

I. EXPERIMENTAL DATA

Table 1 summarizes the experimental evidence for the presence of circulating antibrain antibodies. Reported studies are listed in chronological order. Some of the early studies did not take into consideration the presence of autoantibodies to common cellular components. However, it will become apparent that several of these studies suggest the presence of specific antineuronal antibodies in a subpopulation of AD patients' sera or cerebrospinal fluid (CSF).

Nandy (1,2) probably started this type of investigation in 1978 by reporting

Table 1 Selected Studies Reporting Antibrain Antibodies in AD Sera

Investigator(s)	Study results
Nandy, 1978 (1)	% of reactive cells in mouse brain was higher with AD than control sera.
Watts et al., 1981 (4)	Analysis presented suggesting that it was not possible to detect brain reactive antibodies due to an increase in autoantibodies with aging.
Fillit et al., 1985 (5)	More intense staining of specific areas of normal rat and human brain and reaction on immunoblots of bovine choline acetyltransferase with a subpopulation of AD sera.
D'Angelo and D'Angelo, 1986 (7)	AD sera react with NFT and plaques.
Singh and Fudenberg, 1986 (10)	Absorbed AD sera showed high incidence (57%) of reaction compared to normals (0%) on rat brain tissue.
Fillit et al., 1987 (6)	Antibody against vascular membrane heparan sulfate proteoglycan in 6/16 AD sera.
Chapman et al., 1988, 1989 (11,12)	Antibodies in AD sera and CSF react with cholinergic neurons by binding specifically to 200 kDa neurofilament protein.
Tanaka et al., 1988 (13)	High titer of anti GFAP was found in AD (80%) compared to multiinfarct dementia (9%) and controls (3%).
Sugiura et al., 1989 (9)	A subpopulation (6/25) of AD sera were positive for rabbit cerebellum neurons after absorption by liver acetone powder.
Gaskin and Finley, unpublished data	After absorptions of sera with HeLa cells, reactivities to NFT, astrocytes, and filaments were found in several AD sera and one normal serum.

that AD sera reacted with a higher percentage of cells in mouse brain than control sera. He counted cells. Since no absorptions were done, some or the majority of the staining may not be brain specific. Thus the interpretation of Nandy's study has been challenged, in particular by Watts and co-investigators (3,4). This group of investigators presented an analysis suggesting that it was not possible to detect brain-reactive antibodies due to an increase in autoantibodies in normal aging.

In 1985, a report published by Fillit and colleagues (5) showed more intense staining of specific areas of normal rat and human brain with AD sera. Fillit et al. did immunoblots using bovine choline acetyltransferase as the antigen and found some reactivity with a subpopulation of AD sera. Inhibition studies eliminated this antibody reaction. They also found many other types of antibody reaction. However, specificities of these reactions were not established. In a more recent study (6) Fillit and colleagues demonstrated the presence of antibodies against CNS vascular membrane in 6/16 AD sera. This reactivity was shown to be specific for heparan sulfate proteoglycan.

Neurofibrillary tangles (NFT) and plaques are pathological hallmarks of AD. In 1986, D'Angelo and D'Angelo (7) reported the presence of antibodies to NFT and plaques in AD sera. Again, specificities cannot be ascertained.

Two studies were carried out with sera absorbed by cell homogenates to remove antibodies with common cellular components. Singh and Fudenberg (8) did absorption studies on AD and control sera with pellets from various tissue homogenates. A high incidence of reaction (57%) in the AD group on rat brain tissue and none in the control group were found. More recently, Sugiura et al. (9) reported a subpopulation of AD sera (6/25) to be positive for rabbit cerebellum neurons after absorption with liver acetone powder.

McRae-Degueurce et al. (10) showed that antibodies in 6/8 AD CSF reacted with cholinergic neurons in rat brain. Chapman et al. (11,12) have extended these studies using AD CSF and sera. They found that binding to cholinergic neurons was due to reaction with the 200 kD neurofilament protein (12). A high titer of anti-GFAP in AD sera (80%) compared to multiinfarct dementia (9%) and controls (3%) has also been reported by Tanaka et al. (13).

Over the past several years, our laboratory has spent considerable effort to generate EBV-transformed B-cell lines from AD and age-matched controls. We have considerable experience in dealing with specificities of antibodies for neuronal tissues. We have used cell homogenates from HeLa cells to absorb antibodies reactive to common cellular components. It is important to note that human cell homogenates were used to remove all such antibodies in view of the increasing evidence that many of the circulating antiantibodies may be specific for human epitopes. The staining patterns of the unabsorbed and absorbed serum from a neuropathologically confirmed AD patient are shown in Figure 1. The unabsorbed and absorbed antibody reactions are detected by secondary rhodamine-conjugated goat antibodies to human Ig and NFT. Plaques are recognized by counterstaining with thioflavine S. The unabsorbed serum reacts with NFT, astrocytes, nuclei, and filaments (Fig. 1a and b) and the absorbed serum shows strong selective reactivity with NFT and filaments (Fig. 1c and d).

Thus, HeLa cells absorb out the autoantibody staining recognizing common cellular components. However, in several of the AD sera, HeLa cells do not absorb out the NFT staining. In the case of control sera, we have also found this in one of our controls. In addition, some astrocytes and filaments are still reactive after absorption of certain sera with HeLa cells.

It should be apparent that antineural specific and anti-NFT antibodies can be

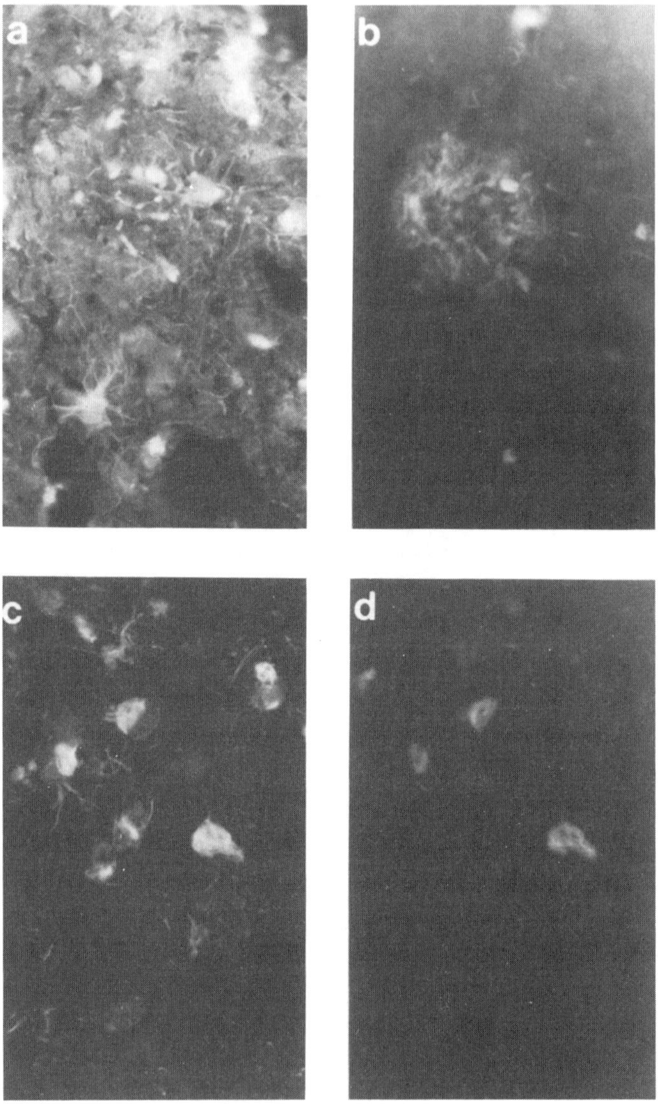

Figure 1 MGO (AD neuropathologically confirmed by biopsy) plasma antibody reaction on AD brain temporal cortex before and after absorption with HeLa cells. (a) Unabsorbed MGO plasma reacts strongly with NFT, astrocytes, nuclei, and filaments. (b) In the same field, a plaque is identified by thioflavine S. (c) Absorbed MGO plasma reacts less with AD tissue but still shows strong reactivity with NFT and filaments. (d) Three NFT are identified by thioflavine S in the same field as (c). (a,c) Red fluorescence of rhodamine-conjugated antibodies. Exposure time 25 sec. (b,d) Thioflavine S counterstaining detected by UV excitation. Exposure time 10 sec.

demonstrated to be present in a subpopulation of AD patients. This demonstration is technically demanding. The titers of these antibodies are low. In order to study these antibodies further, we decided to generate EBV-transformed B-cell lines in an attempt to immortalize the B-cells which secrete these antibodies.

Although the majority of cell lines established by EBV transformation secrete IgM, we consider that these IgM antibodies are a part of the repertoire of the circulating antibodies. Thus, we have taken B-cells from patients with Alzheimer's disease, from age-matched controls, from a multiple sclerosis patient, from a Gerstmann-Straussler-Scheinker (GSS) syndrome patient who has AD changes in his brain (from a genetic family in Indiana identified by M. Farlow and B. Ghetti), and two stroke patients, and looked at the types of antibodies being secreted by these B-cells (14–18). These B-cell lines were derived from a limited number of B-cells. The resulting lines were either monoclonal or oligoclonal. The screening results show that all these groups generate anti-NFT antibody-producing lines. However, only two of them were identified to be specific.

Table 2 shows the numbers or percentages of antibodies we have that are reacting with NFT in AD tissue. We have a higher percentage: 2.4% ± 1.3% of the cell lines that are secreting antibody reactive with the NFT compared to the age-matched controls (0.8 ± 0.7%). This is significant at $p < .02$. We also found antibody-positive cell lines from the other groups, although the percentages were less.

Not all of these antibodies react just with NFT. They show cross-reactivity with several proteins. We have published data showing two different HeLa cell and normal brain staining profiles of antibodies from two different cell lines from two different patients that react with NFT (14). They have been cloned and so have different antigenic determinants. This suggests that there is more than one epitope being recognized by these anti-NFT antibodies.

Without discussing further at this time the specificities of these anti-NFT antibodies, the question may be asked whether the higher percentage in the AD group

Table 2 Antibodies Reactive with Neurofibrillary Tangles (NFT) in Situ

Patients (N)	NFT-reactive antibodies/ No. cell lines screened (mean %)
Alzheimer's disease (6)	35/1751 (2.4% ± 1.3%)*
Age-matched controls (6)	12/1288 (0.8% ± 0.7%)*
Gerstmann-Straussler-Scheinker syndrome (1)	8/639 (1.3%)
Poststroke (2)	2/382 (0.5%)
Multiple sclerosis (1)	5/604 (0.8%)

*The control values are significant at $p < 0.02$ when compared with AD.

Table 3 Antibodies Reactive with HeLa Cells

Patients (N)	HeLa cell reactive antibodies/ No. cell lines screened (mean %)
Alzheimer's disease (7)	149/866 (16.8% ± 5.5%)
Age-matched controls (7)	75/597 (12.2% ± 4.6%)

$p > 0.05$

is reflective of enhanced autoimmunity in the AD group. If this is indeed the case, one would see an elevated number of autoantibodies to the traditional cellular components to which autoantibodies react. We have used two approaches. One is the staining of HeLa cells; this study suggests that more cell lines from the AD group secrete autoantibodies. However, this difference is not statistically significant. The other is the enzyme-linked immunosorbent assay (ELISA), using several cytoskeletal proteins; we do not see any overall difference in the percentages of autoreactivity.

Table 3 summarizes the data on HeLa cells. We find that 16.8% of the AD cell lines secrete antibodies reactive with HeLa cells, whereas 12.2% do from the age-matched controls. At the 0.05 level, this difference is not significant.

Table 4 is a summary of our ELISAs for which we have assayed for reactivity to tubulin, microtubule-associated proteins including MAP2 and tau, to keratin, myosin, and actin. These proteins were used because many autoantibodies are reactive to many of these proteins. Many of our antibodies show cross-reactivity. There are not differences between the two groups. If we look at the number of antibodies that are reactive to only one antigen and are possibly specific, again we find about the same percentage in the two groups reactive to only one antigen,

Table 4 Percentages of Cell Line Antibodies Reactive to Cytoskeletal Proteins

Group (N tested)	Reactive to one or more of antigens tested		Reactive to only one antigen	
	$A_{405}>3$	$A_{405}>10$	$A_{405}>3$	$A_{405}>10$
AD (515)	5.4%	3.1%	2.8%	1.6%
Controls (432)	5.1%	3.9%	3.5%	1.7%

Table 5 Antibodies Not Reactive With Cultured Cell Lines or in the ELISA but Reactive With AD Brain Temporal Cortex Only and/or Normal Brain Temporal Cortex

Patient/Code	AD brain only		AD and/or Normal Brain	
AD/KKN	3/538	(0.6%)	7/538	(1.3%)
GSS/LDI	4/639	(0.6%)	6/639	(0.9%)
Control/CAN	1/67	(1.5%)	1/67	(1.5%)
Stroke/BLO	2/110	(1.8%)	3/110	(2.7%)
Stroke/JOG	3/142	(2.1%)	4/142	(2.8%)
AD/Others	0/308		0/308	
Control/Others	0/415		0/415	

ELISA = Enzyme-linked immunosorbent assay.
GSS = Gerstmann-Straussler-Scheinker syndrome.
Other abbreviations = Patient codes.

although the actual antigens that they are reactive to are different in the two groups.

Thus, our data indicate that there is no evidence for an increased percentage of B-cells which secrete autoreactive antibodies in our assay systems. The percentage increase in anti-NFT antibodies reactive in situ in AD appears to be significant.

In certin AD, GSS, age-matched controls, and poststroke patients, a considerable number of cell lines secrete antibodies specific for AD brain or neuronal tissue. This observation has the implication that the immune response precedes the clinical ramifications of AD.

Table 5 is a summary of the specific antibodies that we have found. These antibodies are not reactive with cultured cell lines including HeLa cells, human fibroblasts, and human neuroblastoma cell lines, and they are not reactive in the ELISA with several cytoskeletal proteins. We have three antibodies from a patient with AD that are reactive only on AD brain (14,15) and an additional four that react just with brain, making a total of seven antibodies that are reactive. With the GSS patient, we found about the same percentage as with the AD patient. We also have an antibody from a control, a 65-year-old female with no history of senility, which was specific for AD brain (15,16). In addition, we have found brain- and AD-specific antibodies from two stroke patients (18).

The staining patterns of these neural-specific antibodies are diverse. The AD brain-specific antibodies stain primarily NFT, plaque neurites, neuritic processes, astrocytes, and/or filaments. The brain-specific antibodies react with astrocytes, nuclei, and/or filaments.

Thus far, we have screened approximately 2,200 cell lines and found 13 secreting antibodies reactive only with AD brain and eight reactive with epitopes shared between AD and normal brains. This is not a large number of antibodies. However, we do not expect to have a lot of antibodies which are highly specific; otherwise, these antibodies would have been identified previously by screening patients' sera. Our studies do show that, with considerable effort, one can identify specific antibodies. These data corroborate the results when AD and normal sera are studied as outlined above.

II. CONCLUSION

Our studies and those of others suggest that there are circulating antibodies which are specific for antigens in AD brain. We have shown that there are more B-cell lines reactive with NFT in situ in the AD group. We have AD brain-specific antibodies from cell lines from both AD and non-AD patients and normals without clinical symptoms of AD. This latter finding is significant with the one possible implication that AD is caused by an environmental agent to which a large population is exposed and that the disease manifests itself later as the population ages. Whether this agent is transmissible is beyond the scope of this chapter.

Accumulating evidence indicates that there is an immune response to an unidentified antigen(s) in AD brain. We do not have evidence to suggest that this represents an immune defect. The identification of the inciting antigen would add credence to our hypothesis and yield important information on the pathogenesis of AD.

REFERENCES

1. Nandy K. Brain-reactive antibodies in aging and senile dementia. In Katzman R, Terry RD, Bick KL (eds): *Alzheimer's Disease: Senile Dementia and Related Disorders (Aging)*, Vol. 7. Raven Press, New York, 1978, pp. 503–514.
2. Nandy K, Nandy LK. Immunological and autoimmune phenomena in senile brain disease. In Scheibel AB (ed). *The Biological Substrates in Alzheimer's Disease*. Academic Press, New York, 1986, pp. 167–176.
3. Watts H, Kennedy PGE, Thomas M. The significance of anti-neuronal antibodies in Alzheimer's Disease. J Neuroimmunol 1:107–116, 1981.
4. Watts HF. Investigations into an immunological component in Alzheimer's Disease. Interdiscipl Topics Gerontol 19:54–61, 1985.
5. Fillit H, Luine VN, Reisberg B, et al. Studies of the specificity of antibrain antibodies in Alzheimer's Disease. In Hutton JT, Kenny AD (eds): *Senile Dementia of the Alzheimer Type*. Alan R. Liss Inc, New York, 1985, pp. 307–318.
6. Fillit HM, Kemeny E, Luine V, et al. Antivascular antibodies in the sera of patients with senile dementia of the Alzheimer's type. J Gerontol 42:180–184, 1987.
7. D'Angelo C, D'Angelo GB. Autoantibodies similar to neurofilament antibodies, di-

rected against tangles and senile plaques are present in patients with presenile and senile dementia or with Down's Syndrome. EOS Riv Immunol 6:8-12, 1986.
8. Singh VK, Fudenberg HH. Detection of brain autoantibodies in the serum of patients with Alzheimer's Disease but not Down's Syndrome. Immunol Lett 12:277-280, 1986.
9. Sugiura M, Yokoi Y, Maruyama S, et al. Detection of anti-cerebral autoantibodies in schizophrenia and Alzheimer's disease. J Clin Lab Immunol 28:1-3, 1989.
10. McRae-Degueurce A, Booj S, Haglid K, et al. Antibodies in cerebrospinal fluid of some Alzheimer disease patients recognize cholinergic neurons in the rat central nervous system. Proc Natl Acad Sci USA 84:9214-9218, 1987.
11. Chapman J, Bachar O, Korczyn AD, et al. Antibodies to cholinergic neurons in Alzheimer's disease. J Neurochem 51:479-485, 1988.
12. Chapman J, Bachar O, Korczyn AD, et al. Alzheimer's Disease antibodies bind specifically to a neurofilament protein in torpedo cholinergic neurons. J Neurosci 9:2710-2717, 1989.
13. Tanaka J, Murakoshi K, Takeda M, et al. A high level of anti-GFAP autoantibody in the serum of patients with Alzheimer's Disease. Biomed Res 9:209-216, 1988.
14. Gaskin F, Kingsley BS, Fu SM. Autoantibodies to neurofibrillary tangles and brain tissue in Alzheimer's Disease. The establishment of Epstein-Barr virus-transformed antibody-producing cell lines. J Exp Med 165:245-250, 1987.
15. Gaskin F, Kingsley BS, Fu SM. Autoantibodies to neurofibrillary tangles and brain tissue in Alzheimer's Disease and Aging. In Davies P, Finch CE (eds): *Banbury Report 27: Molecular neuropathology of Aging*. Cold Spring Harbor Laboratory, New York, 1987, pp. 321-334.
16. Kingsley BS, Gaskin F, Fu SM. Human antibodies to neurofibrillary tangles and astrocytes in Alzheimer's disease. J Neuroimmunol 19:89-99, 1988.
17. Gaskin F, Hart MA. Antibodies to cytoskeletal proteins in Alzheimer's disease. J Cell Biol 107:368a, 1988.
18. Gaskin F, Farlow MR, Fu SM. Human antibodies preferentially reactive with brain or with temporal cortex in Alzheimer's Disease. Soc for Neurosci Abs 15:330, 1989.

11

Immune-Related Mechanisms of Alzheimer's Disease Pathogenesis

Joseph Rogers, W. Harold Civin, and Scot D. Styren
Institute for Biogerontology Research, Sun City, Arizona
Patrick L. McGeer
University of British Columbia, Vancouver, British Columbia, Canada

I. INTRODUCTION

The central nervous system was long believed to be immunologically privileged. Although this may be the case for young, normal adult animals, research over the last decade has shown that it is definitely not true for older patients with Alzheimer's disease (AD) (1-11). This chapter reviews data from our laboratories and others demonstrating that with few exceptions all the elements of chronic inflammation are present in AD brain tissue, and that they co-localize with the classic hallmarks of AD pathology.

II. OVERVIEW OF THE IMMUNE RESPONSE AND INFLAMMATION

A simplified overview of the immune response and inflammation might begin with scavenger cells, which phagocytize infected or damaged cells and the detritus of inflammatory responses. If the scavenger cells bear major histocompatibility complex (MHC) type II antigens on their surface, they can present processed fragments of their phagocytic activity, antigens, to T- and B-lymphocytes. T-helper lumphocytes are activated by such presentation and express cytokines which activate other immune cells, particularly B-cells that have also been presented with antigen. The B-cells proliferate and produce antibodies (Ig) specifically directed against the original antigenic stimulus. Ig then binds to antigen in the tissue. Scavenger cells are redirected to sites of Ig binding by means of receptors to an epitope on the Fc region of Ig. Classical pathway complement proteins also begin to attach to the antigen-antibody complex, beginning with Clq at an Fc site on Ig. The other complement proteins follow, culminating with the membrane attack complex (C5–C9), which inserts pores in the cell wall. Cell lysis and phagocytic activity follow, with additional attraction of scavenger cells by means of binding sites on C3 and C5 (12,13).

III. IMMUNOLOGIC PARALLELS IN AD PATHOGENESIS

With few exceptions, recent data suggest that most of the basic processes of the immune response and inflammation can be observed in the AD brain. These parallels are considered below using the same simplified outline of immune mechanisms given in the overview.

A. Scavenger Cells Phagocytize the Products of Pathology

Gray matter is the site of the classic elements of AD pathology: neuron loss, neurofibrillary tangle accumulation, and senile or neuritic plaque formation (14). Similarly, gray matter of AD brain tissue is characterized by increased numbers and reactivity of glia, namely, astrocytes (15,16) and microglia (2–4,6–10). Although there is controversy about the phagocytic capabilities of astrocytes, there is little with regard to microglia. Both cell types co-localize particularly well with senile plaques—astrocytes more toward the plaque rim, and microglia more toward the plaque core (4). Microglia are close cousins to (if not transformed examples of) macrophages, the prototypical scavenger cells of the body (12,13). Thus, it is not surprising that electron microscopy clearly shows microglia within plaques to contain B-amyloid fibrils and other neuropil debris (5,17–19) (Fig. 1).

B. Scavenger Cells Process and Present Antigen

In addition to scavenging activities, microglia may also be involved in antigen presentation. In AD, microglia, particularly those that co-localize with AD pathology (Fig. 2), are immunoreactive for HLA-DR (2–4,6,10), HLA-DP (2), and HLA-DQ (2). White matter microglic but not gray matter microglia are HLA-DR positive in nondemented (ND) elderly patients. Consistent with this, Western blot analyses suggest highly elevated levels of HLA-DR in AD gray matter compared to ND gray matter (4) (Fig. 3).

HLA-DR, HLA-DP, and HLA-DQ are the human MHC type II antigens that confer antigen-presenting capabilities (12,13). Peripheral cells with these capa-

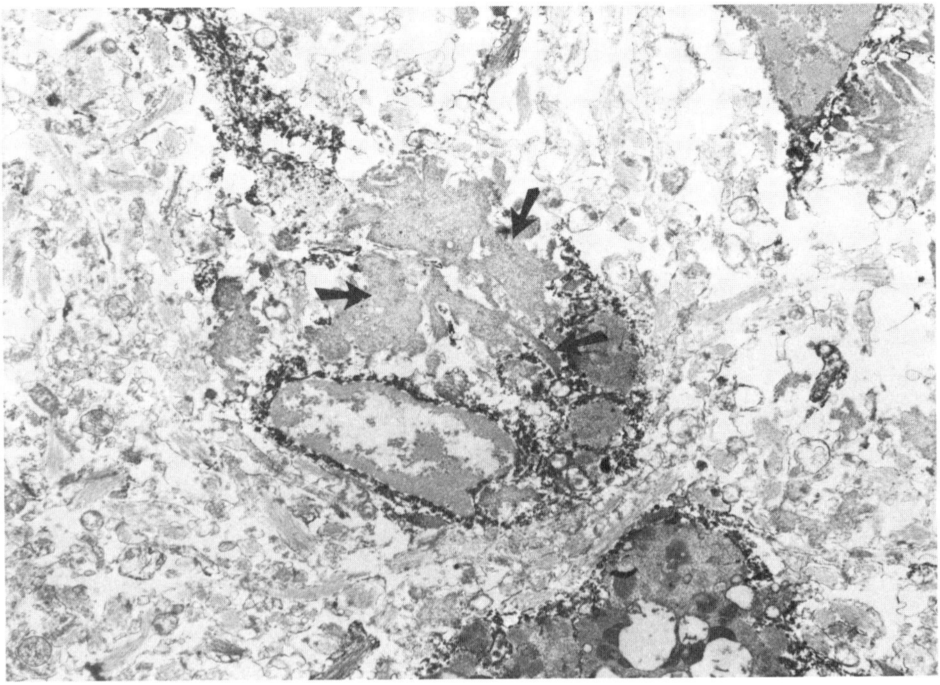

Figure 1 Electron micrograph of a representative microglial cell in AD brain. Note the highly reactive appearance, much more typical of AD than ND brain. Arrows denote fibrillar material with the ultrastructural properties of B-amyloid in the microglial cytoplasm. (X7,000; HLA-DR immunoelectron microscopy.)

bilities, such as macrophages, phagocytize target tissues and then process the debris. Processed fragments associate with MHC II and are transported to the cell surface for presentation (12,13). As mentioned above, ultrastructural studies of AD brain samples show that microglia contain presumably phagocytized cellular detritus, including B-amyloid fibrils (4,17–19). Since they also express MHC II markers on their surfaces, conventional immunology theory (12,13) strongly suggests that the products of microglial processing can become antigenic stimuli. Indeed, they may be especially good antigens given that the nervous system contains unique proteins which the immune system may never have encountered previously.

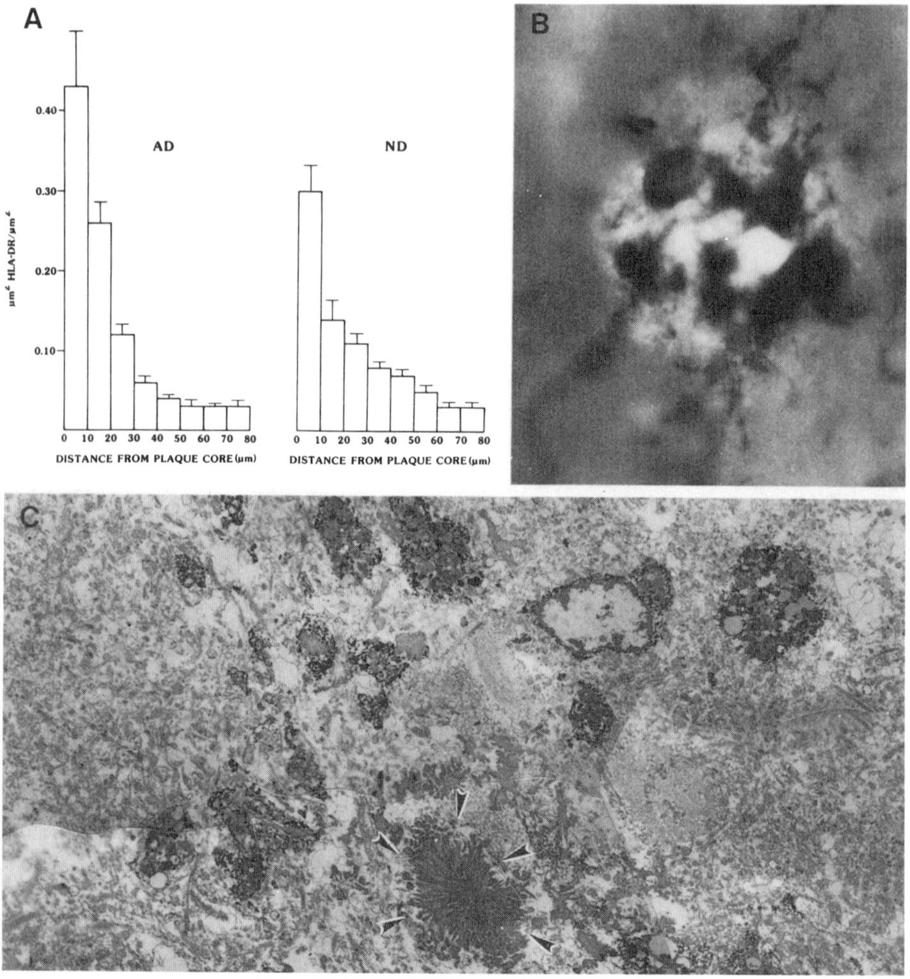

Figure 2 (A) A real density of HLA-DR immunoreactivity at progressive 10-μm diameter distances from the plaque core or approximate plaque center in AD and ND gray matter. (B) This HLA-DR immunoreactivity is carried by clusters of microglia that co-localize with thioflavin-positive amyloid deposits (X400) (HLA-DR immunoreactivity/thioflavin counterstain in dim bright field and fluorescence). (C) Co-localization with B-amyloid deposits (arrowheads) can be seen to particular advantage in electron micrograph montages of plaques with HLA-DR immunoreactivity. Profiles labeled by black DAB reaction product have ultrastructural characteristics of microglia and their processes. Note typical absence of HLA-DR immunoreactivity on astrocytic processes that permeate the plaque from cell bodies on the plaque rim. (From Reference 4.)

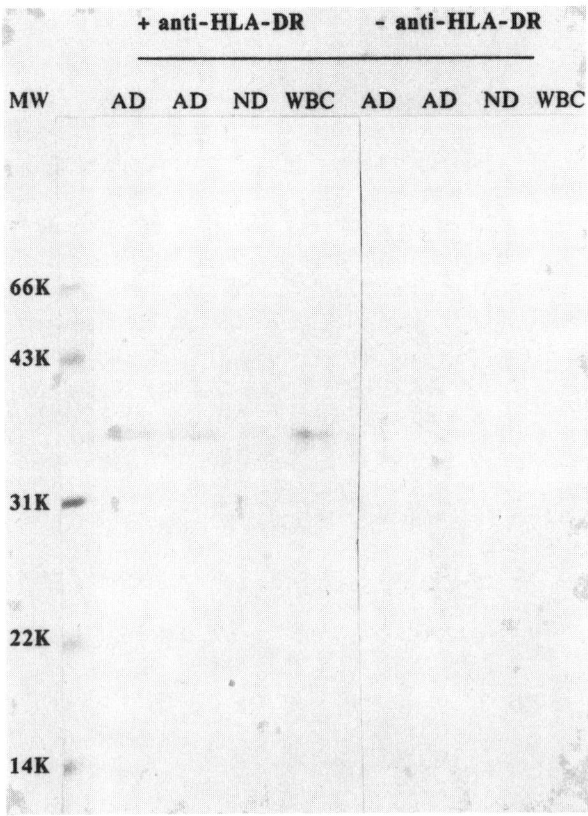

Figure 3 Typical Western blot for HLA-DR comparing AD and ND gray matter samples, as well as peripheral white blood cells (WBC). Note that a single band running at the appropriate molecular weight for HLA-DR is detected in both brain and peripheral blood (left panel). It is unlikely, therefore, that the immunoreactivity detected on microglia in immunohistochemical experiments is due to cross-reactivity, since the cross-reactive antigen would show up as a second band in the Western blots. Control lanes based on deletion of primary antibody (right panel) or use of a nonspecific mouse serum are uniformly negative. (From Reference 4.)

C. T-Lymphocytes Are Present and Are Activated by Antigen Presentation

Through appropriate receptors, T-lymphocytes recognize antigens presented to them by other cells in the context of MHC restriction (12,13). The T-helper subset, characterized by its CD4 marker, then assists in the activation of appropriate B-lymphocytes using cytokine and other mechanisms (12,13). $CD4^+$ T-lymphocytes have been observed in AD and ND cortical neuropil by our laboratories (2,3,6), consistent with previous neuroscience reports on T-cells generally (20). These cells can be found both within and outside clearly patent blood vessels (3,5,6,20) (Fig. 4). $CD8^+$ T-lymphocytes, which serve to damp the immune response, are also present in AD brain (3,6). Instances of physical apposition, necessary for antigen presentation, have been observed in AD cortex between cells with the ultrastructural characteristics of lymphocytes and HLA-DR positive cells (i.e.,

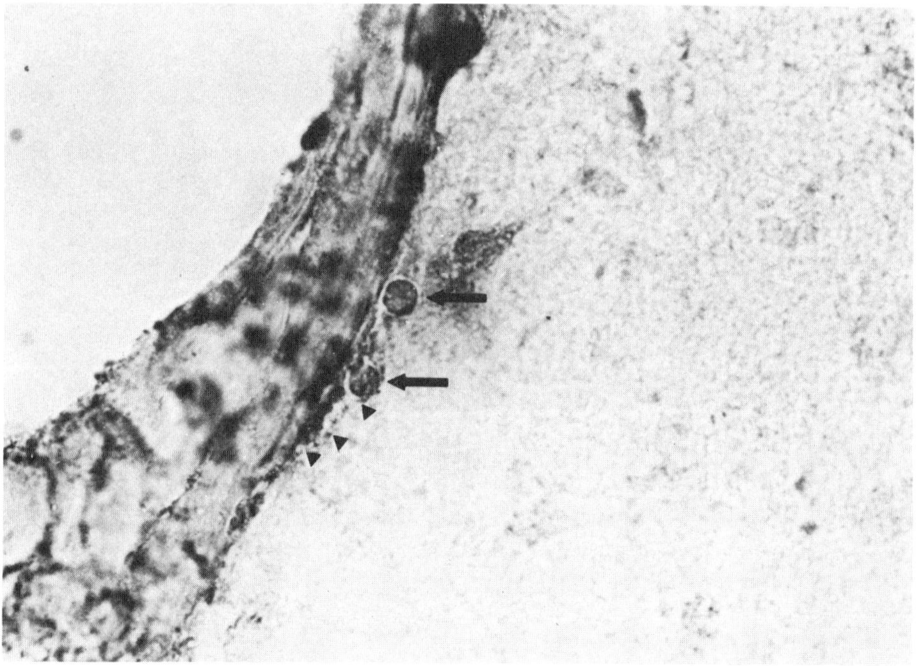

Figure 4 Two putative lymphocytes within the cortical neuropil outside an apparently patent blood vessel. These cells exhibit the small size, round shape, lack of processes, and CD4 cell surface immunoreactivity characteristic of the T helper lymphocyte subset. A hint of basement membrane through which one of the lymphocytes may be emerging is suggested at close inspection (arrowheads). (X1,000.) (From Reference 3).

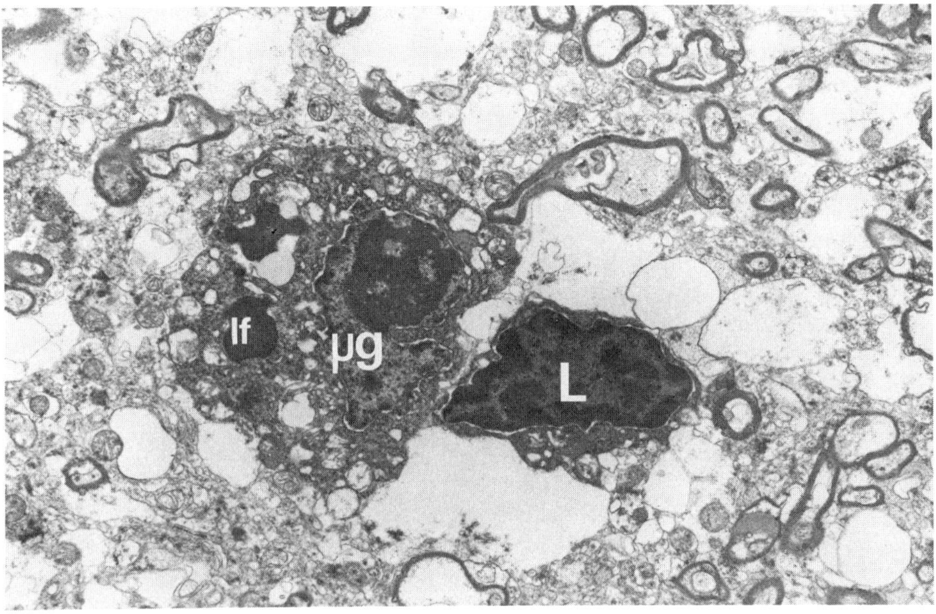

Figure 5 Electron micrograph from AD gray matter showing a cell with the ultrastructural characteristics of microglia (μg) in apposition to a cell with the ultrastructural characteristics of the T or, possibly, B lymphocyte (L). Such apposition occurs in the course of antigen presentation but does not necessarily prove that antigen presentation has occurred. lg - lipofuscin granules, large quantities of which are present in reactive microglia (X15,000). (From Reference 3).

antigen-presenting cells) with the ultrastructural characteristics of microglia (3) (Fig. 5). Thus, to summarize so far, in the AD brain, scavenger cells co-localize with AD pathology. They contain the detritus of AD pathology. They bear the requisite markers for antigen presentation. Antigen-accepting cells, T-cells, are present and can sometimes be observed in apposition to the antigen-presenting cells.

D. B-Lymphocytes Are Present

Antigen presentation may ultimately lead to activation and proliferation of those B-lymphocytes making antibody to the particular antigen (12,13). Using an antibody developed to label peripheral B-lymphocytes (21), we have recently demonstrated that cells with the antigenic and morphologic properties of B-lymphocytes can also be labeled in AD and ND brain (5). Although the possibility exists that these cells (and T-cells as well) are present in the neuropil as an artifact of sectioning, much data now exist to suggest that they infiltrate the brain through the vasculature (20). For example, at the light level cells with the antigenic and morphologic characteristics of T- or B-lymphocytes can be visualized outside clearly patent blood vessels (3,5,6,20), and our light level and ultrastructural studies provide instances in which lymphocytes appear to be squeezing through the vascular wall (Rogers and Styren, unpublished data), much as they do in the periphery.

E. Activated Immune Cells Express Cytokines

Cytokines are the intercellular messengers of the immune response and inflammation. They are secreted by several cell types with the general end of signaling proliferation, activation, and further inflammation (12,13). One important cytokine-dependent mechanism, for example, is the production of cytokines by T-helper lymphocytes which have received antigen from scavenger cells. Among other things, these cytokines induce clonal proliferation of B-lymphocytes that have also been stimulated by antigen presentation (12,13).

Griffin and colleagues (22) have reported that levels of the cytokine IL-1β are elevated in AD brain; preliminary results from studies we are currently pursuing suggest that IL-1α, IL-6, and TNF may be elevated as well (23) (Fig. 6). These three cytokines, particularly tumor necrosis factor (TNF) (24), are often associated with vascular damage, and may help account for reports of microvessel abnormalities in AD brain (25,26) as well as our recent finding of vascular epidermal growth factor receptor (EGFR) expression in demented but not nondemented patients (27) (Fig. 7).

Although studies on cytokine receptors in AD brain have so far been limited, we (2,10) have shown that IL-2 receptors are present on gray and white matter microglia of AD cortex, but only white matter microglia of ND cortex. This may likely account for the more reactive appearance of microglia in AD gray matter (3,4).

F. Antibody (Ig) Is Produced

Activated, clonally proliferating B-lymphocytes produce antibodies to antigens processed and presented by scavenger cells (12,13). Such antibodies constitute the most important missing element in a full characterization of neuroimmune mechanisms in AD. Several studies have reported detecting brain-reactive antibodies in AD serum samples 91), as well as antibodies, presumably from the patient and bound before the patient's death, co-localized with AD pathology (28,29). These studies, however, are technically very difficult, and conflicting reports exist (30,31).

One possible source of difficulty in detecting AD-specific antibodies is com-

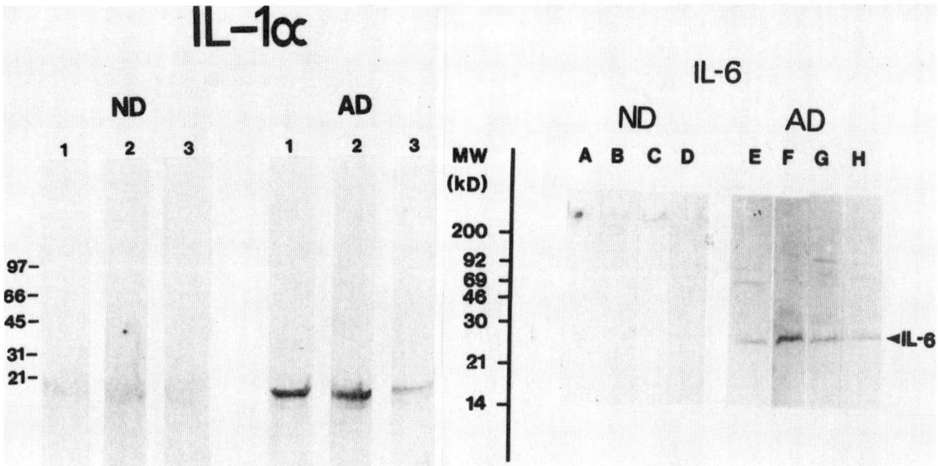

Figure 6 Western blots for IL1-α and IL-6 in AD and ND brain samples. This cytokine elevation has proven difficult to confirm in additional patients. We believe this is because concentrations of the cytokines may be just at the threshold of sensitivity for colorimetric detection. More sensitive autoradiographic methods have now been applied, and the results are in preparation. (Collaborative research with I. Lieberberg, Athena Neurosciences).

plement. C1q binds to the Fc region of Ig in the antibody-antigen complex. The remaining complement proteins then bind sequentially (12,13) and may render critical epitopes on the Ig molecule inaccessible to anti-Ig antibodies. Moreover, binding affinities within the antigen-antibody-C1 complex are relatively weak, so that specific Ig binding might not survive the rigors of autolysis and tissue preparation. Sternberger (personal communication) has also pointed that during autolysis serum may leak from capillaries, especially in the aged brain. Thus, it is difficult to detect antibodies in AD brain, and even if one does so successfully, it is difficult to be sure the result is not an artifact.

Studies by Gaskin (29), based on antibodies from B-lumphocytes cloned from AD and ND patients, may provide some resolution to the problem of Ig detection. However, this work is obviously very difficult and will require much time and effort for successful completion.

G. Complement Binds to Ig Mediating Inflammation

Complement is a group of some 20 proteins that bind together in sequential steps through serine protease type reactions. In the classic immune response, C1q binds to Ig followed by C1r and C1s, C4, C2, C3, and C5–C9. The latter are referred to as the membrane attack complex because they attach not only to the growing cas-

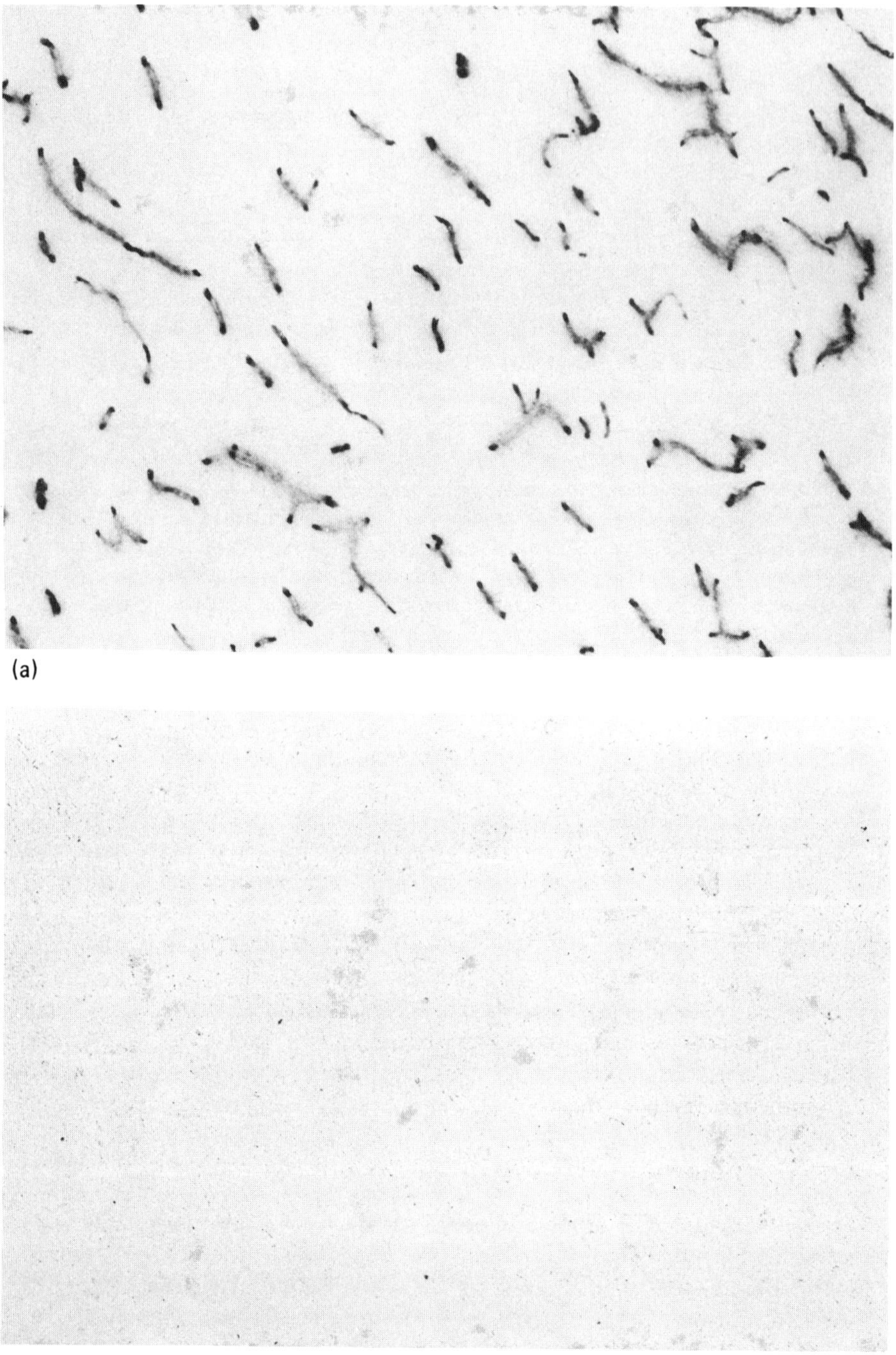

(a)

(b)

Figure 7

cade of complement proteins but also to the cell wall itself. There, a lytic plug is inserted. Reactive lysis of nearby autologous tissue may occur, in addition, by the release of C5b6 and its binding by other members of the membrane attack complex. Although complement can be an initiating point, independent of Ig, for generating an immune response (see below), more commonly it is the final common pathway for inflammation (12,13). For this reason, the finding that complement activation occurs in AD brain (6,11) has considerable importance, for it presupposes and helps explain many of the other immune-related phenomena that have been described above.

When antibodies to complement proteins, including C1q, C4d, C3d, and C5b-9, are applied to nondemented elderly (ND) brain tissue, the sections are typically blank. When they are applied to AD samples, however, intense immunoreactivity is observed in senile plaques, neurofibrillary tangles, and some neurons or dystrophic neurites (Fig. 8). Presence of the membrane attack complex (C5–C9) (6) indicates that the target has been or is about to be lysed (12,13). These data therefore suggest that the loss of neurons (32) and the appearance of plaques and tangles (33) in AD may in part be mediated by immune mechanisms.

H. Antibody Independent Complement Activation

Antibody-dependent mechanisms are not the only means by which complement activation can occur (12,13); and in some rarer cases it has been demonstrated that complement may be activated without prior induction and binding of specific Ig (12,13). The alternative complement pathway, for example, can be initiated by binding of C3b to various substrates in the absence of Ig. However, it seems unlikely that the alternative pathway contributes significantly to inflammation in AD brain, because the classical pathway initiator C1q is so abundantly present in

---

Figure 7 Immunoreactivity for a monoclonal antibody directed against an epitope on epidermal growth factor receptor (EGFR). (A) In AD brain, vascular endothelial cell immunoreactivity is profuse. (B) In ND brain, immunoreactivity is not detectable. In a series of well over 60 cases, EGFR immunoreactivity has proven to be a universal marker for organic dementia. However, it does not discriminate among the organic dementias (e.g., brain tissues from non-AD Parkinson's dementia, Pick's disease, and AD patients stain equally well). Of some 40 clinically nondemented patients, only two have ever shown a positive EGFR response: one of the latter had advanced CNS carcinoma and the other had sufficient AD pathology to otherwise warrant the diagnosis of AD. Among many other phenomena in which EGFR has been implicated, EGFR upregulation is known to occur at sites of vascular regeneration and repair and is stimulated by tumor necrosis factor (TNF). (From reference 27).

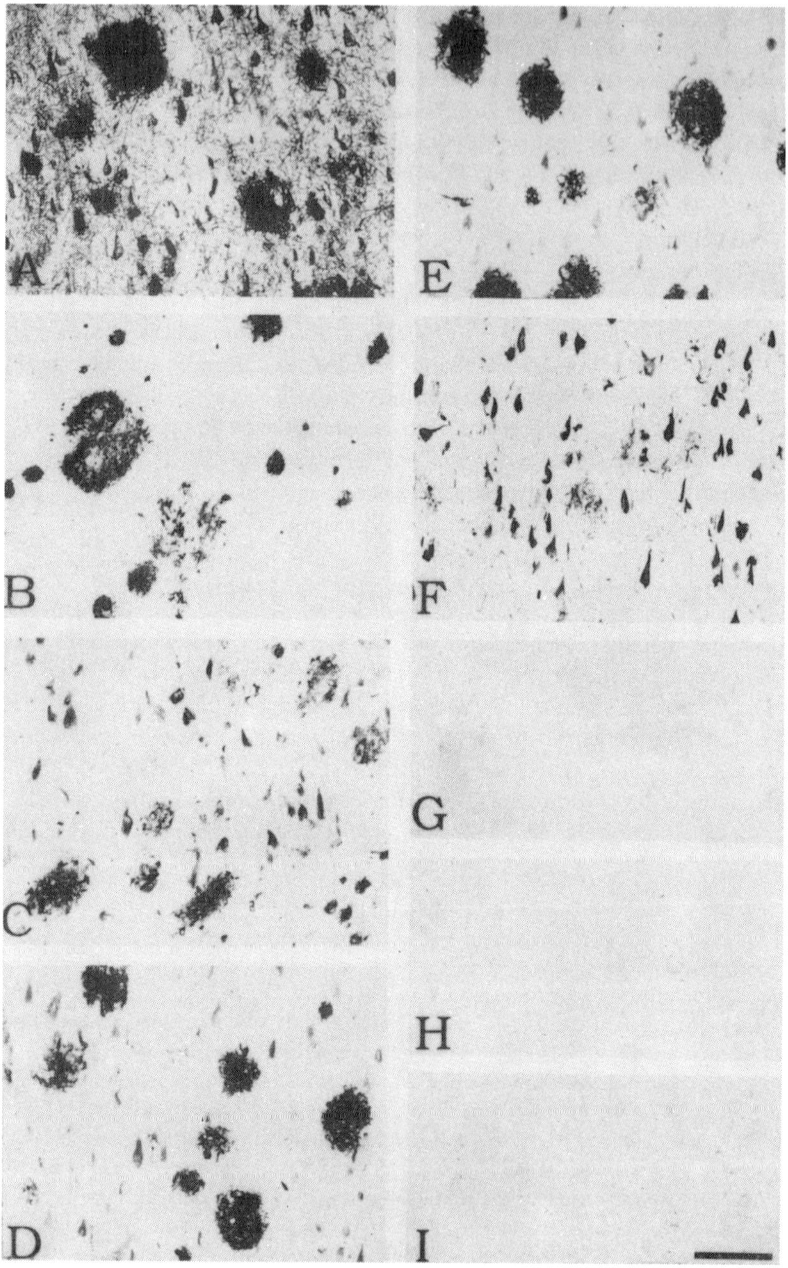

Figure 8

AD and because the alternative pathway elements factor P and the Bb fraction of factor B are not detectable (6).

A second pathway for Ig-independent complement activation follows from the highly cationic charge of C1q, leading to electrostatic binding to a variety of substrates. This process is normally held in check by various endogenous inhibitors of complement activation, such as C1 inhibitor. In patients with cogenital deficiencies of these inhibitors, Ig-independent complement activation occurs and immune-associated pathology ensues (12,13). Given the difficulty in identifying specific Ig in AD, we should continue to entertain the possibility that complement activation co-localized with AD pathology may be an antibody independent event. The β-amyloid region of APP is believed to be highly anionic, so that an intriguing possible target for electrostatic binding of the highly cationic C1q molecule is β-amyloid itself.

I. Phagocytic Chemotaxis to Complement Dependent Lesion Sites

The immune response and inflammation come full circle with the additional recruitment of scavenger cells to the antigen-antibody-complement complex site. As we have seen, these sites are highly co-localized with AD pathology. In the periphery, macrophages are guided to such sites by three principal means: receptors to C3, receptors to C5, and receptors to the Fc chain of Ig (12,13). In AD (and to a lesser extent ND) brain tissue, microglia are found to bear the complement receptors CR3 and CR4 (B-2 integrins) (34) as well as Fc receptors (6). Taken together, these data therefore provide an explanation for the co-localization of re-

---

Figure 8 Immunoreactivity for antibodies directed against classical pathway complement proteins in AD. (A) Typical Bielschowsky silver staining in AD hippocampus. (B) An adjacent section processed for β-amyloid immunoreactivity. As will be seen in the following adjacent sections, complement immunoreactivity is highly co-localized with sites of AD pathology, particularly those that feature concentrated B-amyloid deposits. (C) An adjacent section processed for Clq. (D) An adjacent section processed for C3d. (E) An adjacent section stained with C4d antibody. (F) Staining of an adjacent section with C5b-9 antibody. In contrast to C1q-C4d, which are most closely associated with β-amyloid deposits, the membrane attack complex (C5b-9) is associated with membranous targets such as dystrophic neurites within plaques. Some tangles and swollen neurites not associated with plaques are also stained. (G) Adjacent section showing negative staining for C5b-9 antibody after preabsorption with human serum containing high levels of C5b-9. (H) Adjacent section showing negative staining with a monoclonal antibody directed against the Bb fragment of factor B (a marker for the alternative complement pathway). (I) Absence of staining with a monoclonal antibody to properdin in an adjacent section. All staining was negative in ND tissue. (Calibration bar = 100 μm). (From reference 36.)

active microglia with senile plaques: a chemotactic response to complement. Once drawn to the plaque, the microglia are in position to scavenge the products of complement-dependent lysis, process potential antigens, and reinitiate yet another cycle of the immune response.

It should be noted that independent of an immune response (i.e., in the absence of specific Ig) scavenger cell chemotaxis to complement activation can in and of itself initiate an immune response (rather than simply recycle an existing immune response). For example, antibody-independent complement activation occurs in patients with deficiencies of complement-inhibiting factors. Scavenger cells move in to ingest, process, and present the detritus of this complement-mediated inflammation. Immune responses to autologous tissues are thereby often generated in these patients secondary to antibody-independent complement mechanisms (12,13).

IV. SIGNIFICANCE OF IMMUNE RELATED PHENOMENA TO AD PATHOGENESIS

The immune response and inflammation are vital elements in the body's defense schemes. They protect us from infectious agents and help cleanse regions of tissue damage. The nervous system, however, may be a singularly unreceptive organ for such benefits. Whereas the removal of infected or weakened cells within and around a skin laceration may be a most helpful product of inflammatory mechanisms, it might not be so in brain. New skin cells are always available to replace those lost in the inflammatory attack, but neurons are postmitotic. Thus, an important question is whether immune mechanisms in AD merely reflect natural processes to help heal the brain damage of AD or whether these immune mechanisms may actually be a pathogenetic source of damage.

The only certain way to assess the pathogenetic significance of immune-related phenomena in AD is to treat patients with appropriate immune-related drugs such as anti-inflammatory agents. As a conservative step in this direction, we have conducted a preliminary retrospective study in which computer records of over a million patients in general hospitals, arthritis clinics, and AD clinics were screened (35). The results covered in detail in Chapter 12, suggest that chronic anti-inflammatory therapy in patients over 65 years of age may lessen or postpone the expression of AD symptomology. Although these data have all the caveats of any retrospective study and can only be regarded as preliminary, they do provide a rationale for further clinical research.

V. FUTURE DIRECTIONS

Presently, there is no therapy or therapeutic agent with proven efficacy for AD. The patients are doomed to an implacable decline in mental status lasting, on the average, 8–9 years. The families of patients will suffer as much or more, though in other ways.

Although there are many unanswered basic research questions concerning neuroimmune mechanisms in AD, to one acquainted with the human impact of this terrible disorder the questions sometimes begin to appear more and more esoteric. Our laboratories have found (2–11,15,23,27,34–35; see also chapter 12) and will doubtless continue to find additional peripheral markers of immune function in AD brain—certainly many more than have been covered in this brief review. But, given that we now have substantial, widely replicated evidence of inflammation in AD brain, the question can no longer be whether immune mechanisms exist there. Rather, we must begin to ask, through clinical trials, what significance they have.

ACKNOWLEDGMENTS

This work was supported by NIA AGO 7367 to J.R., a grant from the American Health Assistance Foundation to P.L.M., and a grant from the Arizona Disease Control Research Commission to W.H.C. Gisele Styren, Margaret Chesinski, Frenchelle Martin, Susan Allen, Ivan Lieberberg, Dora Games, and Scott Webster provided significant technical and/or critical assistance.

REFERENCES

1. Lal H, Forster MJ. Autoimmunity and age-associated cognitive decline. Neurobiol Aging 9:733–743, 1988.
2. Luber-Narod J, Rogers J. Immune system associated antigens expressed by cells of the human central nervous system. Neurosci Lett 94:17–22, 1988.
3. Rogers J, Luber-Narod J, Styren S, et al. Expression of immune system-associated antigens by cells of the human central nervous system: relationship to the pathology of Alzheimer's disease. Neurobiol Aging 9:339–349, 1988.
4. Styren SD, Civin WH, Rogers J. Molecular, cellular and pathologic characterization of HLA-DR immunoreactivity in normal elderly and Alzheimer's disease brain. Exp Neurol 110:93–105, 1990.
5. Styren SD, Moon G, Eng L, et al. Immunoreactivity for LN-1 a B-lymphocyte marker in Alzheimer's disease and nondemented elderly brain. Neurobiol Aging 1990 (in submission).
6. McGeer PL, Akiyama H, Itagaki S, et al. Immune system response in Alzheimer's disease. Can J Neurol Sci 16:516–527, 1989.
7. McGeer PL, Itagaki S, Tago H, et al. Reactive microglia in patients with senile dementia of the Alzheimer type are positive for the histocompatibility glycoprotein HLA-DR. Neurosci Lett 79:195–200, 1987.
8. McGeer PL, Itagaki S, Boyes BE, et al. Reactive microglia are positive for HLA-DR in the substantia nigra of Parkinson's and Alzheimer's disease brains. Neurology 20: 1285–1291, 1988.

9. McGeer PL, Itagaki S, McGeer EG. Expression of the histocompatibility glycoprotein HLA-DR in neurological disease. Acta Neuropathol 76:550–557, 1988.
10. Itagaki S, McGeer PL, Akiyama H, et al. Relationship of microglia and astrocytes to amyloid deposits of Alzheimer's disease. J Neuroimmunol 24:173–182, 1989.
11. Yamada T, Akiyama H, McGeer PL. Complement-activated oligodendroglia: A new pathogenic entity identified by immuno-staining with antibodies to human complement proteins C3d and C4d. Neurosci Lett 112:161–166, 1990.
12. Roitt I, Brostoff J, Male D (eds): *Immunology*, 2nd ed. CV Mosby Co, St Louis, Mo, 1985.
13. Colman RM, Lombard MF, Sicard RE, et al. *Fundamental Immunology*, Wm C Brown Publihsers, Dubuque, Iowa, 1990.
14. Khachaturian Z. Diagnosis of Alzheimer's disease. Arch Neurol 42:1097–1105, 1985.
15. Beach TG, Walker R, McGeer EG. Patterns of gliosis in Alzheimer's disease and aging cerebrum. Glia 2:420–436, 1989.
16. Schechter R, Yen S-H, Terry RD. Fibrous astrocytes in senile dementia of the Alzheimer type. J Neuropathol Exp Neurol 40:95–101, 1980.
17. Moretz RC, Wisniewski HM, Loswsinsky AS. Pathogenesis of neuritic and amyloid plaques in scrapie: ultrastructural study of early changes in the cortical neuropil. In Samuel D (ed): *Aging of the Brain*. Raven Press, New York, 1983, pp. 61–79.
18. Wisniewski HM, Terry RD. Reexamination of the pathogenesis of the senile plaque. In Zimmerman HM (ed): *Progress in Neuropathology*. Vol 2. Grune & Stratton, New York, 1973, pp. 1-26.
19. Wisniewski HM, Vorbrodt AW, Moretz RC, et al. Pathogenesis of neuritic (senile) and amyloid plaque formation. In Hoyer S (ed): *The Aging Brain—Physiological and patho-Physiological Aspects.* Suppl 5, Springer-Verlag, New York, 1982, pp. 3–9.
20. Wekerle H, Linington C, Lassmann H, et al. Cellular immune reactivity within the CNS. Trends Neurosci 9:271–277, 1986.
21. Epstein A, Marder R, Winter J, et al. Two new monoclonal antibodies (LN-1, LN-2) reactive in B5 formalin fixed, paraffin embedded tissues with follicular center and mantle zone human B lymphocytes and derived tumors. J Immunol 133:1028–1036, 1984.
22. Griffin WST, Stanley LC, Ling C, et al. Brain interleukin 1 and S-100 immunoreactivity are elevated in Down Syndrome and Alzheimer disease. Proc Nat Acad Sci USA 86:7611–7615, 1989.
23. Allen SA, Styren SD, Rogers J. Molecular and cellular characterization of cytokines in Alzheimer's disease. Soc for Neurosci Abstr 15:329, 1989.
24. Yoshimura T, Sone S, Ogira T. Membrane perturbation as a possible cytotoxic mechanism of TNF and interferons. In Bonavida B, Granger G (eds): *Tumor Necrosis Factor: Structure Mechanism of Action, Role in Disease Therapy*, S Karger, Basel, Switzerland, 1990, pp 70–76.
25. Hassler O. Vascular changes in senile brains. A Micro-angiographic study. Acta Neuropathol 5:40–53, 1965.
26. Mooradian AD. Effect of aging on the blood-brain barrier. Neurobiol Aging 9:31–39, 1988.

27. Styren SD, Mufson EJ, Styren GC, et al. Epidermal growth factor receptor expression in demented and aged human brain. Brain Res. 347:347-352, 1990.
28. Bahmanyer S, Moreau-Dubois M, Brown P. et al. Serum antibodies to neurofilament antigens in patients with neurological and other diseases and in health controls. J Neuroimmunol 5:191-196, 1983.
29. Gaskin F, Kingsley BS, Fu SM. Autoantibodies to neurofibrillary tangles and brain tissue in Alzheimer's disease. J Exp Med 165:245-250, 1987.
30. Rosemuller JM, Eikelenboom P, Kamphorst W, et al. Lack of evidence for dysfunction of the blood-brain barrier in Alzheimer's disease: An immunohistochemical study. Neurobiol Aging 9:383-391, 1988.
31. Watts H, Kennedy PGE, Thomas M. The significance of antineuronal antibody in Alzheimer's disease. J Neuroimmunol 1:107-116, 1981.
32. Terry RD, Peck A, DeTeresa R. Some morphometric aspects of the brain in senile dementia of the Alzheimer type. Ann Neurol 10:184-192, 1981.
33. Rogers J, Morrison J. Quantitative morphology and regional and laminar distributions of senile plaques in Alzheimer's disease. J Neurosci 5:2801-2808, 1985.
34. Akiyama, H, McGeer PL. Brain microglia constitutively express B-2 integrins. J Neuroimmunol 1990 (in press).
35. McGeer PL, McGeer EG, Rogers J, et al. Anti-inflammatory drugs and Alzheimer's disease. Lancet 335:1037, 1990.
36. McGeer PL, Akiyama H, Itagaki S, McGeer EG. Activation of the classical complement pathway in brain tissue of Alzheimer's patients. Neurosci Lett 107:341-346, 1989.

12

Does Anti-Inflammatory Treatment Protect Against Alzheimer's Disease?

Patrick L. McGeer and Edith G. McGeer
University of British Columbia, Vancouver, British Columbia, Canada
Joseph Rogers
Institute for Biogerontology Research, Sun City, Arizona
John Sibley
University of Saskatechewan, Saskatoon, Canada

Recent immunohistochemical investigations indicate that Alzheimer's disease produces a chronic inflammatory state of the brain. T4 and T8 lymphocytes (1-4), as well as large numbers of reactive microglia which strongly express major histocompatibility complex (MHC) surface glycoproteins (2-5), are found in areas of plaque and tangle pathology. Cell membranes of reactive microglia are densely occupied by complement receptors (4,6). Degenerating elements in affected tissue are stained by antibodies to various complement proteins (4,7,8), including the membrane attack complex. Active cell lysis, as well as opsonization of tissue debris, may therefore be taking place (4,8).

These data imply that anti-inflammatory therapy, taken over long periods of time, might retard the development of Alzheimer's disease. One retrospective means of testing such a hypothesis would be to compare the prevalence of Alzheimer's disease among patients receiving chronic anti-inflammatory medication against the prevalence in the overall population. Patients with rheumatoid arthritis provide a test population, since such patients generally receive anti-inflammatory therapy and many contract their disease between the ages of 35 and 50, well before the age of risk for Alzheimer disease.

I. METHODS AND RESULTS

We explored this question by analyzing data of four types from multiple centers: 1) the prevalence of rheumatoid arthritis in autopsied Alzheimer's cases; 2) the prevalence of Alzheimer's disease in rheumatoid arthritis clinic cases; 3) the prevalence of rheumatoid arthritis among Alzheimer's clinic patients; and 4) the prevalence of coexisting diagnoses of rheumatoid arthritis and Alzheimer's disease in cases at discharge from general hospitals.

We compared these data with published prevalence figures for the two conditions in the general population. The comparisons suggest that Alzheimer's disease is far less likely to develop in the rheumatoid arthritic population than in the general population. Moreover, many of the cases diagnosed as having both diseases had not been receiving anti-inflammatory therapy at the time of onset of Alzheimer's disease.

We first examined the records of 290 postmortem cases of dementia where there was some evidence of plaque and tangle pathology. Only two had an antecedent history of rheumatoid arthritis (Table 1). They were included in a series of 107 consecutive dementia cases (age, 77.06 ± 8.62; average duration of illness, 6.45 ± 2.9 years) that had been referred to the Kinsmen Laboratory of Neurological Research in British Columbia. Both had only mild-to-moderate plaque and tangle pathology and both had choline acetyltransferase (ChAT) levels in the normal range. This meant they were not typical Alzheimer's cases since the average cortical ChAT of the Alzheimer's group was approximately one third that of age-matched normals (0.20 vs. 0.59 μm/h–100 mg protein). Moreover, one of the cases had multi-infarcts causing hippocampal cell loss.

We next reviewed data from rheumatoid arthritis clinics in Saskatchewan and Arizona where patients had been followed with regular examinations over long periods of time and changes in the history had been carefully noted. Of 923 patients over 64 years of age, only four developed clinical signs of Alzheimer's disease, giving a prevalence of 0.43% (Table 1). All four are still living, so there has not been confirmation of the clinical diagnoses.

We then reviewed data from Alzheimer's clinics in British Columbia, Arizona, and Quebec. Of 567 cases diagnosed clinically as Alzheimer's disease, only two had a coexisting diagnosis of rheumatoid arthritis, giving a prevalence of 0.35% (Table 1). One of these cases had developed rheumatoid arthritis concomitantly with Alzheimer's disease, while the other was the atypical autopsy case noted above with a multi-infarct component.

Finally, we reviewed separation statistics of patients over age 64 from general hospitals in British Columbia, Ontario, Alberta, and Arizona for diagnoses of Alzheimer's disease (DS-9 331.0), rheumatoid arthritis (DS-9 714.0), or both (9). Of 7,490 patients with the diagnosis of rheumatoid arthritis, 29 were recorded as having Alzheimer's disease (0.39%). Of 5,756 patients diagnosed as having prob-

Table 1 Patients Over Age 64 with Diagnosis of Rheumatoid Arthritis and Alzheimer's Disease

Source of data	Rheumatoid arthritis	Alzheimer's	Both diseases
Postmortem			
British Columbia	na	107	2
Arizona	na	62	0
Quebec	na	121	0
Total		290	2
Arthritis clinics			
Saskatchewan	818	na	4
Arizona	105	na	0
Total	923		4
Alzheimer's clinics			
British Columbia	na	317	1
Arizona	na	92	1
Quebec	na	158	0
Total		567	2
General hospitals			
British Columbia	2,261	1,960	16
Ontario	3,987	3,073	12
Alberta	375	30	0
Arizona	867	693	1
Total	7,490	5,756	29

able Alzheimer's disease, the same 29 were recorded as having rheumatoid arthritis (0.50%) (Table 1).

Studies of the prevalence of Alzheimer's disease in different areas of the world in the general population over 64 years of age have varied somewhat, but all have recorded prevalence rates that are many-fold higher than has been found for the rheumatoid arthritic population. Evans et al. (10), in their recent East Boston survey, reported a prevalence of probable Alzheimer's disease of 10.3% in the over-65 population. This value is substantially higher than that recorded in several other studies. Sulkava et al. (11) reported a figure of 3.6% for Finland in this age group, Shibayama et al. (12) 2.4% for Japan, and Mortimer et al. (13) 2.5% for North America. Zhang et al. (14) reported a dementia prevalence of 4.6% in Shanghai, 65% of whom had clinically diagnosed Alzheimer's disease. Jorm et al.

(15) reviewed 47 studies of dementia in the elderly and estimated the overall prevalence to rise from 1.4% in the 65–69-year age group to 38.6% in the 90–95-year age group.

In order to carry out statistical probability analysis, the prevalence of Alzheimer's disease in the over-64 population was averaged from several studies, excluding the East Boston survey, and taken to be 2.9%. This compares with our overall prevalence figures for Alzheimer's disease of only 0.43% (4/923) for the rheumatoid arthritis clinic population and 0.39% (29/7490) for the general hospital population with a diagnosis of rheumatoid arthritis (Table 1). The difference is highly significant at $p < 0.001$ in each case ($z = 4.47$ and 12.75, respectively).

Epidemiological data on rheumatoid arthritis are less extensive. The Minnesota survey (16) quoted an adult prevalence of 0.54% for males and 1.34% for females, but the figure is generally considered to increase with age. Hochberg (17), in reviewing numerous studies, quoted values approaching 2% in males and 5% in females over age 55. Engel et al. (18) reported a prevalence of definite rheumatoid arthritis of 4.1% in the 65–74-year age group and 6.2% in the 75–79-year age group, while Bergstrom et al. (19) reported a prevalence of 10% in a survey of 79-years-olds. Thus, there is no widely accepted prevalence of rheumatoid arthritis in the general population to compare with our observed prevalence of 0.35% (2/567) for the Alzheimer clinic population, and 0.50% (29/5756) for the general hospital population with a diagnosis of Alzheimer's disease (Table 1). However, the differences would be significant at the 0.05 level if the prevalence of rheumatoid arthritis in the over-64 general population was, respectively, ≥1.41% or ≥0.73%.

II. DISCUSSION

There are several possible interpretations for the observed low prevalence of coexisting Alzheimer's disease and rheumatoid arthritis. One explanation is that the reported prevalences for both diseases in the general population are several-fold too high. However, this explanation is inconsistent with multiple epidemiological studies. A second explanation is that only a small minority of those patients having coexisting disease were diagnosed as suffering from the two diseases. Since Alzheimer's disease and rheumatoid arthritis are major illnesses with prominent symptoms, it seems unlikely that this would occur in clinic populations where patients are carefully diagnosed and followed over long periods of time. Separation statistics from general hospitals are much more suspect, since the various illnesses precipitating entry are the main focus of diagnostic attention. Furthermore, hospital populations may not represent a proper sample of the general population. However, prevalence statistics from clinics and general hospital populations were comparable. A third explanation is that genuinely less Alzheimer's disease develops in the rheumatoid arthritic population, but for reasons unrelated to the administration of anti-inflammatory drugs. This interpretation of the data cannot be discounted.

The fourth and most interesting interpretation is that anti-inflammatory therapy confers some protection against Alzheimer's disease. To assess this possibility further, a more detailed review of the charts of all patients in British Columbia and Saskatchewan reported to have coexisting disease was carried out. Of the 22 case histories reviewed, six had onset of dementia at ages 62, 66, 79, 86, 93 and 96, many years after discontinuing anti-inflammatory medication. One developed rheumatoid arthritis in the left knee after the onset of dementia, and another, with no history of anti-inflammatory treatment, developed concurrent disease at age 79. In seven others, no clear records were available, while seven were receiving long-term anti-inflammatory treatment. One additional patient, who was under long-term treatment with steroids for rheumatoid arthritis and had been clinically diagnosed as having Alzheimer's disease, showed no evidence of plaques and tangles on autopsy and had ChAT levels within the normal range. Thus, the numbers of patients developing Alzheimer's disease while on anti-inflammatory medication for rheumatoid arthritis may be substantially fewer than the numbers recorded as having coexisting disease.

In conclusion, the data available to us suggest a relative exclusion between Alzheimer's disease and rheumatoid arthritis. This apparent exclusion may be related to anti-inflammatory therapy. It will be important to establish whether this is generally observed, since new therapeutic approaches to Alzheimer disease would be opened up (20).

ACKNOWLEDGMENTS

We thank Dr. Cyril Nair, Chief, Health Care Statistics Canada, for searching data from the Ontario hospitals; Dr. David Yocum for those from the Arizona Rheumatoid Arthritic Clinic; Dr. Jack Boyer for data from the University of Arizona Alzheimer Clinic; Dr. N.P.V. Nair for data from the Douglas Research Hospital of Verdun, Quebec; Dr. Lynne Beattie, Ms. Janine Weir, and Ms. Margaret Druhan for data from the University of British Columbia (U.B.C.) Alzheimer Clinic; Ms. Elke Lewis and Ms. Jan Weedman for data from Boswell Memorial Hospital, Sun City, Arizona; and Dr. Paul Davies for those from the University Hospital, Edmonton, Alberta. Dr. Michael Schulzer, Dept. of Statistics, U.B.C., helped greatly with the statistical analyses.

This research was supported by grants from the Alzheimer Society of British Columbia, Friends of U.B.C., Mr. Guy Mills, the Jack Brown Estate, and the National Institute of Health.

REFERENCES

1. Itagaki S, McGeer PL, Akiyama H. Presence of T-Cytotoxic suppressor and leucocyte common antigen positive cells in Alzheimer's disease brain tissue. Neurosci Lett 91:259–264, 1988.
2. Lunber-Narod J, Rogers J. Immune system associated antigens expressed by cells of the human central nervous system. Neurosci Lett 94:17–22, 1988.
3. Rogers J, Lunber-Narod J, Styren SD, et al. Expression of immune system-associated antigen by cells of the human central nervous system. Relationship to the pathology of Alzheimer's disease. Neurobiol Aging 9:330–349, 1988.
4. McGeer PL, Akiyama H, Itagaki S, et al. Immune system response in Alzheimer's disease. Can J Neurol Sci 16:516–527, 1989.
5. McGeer PL, Itagaki S, Tago H, et al. Reactive microglia in patients with senile dementia of the Alzheimer's type are positive for the histocompatibility glycoprotein HLA-DR. Neurosci Lett 79:195–200, 1987.
6. Eikelenboom P, Hack CE, Rozemuller JM, et al. Complement activation in amyloid plaques in Alzheimer's dementia. Virchows Arch (Cell Pathol) 56:259–262, 1989.
7. Rozemuller JM, Eikelenboom P, Pals ST, et al. Microglial cells around amyloid plaques in Alzheimer's disease express leucocyte adhesion molecules of the LFA-1 family. Neurosci Lett 101:288–292, 1989.
8. McGeer PL, Akiyama H, Itagaki S, et al. Activation of the classical complement pathway in brain tissue of Alzheimer patients. neurosci Lett 107:341–346, 1989.
9. *International Classification of Diseases*, 9th revision. World Health Organization, Geneva, 1977.
10. Evans DA, Funkenstein HH, Albert MS, et al. Prevalence of Alzheimer disease in a community population of older persons. JAMA 262:2551–2556, 1989.
11. Sulkava R, Wikstrom J, Aromaa A, et al. Prevalence of severe dementia in Finland. Neurology 35:1025–1029, 1985.
12. Shibayama H, Kasahara Y, Kobayashi H. Prevalence of dementia in a Japanese elderly population. Acta Psychiatr Scand 74:144–151, 1986.
13. Mortimer JA. Alzheimer's disease and dementia: Prevalence and incidence. In Reisberg B (ed): *Alzheimer's Disease*. Free Press, Glencoe, 1983.
14. Zhang M, Katzman R, Salmon D, et al. The prevalence of dementia and ALzheimer's disease in Shanghai, China: Impact of age, gender and education. Ann Neurol 27:428–437, 1990.
15. Jorm AF, Korten AE, Henderson AS. The prevalence of dementia: A quantitative integration of the literature. Acta Psychiatr Scand 76:465–479, 1987.
16. Linos A, Worthington JW, O'Fallon WM, et al. The epidemiology of rheumatoid arthritis in Rochester, Minnesota: A study of incidence, prevalence, and mortality. Am J Epidemiol 111:87–98, 1980.
17. Hochberg MC. Adult and juvenile rheumatoid arthritis: Current epidemiological concepts. Epidemiol Rev 3:27–44, 1981.
18. Engel A, Roberts J. Rheumatoid arthritis in adults. Vital and Health Statistics Data from the National Health Survey (National Center for Health Statistics) 17:1–43, 1966.

19. Bergstrom G, Bjelle A, Sorensen LB, et al. Prevalence of rheumatoid arthritis at age 79. J Rheumatol 13:527–534, 1986.
20. McGeer PL, McGeer EG, Rogers J, et al. Anti-inflammatory drugs and Alzheimer disease. Lancet 335:1037, 1990.

Part V

Other Innovative Approaches

13

A Cell Biological Approach to the Therapy of Alzheimer-Type Cerebral β/A4-Amyloidosis

Samuel E. Gandy
The Rockefeller University and New York University, New York, and New York State Office of Mental Health, Orangeburg, New York

Joseph D. Buxbaum and Paul Greengard
The Rockefeller University, New York, New York

Cerebral β/A4-amyloidosis is characteristic of several apparently related human conditions: Alzheimer's disease (1), Down's syndrome (2), hereditary cerebral hemorrhage with amyloidosis, Dutch type (HCHWAD; ref. 3), and, to a lesser extent, normal aging. Like other organ-specific amyloidoses, the pathology of these conditions includes the accumulation of extracellular protein precipitates which form β-pleated sheets and bind Congo red dye (4). Unlike other amyloidoses, however, in which the deposited peptide seems clearly derived from a hydrophilic domain in a circulating serum precursor (4), deposited β/A4-amyloid includes a portion of the intramembranous domain of an integral transmembrane protein, the Alzheimer β/A4 amyloid precursor protein (APP) (5–14). This raises several novel questions about how APP is processed within the cell and about how β/A4 is released into the extracellular space. Synthetic β/A4 spontaneously aggregates and precipitates (15), thus demonstrating that the primary amino acid sequence of this domain of APP encodes sufficient structural information to determine its amyloidogenicity. Further understanding of the cell biological mechanisms which underlie APP trafficking and its normal and abnormal processing pathways should enable rational design of therapeutic agents aimed at modifying the process of amyloidogenesis.

I. MECHANISMS

APP is synthesized as an integral transmembrane protein (Fig. 1), probably on membrane-bound ribosomes or rough endoplasmic reticulum (ER) to allow for cotranslational insertion into the vesicle lumen (16; Fig. 2). Such membrane vesicles typically contain a signal sequence receptor (17), which recognizes a hydrophobic signal sequence on the NH_2-terminus of the nascent polypeptide chain (18), and an intraluminal (intravesicular) signal peptidase activity (19), which cleaves off the hydrophobic signal peptide. Such a signal peptide sequence is present at residues 1–17 of nascent APP (7–14). Direct sequencing of the NH_2-terminus of secreted APP has revealed that the first residues are LEVPT (one-letter amino acid code; ref. 20), corresponding to predicted residues 18–22 of APP, and

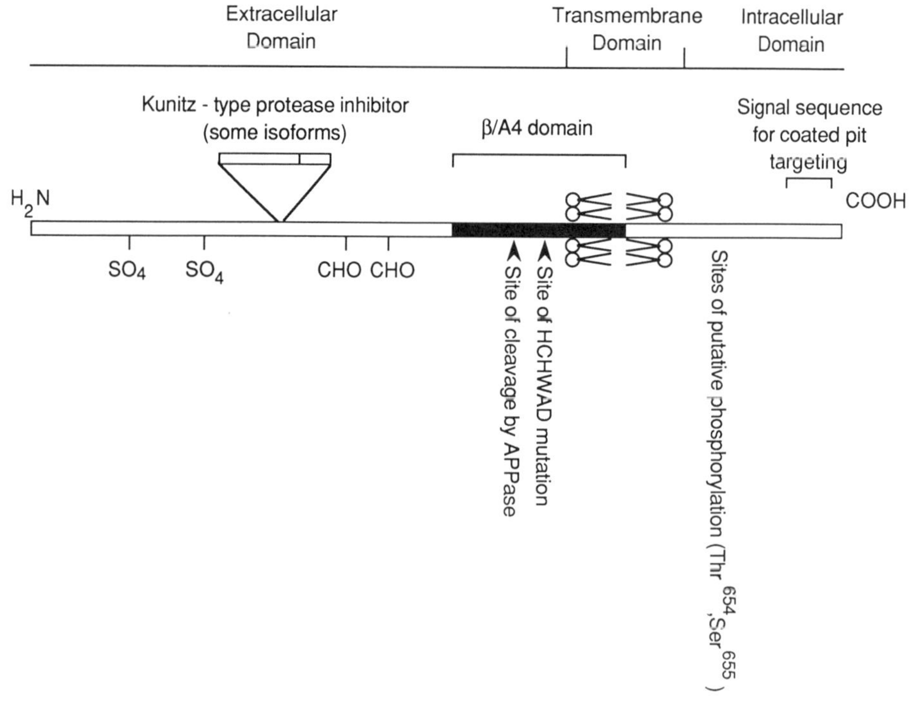

Figure 1 Domain model of transmembrane APP isoforms (APP_{695}, APP_{714}, APP_{751}, APP_{770}; refs. 7–13. (Courtesty of John Wiley & Sons, Chichester, England.)

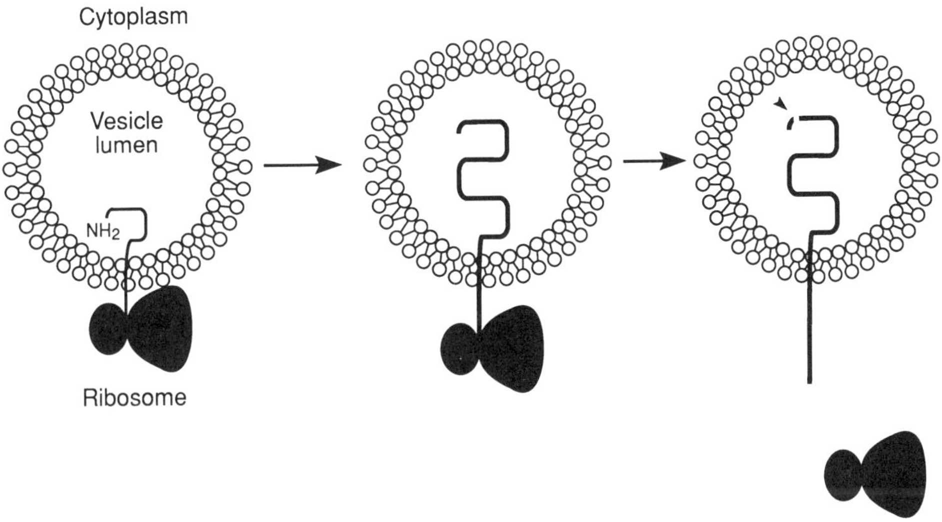

Figure 2 Presumed pathway for APP synthesis, cotranslational membrane insertion, and signal sequence cleavage.

consistent with the predicted NH_2-terminal sequence following cleavage of the signal peptide.

Following synthesis, the APP polypeptide is subjected to several posttranslational modifications. In the Golgi, sulfate groups and carbohydrates are added to the extracellular or intraluminal domain (21; Fig. 1). Sulfate is added to tyrosyl residues, and consensus sequence data suggest that the modified residue(s) may be tyrosine^{217} and/or tyrosine^{262} (21,22). N-glycosylation may occur at residues 467–469 and 496–498 (9). O-glycosylation may also occur, but the glycosylation site has not been localized (9,21). Phosphate groups are also added to APP (23,24), presumably in its cytoplasmic domain (Figs. 1 and 3), since protein phosphorylation enzymes (protein kinases) are typically intracellular in location (25).

These posttranslational modifications may offer some clues about the biology of APP. Tyrosine sulfation typically occurs in the domains of proteins which are destined to be released from the cell (22). This has proven to be the case for APP: following a short cellular half-life, the tyrosine sulfated ectodomain is released into the medium of cultured cells (21). Covalently attached sugar side groups are typical of the ectodomains of cell-surface proteins; indeed, a population of apparently full-length APP holoprotein can be detected on the surface of transfected cells (21).

Phosphorylation of a substrate protein frequently gives clues about the biology of that protein (26). Changes in the phosphorylation state of a protein can produce dramatic changes in the trafficking, processing, or biological activity of the protein. Certain cell-surface receptors are phosphorylated in their cytoplasmic domains as a mechanism of modifying sensitivity to ligand-induced effects (27). Cell adhesion molecules (CAMs) and extracellular matrix receptors are phosphorylated in their cytoplasmic domains, and the state of phosphorylation of CAMs may regulate interactions with the cytoskeleton (28). Endocytosis of the epidermal growth factor (EGF) receptor and interleukin-2 (IL-2) receptor is induced by protein kinase C-mediated phosphorylation in their respective cytodomains, at residues near the transmembrane domain (29-33). Of note, an APP phosphorylation site is rapidly phosphorylated by protein kinase C or calcium/calmodiulin-dependent protein kinase II (23; Table 1, Fig. 3) and, like the protein kinase C phosphorylation site on IL-2R or EGFR, is located within 10 residues of the plasma membrane. Several other protein kinases were tested for their ability to phosphorylate $APP^{645-661}$ but were ineffective (Table 1).

Recent evidence (34) demonstrates directly that protein phosphorylation modulates an important event in the biology of APP, i.e., its proteolytic processing. In pulse-chase studies using PC12 cells, phorbol esters (drugs which stimulate protein kinase C) dramatically diminished recovery of mature APP while enhancing recovery of a COOH-terminal fragment of approximately 15 kDa (Figs. 4-6). Okadaic acid (a drug which inhibits protein phosphatases 1 and 2A) had similar effects (Figs. 4-6). When both phorbol ester and okadaic acid were simultaneously applied to cells, in addition to the effects on mature APP and the 15-kDa COOH-terminal fragment, a larger (~19 kDa) COOH-terminal fragment was generated in elevated amounts (Fig. 4). In other experiments, H-7 (an inhibitor of protein kinases including protein kinase C) led to an apparent decrease in the

Table 1 Kinetics of Phosphorylation of the Synthetic Peptide $APP^{645-661}$ by Various Protein Kinases

Protein kinase*	V_{max} (μmol/min/mg)	K_m (μM)	Catalytic efficiency (V_{max}/K_m, $\times 10^3$)
Protein kinase C	7.3	132	55.3
Ca^{2+}/CaM kinase II	1.3	24	54.2
cAMP-dependent protein kinase	0.02	125	0.2
cGMP-dependent protein kinase	<0.01	—	—
Casein kinase II	<0.01	—	—
Insulin receptor	<0.01	—	—

*From Reference 23. Residues numbered according to Reference 9.

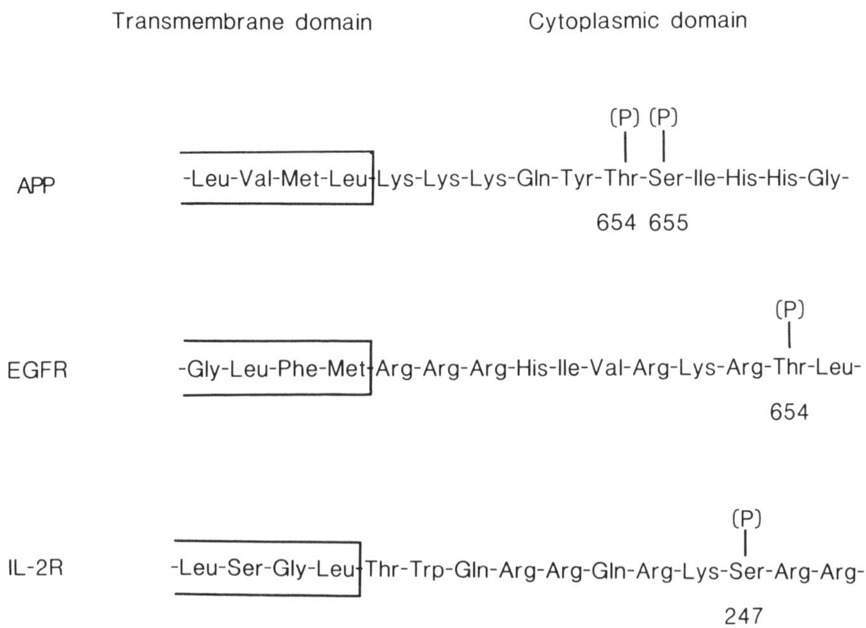

Figure 3 Location of phosphorylatable residues in the putative cytoplasmic domains of APP, epidermal growth factor receptor (EGFR), and interleukin-2 receptor (IL-2R). In each case, the PKC phosphorylation site is within 10 residues of the plasma membrane. (From Reference 23.)

basal rate of processing of APP (Fig. 5), supporting the physiological significance of modulation of APP processing by protein kinase C. These results provide the first direct evidence for regulation of the rate of APP processing by protein phosphorylation. They also raise the possibility that protein phosphorylation can lead to an alternative, i.e., qualitatively different, pathway of APP processing.

The intracellular trafficking pathways involved in APP processing have begun to attract attention, but much remains to be clarified. Following its departure from the trans-Golgi, APP has been localized at two sites: Apparently intact APP holoprotein is detectable on the cell surface (21); and a truncated soluble protein, containing the NH_2-terminal region of the molecule, is released from the cell (21). The cellular location at which APP is cleaved to produce the truncated soluble protein is unknown, but likely candidates include the Golgi, the lysosomal compartment, and/or the cell surface (Fig. 7).

Several lines of evidence suggest that the lysosome is likely to be one way sta-

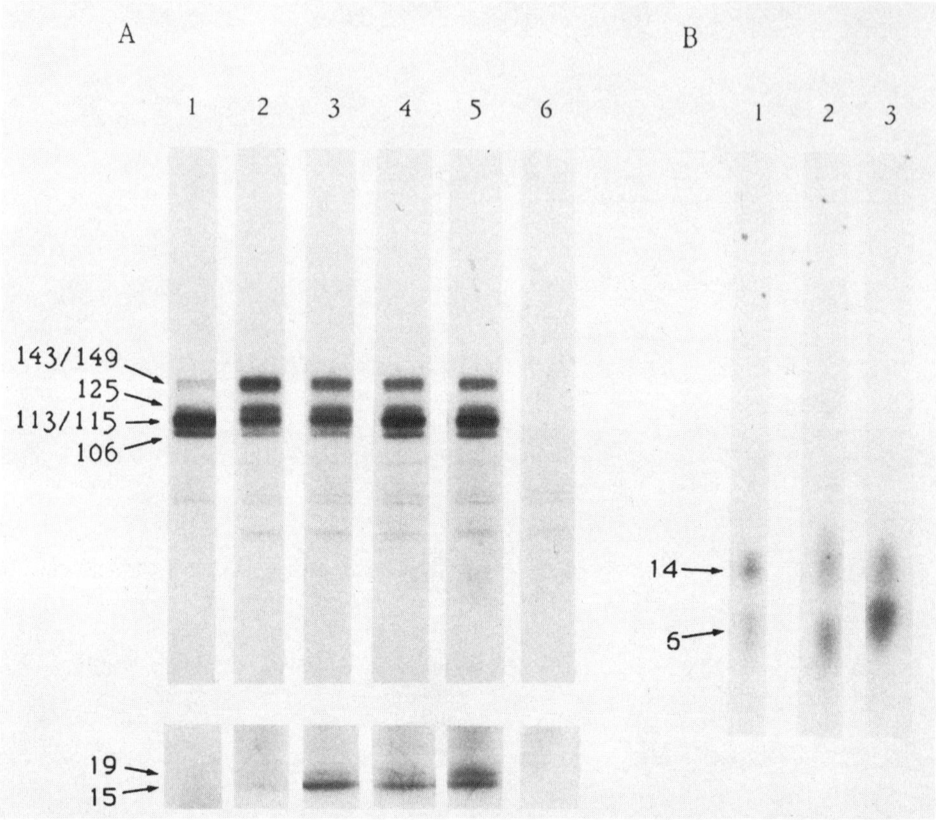

Figure 4 Identification of APP and APP-derived peptides in PC12 cells and regulation of processing by phorbol ester and okadaic acid. (A) Immunoprecipitation of APP and APP-derived peptides using anti-$APP^{645-694}$ antibodies (numbering according to Kang et al; ref. 9, for APP_{695}). Cells were prelabeled with [^{35}S]methionine for 20 min and either harvested immediately (lane 1) or chased for 45 min with unlabeled methionine and then harvested (lanes 2-6). Vehicle alone or a test substance was added at the start of the chase period (time zero). After cell lysis, extracts were subjected to immunoprecipitation, SDS-PAGE, and autoradiography. (Upper) Large molecular mass region of a 6-18% gradient gel; arrows indicate the positions of the six protein bands of 106, 113, 115, 125, 143, and 149 kDa. (Lower) A longer exposure of low-molecular-mass region of the gel; arrows indicate the positions of the 15- and 19-kDa peptides. Lanes: 1, 2, vehicle; 3, 1 μM phorbol ester (PDBu); 4, 1 μM okadaic acid; 5 and 6, 1 μM PDBu and 1 μM okadaic acid. For lane 6, 100 μM $APP^{645-694}$ peptide (9) was present during immunoprecipitation. (B) Limited proteolysis of the putative APP isoforms in levels of the 106-kDa band and the 113/115 kDa doublet were maximal at time zero and decreased thereafter with a half-life of 30-40 min. Levels of the 125-kDa band and the 143/149 kDa doublet were minimal at time zero,

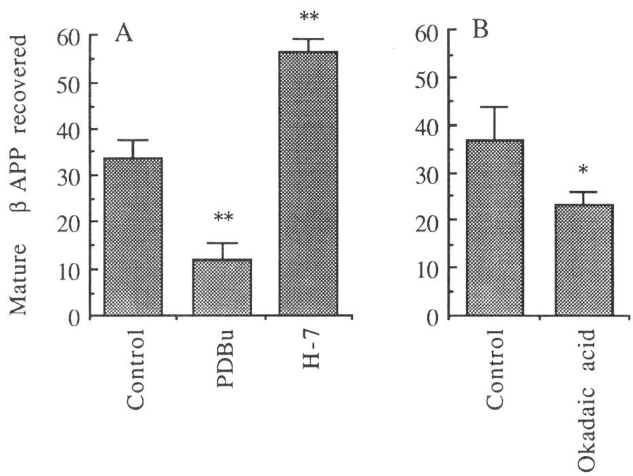

Figure 5 Regulation of levels of mature $APP_{751/770}$ by PDBu, by H-7, and by okadaic acid. PC12 cells were incubated with the indicated agents and processed as described in the legend to Figure 4. Mature $APP_{751/770}$ was quantified by densitometric scanning of the 143/149-kDa doublet of the autoradiogram. The results shown are the means ± SEM of four experiments. Data were normalized to the total $APP_{751/770}$ recovered (100 units) at time zero. Data were corrected for the amount of mature $APP_{751/770}$ present at time zero (10 units in A, 6 units in B). PDBu, 1 μM; H-7, 100 μM; okadaic acid, 1 μM. *, $p < 0.05$ compared to control; **, $p < 0.01$ compared to control. (From Reference 34.)

---

increased to a maximum by 45 min of chase, and decreased thereafter. The 15- and 19-kDa peptides were detectable by 15 min of chase and the levels of these peptides remained elevated throughout the 135 min of chase (see also Fig. 6). These data suggest a precursor-product relationship between the doublets of 113/115 and 143/149 kDa, as well as between the bands of 106- and 125-kDa. Based on these observations and on the results of Wiedemann et al. (21), we made the following tentative assignments: 106-, 113-, and 115-kDa bands represent the immature (N-glycosylated) forms of APP_{695}, APP_{751}, and APP_{770}, respectively; 125-, 143-, and 149-kDa bands represent the mature (sulfated, and N- and O-glycosylated) forms of APP_{695}, APP_{751}, and APP_{770}, respectively. Since the antibodies used were prepared against COOH-terminal regions of APP, we concluded that the 15- and 19-kDa peptides were COOH-terminal fragments of APP. PC12 cells and of human APP_{695}. The 113/115-kDa doublet (from A, lane 1) and the 143/149-kDa doublet (from A, lane 2) were excised, subjected to limited proteolytic digestion with V8 protease, electrophoresed, and compared with similarly treated in vitro transcribed and translated human APP_{695}. Lanes: 1, 113/115-kDa doublet; 2, 143/149-kDa doublet; 3, human APP_{695}. Arrows indicate the positions of 14- and 6-kDa digestion products. (From Reference 34.)

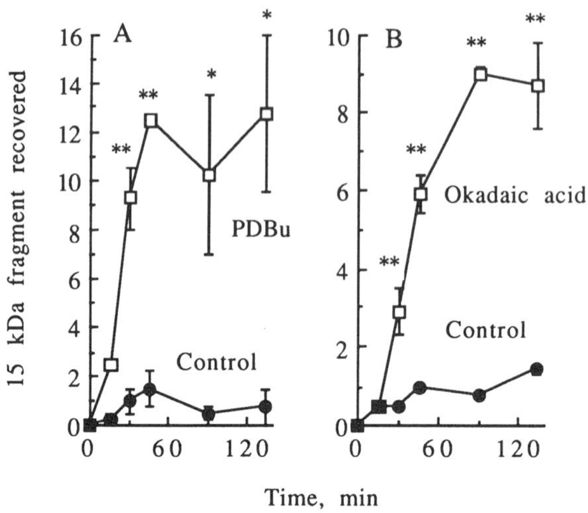

Figure 6 Regulation of levels of 15-kDa putative COOH-terminal fragment of APP by PDBu and by okadaic acid. PC12 cells were metabolically labeled for 20 min with [^{35}S]methionine followed by a chase with complete medium for periods ranging from 0–135 min. After cell lysis, extracts were subjected to immunoprecipitation, SDS-PAGE, and autoradiography. The 15-kDa fragment was quantified by densitometric scanning of the autoradiogram. Data were normalized as described in the legend to Figure 5. Incubation was carried out in the presence of vehicle alone (Control), 1 μM PDBu (A) or 1 μM okadaic acid (B). Test substances were added at the start of the chase period. Results are means ± SEM of four experiments. * $p < 0.05$ compared to control; ** $p < 0.01$ compared to control. (From Reference 34.)

tion of APP during its intracellular itinerary. Neuronal lipofuscin, formed by the age-dependent accumulation of incompletely degraded lysosomal by-products, is characterized by the presence of APP-like immunoreactivity in association with intracellular vesicular lipofuscin granules (35). Using immunocytochemistry of brain, APP-like immunoreactivity appears as an intracellular vesicular staining pattern, interpreted as possibly representing association of APP immunoreactivity with lysosomes (36). Various protease inhibitors, including the lysosome acidification inhibitors ammonium chloride and chloroquine, have been suggested to slow APP processing (37). A signal sequence, asparagine-proline-X-tyrosine (or NPXY in one-letter code, ref. 38; Fig. 1), has recently been identified. It is believed to target transmembrane proteins (including the low-density lipoprotein receptor, EGF receptor, and insulin receptor) to coated pits to initiate their endocytosis. These converging lines of evidence strongly suggest that at least some step in APP processing may occur in lysosomes. Such evidence would not necessarily preclude cell surface cleavage or the possibility that lysosomal residence occurs late in trafficking of COOH-terminal APP fragments rather than in the initial processing of APP holoprotein. Likewise, one cannot discern from the data currently available whether the proposed early lysosomal residence occurs after residence at the cell surface or along a pathway that delivers APP directly to the lysosome after it emerges from the trans-Golgi. Some of these possibilities are illustrated in Figure 7.

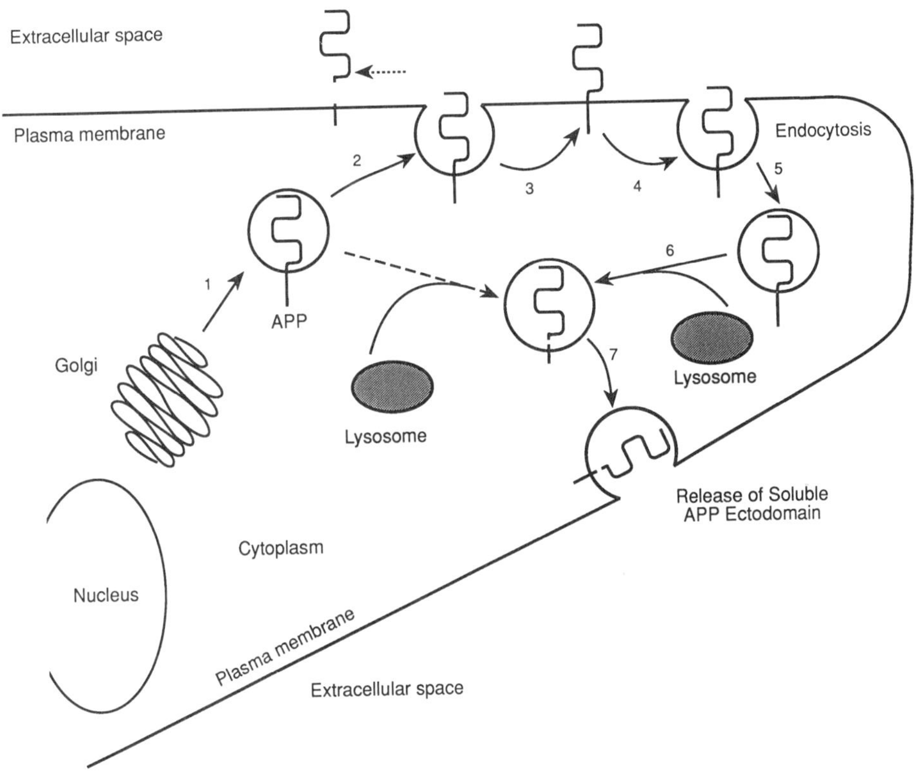

Figure 7 Possible pathways for initial cleavage of APP following exit from the trans-Golgi (step 1). In one possible scenario, APP may be directed initially to the cell surface (step 2). APP cleavage may occur either due to ectoproteases (dotted arrow) or within lysosomes following endocytosis (steps 3–5). Alternatively, or in a parallel fashion, a population of APP-bearing vesicles may fuse with lysosomes upon exit from the trans-Golgi (dashed arrow), followed by cleavage and release of the truncated soluble APP ectodomain from the cell surface (step 6). For simplicity, processing of the COOH-terminal fragment is not shown.

II. EXPERIMENTAL RESULTS

The site within APP at which the initial cleavage occurs has recently been determined by molecular biological (39) and protein chemical methods (40). These data reveal that in cultured, transfected cells, the initial constitutive cleavage of APP occurs within the β/A4 domain, hence precluding amyloidogenesis. These studies, then, serve to define a major pathway of APP processing and to demonstrate that this major pathway is nonamyloidogenic. Alternate pathways, preserving β/A4 intact within either the released APP ectodomain or the remaining cell-associated COOH-terminal fragments, are currently being sought. Selkoe (41), using an APP COOH-terminal antiserum for Western blotting of brain homogenate and APP-transfected cells, resolved the COOH-terminal fragments into a doublet of ~11 kDa. Wolf et al. (42) observed production of 12-and 16-kDa COOH-fragments of APP following high-level overexpression of APP holoprotein. High-level overexpression of the last 99 residues of APP (beginning with the NH_2-terminus of β/A4) yielded a 16-kDa protein (as well as higher molecular mass aggregated multimers) (42). Several tryptic-like potential cleavage sites, following lysine^{595}, lysine^{612}, and lysine^{624}, have been suggested as alternative sites for producing heterogenous cleavage in the β/A4 region of APP (43).

We obtained the above data using phorbol ester and okadaic acid for the production of 15- and 19-kDa COOH-terminal fragments of APP. One possible interpretation of these observations is that the 15-kDa COOH-terminal fragment represents constitutive intra-β/A4 cleavage while the 19 kDa COOH-terminal fragment represents processing via an alternative and potentially "β/A4-preserving" amyloidogenic pathway, perhaps by cleavage at or near the β/A4 NH_2-terminus (Fig. 8). (Although we think it likely that phorbol esters and okadaic acid increase the formation of the 15 kDa and 19 kDa peptides, we cannot exclude the possibility that the effects observed are due to decrease degradation of these peptides.) Our results suggest the possible existence of a subpopulation of cell-associated COOH-terminal fragments containing intact β/A4, and that this subpopulation is a likely source for β/A4 which is deposited. Direct sequencing of these COOH-terminal fragments will be required to evaluate this possibility.

Another conceivable source for amyloidogenic APP or APP fragments would be circulating APP holoprotein. In addition, we cannot rule out the possibility that intramembranous or intracytoplasmic cleavage could liberate APP ectodomain containing intact β/A4. Such pathways, if proven to exist, would argue for a potential circulating or serum source for deposited β/A4, as has been proposed (44,45). Such a source cannot be definitively supported or refuted based on the current data. However, several lines of investigation raise questions about the possibility of a serum source. The kidney is a typical site of amyloid deposition in other amyloidoses in which the deposited protein is derived from a circulating serum precursor (4), but β/A4 deposition in kidney has not been reported as a feature of

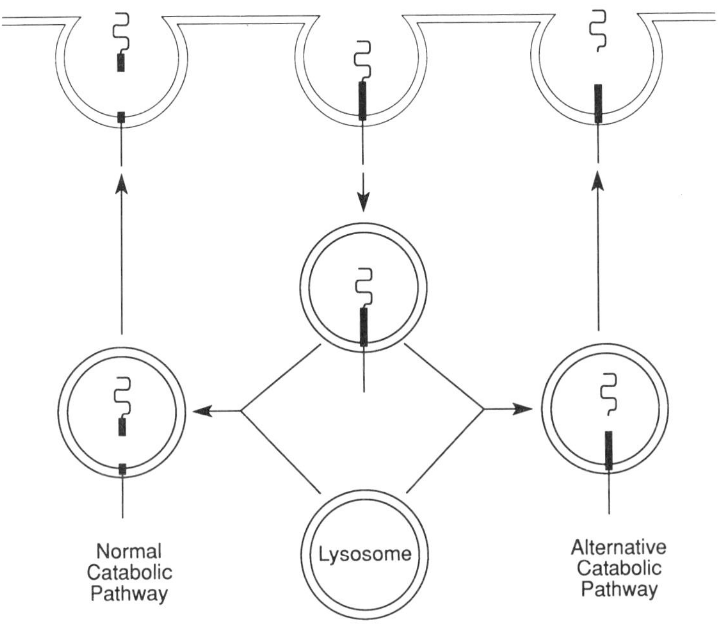

Figure 8 Schematic representation of possible APP processing pathways, including normal intra β/A4 cleavage (left) and postulated alternative cleavage at the NH_2 terminus of β/A4 (right). Solid boxed domain is β/A4; top of figure is extracellular space. For simplicity, processing of the COOH-terminal fragment to form β/A4 is not shown. (Courtesy of John Wiley & Sons, Chichester, England.)

any of the β/A4-amyloidoses. Circulating serum APP has been detected (46) but appears to be truncated at the COOH-terminus, presumably in the same position as APP released from the surface of cultured cells. However, intact platelet alpha granules, which have been shown to contain APP (47), may be released from ruptured platelets in the circulation and could thus provide one potential source of circulating APP holoprotein.

Intramembranous or intracytoplasmic cleavage of an integral membrane protein, followed by release of the protein from the cell surface, would be a novel event. The thermodynamic constraints of displacing a hydrophobic transmembrane domain from the lipid bilayer would appear to be prohibitive. Indeed, small hydrophobic moieties (e.g., myristate; ref. 48) can serve as highly effective anchors, securing large proteins to plasma or organellar lipid membranes. Membrane damage has been suggested as a possible etiologic or early pathogenetic event in amyloidogenesis in Alzheimer's disease, but studies of a rare form of

β/A4-amyloidosis, i.e., HCHWAD, have proven that cerebral vascular and parenchymal β/A4-amyloidosis may occur in the absence of a primary defect in plasma membrane structure. Unlike some other β/A4-amyloidoses, HCHWAD (3) appears to be caused by a mutation within the APP coding sequence. The mutation, substituting glutamine for glutamate, occurs a few residues COOH-terminal to the site of intra-β/A4 cleavage (Fig. 1). The putative changes in APP processing consequent to this mutation have not yet been defined but are likely to illuminate the question of the source of deposited β/A4.

III. FUTURE DIRECTIONS

It is worth considering whether there exists a pathway for discharging β/A4-containing COOH-terminal fragments of APP into the extracellular space. Current cell biological concepts of the trafficking of transmembrane proteins suggests that such a pathway might well exist, although direct evidence is lacking (49). Such a pathway might include endocytosis and proteolysis in lysosomes. This pathway is shown schematically in Figure 9. Following internalization, an endosome containing an amyloidogenic APP holoprotein or COOH-terminal fragment could be surrounded to form a "multivesicular body," and the contents subsequently degraded by the combined action of lipases and proteases. Lipases could degrade the endosomal membrane, liberating the amyloidogenic fragment into the lysosomal lumen. If proteolysis were incomplete, then fusion of the multivesicular body with the plasma membrane could release β/A4-containing fragments into the extracellular space, where spontaneous aggregation might occur. The data of Wolf et al. (42) support the possibility that amyloidogenic fragments might be poorly catabolized, since overexpression of a COOH-terminal construct led to accumulation of a 16 kDa fragment but no detectable 12 kDa fragment (the major COOH-terminal catabolite following overexpression of APP holoprotein).

The observations of Wolf et al. (42) may facilitate interpretation of the effects of phorbol esters and okadaic acid on APP processing. As described (Fig. 3, refs. 23,29–33), there exists a striking homology between an APP phosphorylation site and phosphorylation sites of the EGF receptor and the IL-2 receptor. In each of the latter cases, phosphorylation at this homologous site induces endocytosis of those proteins. As a further analogy, protein kinase C is implicated in regulating the phosphorylation of the juxtamembrane sites in EGFR, IL-2R, and APP (23,29–33). Acceleration of APP endocytosis, mediated via APP phosphorylation,could be expected to lead to the increased delivery of APP to lysosomes. This suggests that the 15- and 19-kDa COOH-terminal peptides produced by the combination of phorbol and okadaic acid (34) may be identical with the 12- and 16-kDa COOH-terminal peptides produced by overexpression (42). Such a scenario suggests that saturation of the intra-β/A4 processing pathway may occur in certain situations of excessive APP processing, hence "activating" an alternate pathway which cleaves

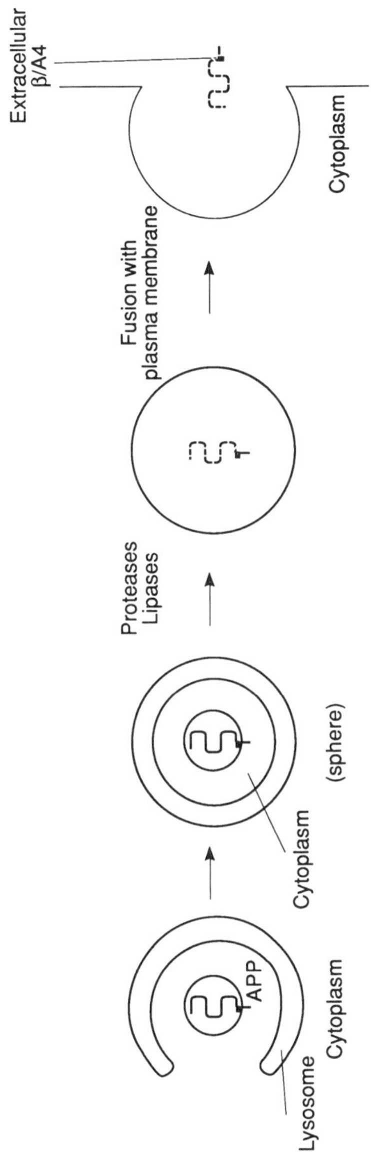

Figure 9 One possible mechanism by which amyloidogenic APP fragments may be released from membranes and discharged into the extracellular space. Thick segment of APP identifies the position of β/A4.

at or near the NH_2-terminus of β/A4. This mechanism might also explain the cerebral β/A4-amyloidosis of Down's syndrome, which is accompanied by APP overexpression in association with triplication of chromosome 21, where the APP gene resides (7).

Identification of amyloidogenic pathways and their regulation could lead to rational antiamyloid therapy for the β/A4-amyloidoses. Based on information summarized here, phosphorylation-sensitive pathways appear to be potential targets for the design of such agents. We have demonstrated that stimulation of protein phosphorylation accelerates APP processing and that hyperstimulation of protein phosphorylation may activate alternate pathways of processing. This suggests the possibility that Alzheimer's disease could be due to a primary abnormality in the regulation of protein phosphorylation. Evidence has accumulated that protein phosphorylation abnormalities are a hallmark of Alzheimer's disease (50–56). In any event, the data raise the possibility that compounds which alter protein phosphorylation could be useful in the therapy of Alzheimer's disease.

If acceleration of APP processing leads to activation of amyloidogenic catabolism, then agents which inhibit protein phosphorylation might be beneficial by slowing APP processing to such a rate that the nonamyloidogenic pathway could process the substrate presented to it. Inhibitors of protein phosphorylation might also prevent the aberrant phosphorylation of the cytoskeleton which is characteristic of Alzheimer's disease (50–55). Further, by mechanisms not discussed in this Chapter, protein phosphorylation has been observed to be a potent stimulus for APP transcription (57). Inhibition of protein phosphorylation, then, may have beneficial antiamyloidogenic actions at both the transcriptional and posttranslational levels (57–59).

Basic investigations could be undertaken in neuronal and peripheral tissues to define which protein phosphorylating enzymes (protein kinases) and dephosphorylating enzymes (protein phosphatases) are implicated in regulating APP catabolic pathways. Knowledge of the exact isoform of the enzyme would also provide useful information. Once the relevant protein kinases/phosphatases have been identified and their regulatory roles defined with regard to APP processing, drug design could begin, aimed at the development of selective potent inhibitors and activators.

Though speculative at this point, there exist no theoretical obstacles to such a line of investigation, targeted toward development of drugs useful for the treatment of Alzheimer's disease. Successfully designing agents with appropriate specificity and acceptable side effects are likely to be difficult steps in the process, since signal transduction via protein phosphorylation is a ubiquitous and important regulatory event. Not surprisingly, however, similar strategies are being employed to develop antineoplastic agents (60,61), based on the identification of several protein kinase oncogenes as etiologic in certain cancers (62). Information derived from these antineoplastic studies could be of great interest to investigators seeking to arrest, via modulation of protein phosphorylation, the pathogenetic events which accompany Alzheimer's disease.

ACKNOWLEDGMENTS

Portions of the text and figures are from Gandy SE, Buxbaum JD, and Greengard P. Signal transduction and the pathobiology of Alzheimer's disease. In *Alzheimer's Disease: Basic Mechanisms, Diagnosis and Therapeutic Strategies.* Iqbal K, Crapper-McLachlan D, Winblad B, et al. (eds): John Wiley & Sons, Chichester, pp. 155-172, and are reproduced with permission of John Wiley & Sons, Chichester.

We thank Carol Ebbecke for secretarial assistance. This work was supported by U.S. Public Health Service Grants NS-01095 (S.E.G.), MH-39327 and MH-40899 (P.G.). J.D.B. was the recipient of a postdoctoral fellowship from the Rothschild Foundation and is the recipient of Individual National Research Award NS-08523.

REFERENCES

1. Tomlinson BE, Corsellis JAN. Aging and the dementias. In Adams JH, Corsellis JAN, Duchen LW (eds): *Greenfield's Neuropathology.* Arnold, London, 1984, pp. 951-1025.
2. Wisniewski KE, Dalton AJ, Crapper McLachlan DR, et al. Alzheimer's disease in Down's syndrome: Clinicopathologic studies. Neurology 35:957-961, 1985.
3. Levy E, Carman MD, Fernandez-Madrid IJ, et al. Mutation of the Alzheimer's disease amyloid gene in hereditary cerebral hemorrhage, Dutch type. Science 248:1124-1126, 1990.
4. Cotran RS, Kumar V, Robbins SL. Robbins' Pathologic Basis of Disease. 4th ed. WB Saunders, Philadelphia, 1984.
5. Glenner GG, Wong CW. Alzheimer's disease: Initial report of the purification and characteristics of a novel cerebrovascular amyloid protein. Biochem Biophys Res Commun 122:885-890, 1984.
6. Masters CL, Simms G, Weinmann NA, et al. Amyloid plaque protein in Alzheimer's disease and Down's syndrome. Proc Natl Acad Sci USA 82:4245-4249, 1985.
7. Goldgaber D, Lerman MI, McBride OW, et al. Characterization and chromosomal localization of a cDNA encoding brain amyloid of Alzheimer's disease. Science 235:877-880, 1987.
8. Tanzi R, Gusella JF, Watkins PC, et al. Amyloid β protein gene: cDNA, mRNA distribution, and genetic linkage near the Alzheimer locus. Science 235:880-884, 1987.
9. Kang J, Lemaire HF, Unterbeck A, et al. The precursor of Alzheimer's disease amyloid A4 protein resembles a cell-surface receptor, Nature 325:733-736, 1987.
10. Robakis NK, Ramakrishna N, Wolfe G, et al. Molecular cloning and characterization of a cDNA encoding the cerebrovascular and the neuritic plaque amyloid peptides. Proc Natl Acad Sci USA 84:4190-4194, 1988.

11. Tanzi RE, McClatchey AI, Lamperti ED, et al. Protease inhibitor domain encoded by an amyloid protein precursor mRNA associated with Alzheimer's disease. Nature 331:528–530, 1988.
12. Ponte P, Gonzales-DeWhitt P, Schilling J, et al. A new A4 amyloid mRNA contains a domain homologous to serine proteinase inhibitors. Nature 331:525–527, 1988.
13. Kitaguchi N, Takahashi Y, Tokushima Y, et al. Novel precursor of Alzheimer's disease amyloid protein shows protease inhibitory activity. Nature 331:530–532, 1988.
14. De Sauvage F, Octave J-N. A novel mRNA of the A4 amyloid precursor gene coding for a possibly secreted protein. Science 245:651–656, 1989.
15. Kirschner DA, Inouye H, Duffy LK, et al. Synthetic peptide homologous to β protein from Alzheimer disease forms amyloid-like fibrils in vitro. Proc Natl Acad Sci USA 84:6953–6957, 1987.
16. Walter P, Gilmore R, Blobel G. Protein translocation across the endoplasmic reticulum. Cell 38:5–8, 1984.
17. Siegel V, Walter P. Functional dissection of the signal recognition particle. Trend Biochem Sci 13:314–316, 1988.
18. Gierasch LM. Signal sequences. Biochemistry 28:923–930, 1989.
19. Evans EA, Gilmore R, Blobel G. Purification of microsome signal peptidase as a complex. Proc Natl Acad Sci USA 83:581–585, 1986.
20. Palmert MR, Podlisny MD, Witker DS, et al. The β-amyloid protein precursor of Alzheimer disease has soluble derivatives found in human brain and cerebrospinal fluid. Proc Natl Acad Sci USA 86:6338–6342, 1989.
21. Weidemann A, Konig G, Bunke D, et al. Identification, biogenesis, and localization of precursors of Alzheimer's disease A4 amyloid protein. Cell 57:115–126, 1989.
22. Huttner WB. Tyrosine sulfation and the secretory pathway. Ann Rev Physiol 50:363–376, 1988.
23. Gandy SE, Czernik AJ, Greengard P. Phosphorylation of Alzheimer disease amyloid precursor peptide by protein kinase C and Ca^{2+}/calmodulin-dependent protein kinase II. Proc Natl Acad Sci USA 85:6218–6221, 1988.
24. Oltersdorf T, Ward PJ, Henriksson T, et al. The Alzheimer amyloid precursor protein: Identification of a stable intermediate in the biosynthetic/degradative pathway. J Biol Chem 265:4492–4497, 1990.
25. Nairn AC, Hemmings HC Jr, Greengard P. Protein kinases in the brain. Ann Rev Biochem 54:931–976, 1985.
26. Nestler EJ, Greengard P. Protein Phosphorylation in the Nervous System. New York: Wiley, 1984.
27. Huganir RL, Greengard P. Regulation of receptor function by protein phosphorylation. Trends Pharmacol Sci 8:472–477, 1987.
28. Mackie K, Sorkin BC, Nairn AC, et al. Identification of two protein kinases that phosphorylate the neural cell-adhesion molecule, N-CAM. J Neurosci 9:1883–1896, 1989.
29. Hunter T, Ling N, Cooper JA. Protein kinase C phosphorylation of the EGF receptor at a threonine residue close to the cytoplasmic face of the plasma membrane. Nature (London) 311:450–453, 1984.
30. Gallis B, Lewis A, Wignall J, et al. Phosphorylation of the human interleukin-2 recep-

tor and a synthetic peptide identical to its C-terminal, cytoplasmic domain. J Biol Chem 261:5075–5080, 1986.
31. Beguinot L, Hanover JA, Ito S, et al. Phorbol esters induce transient internalization without degradation of unoccupied epidermal growth factor receptors. Proc Natl Acad Sci USA 82:2774–2778, 1985.
32. Lin CR, Chen WS, Lazar CS, et al. Protein kinase C phosphorylation at Thr 654 of the unoccupied EGF receptor and EGF binding regulate functional receptor loss by independent mechanisms. Cell 44:839–848, 1986.
33. Shackelford DA, Trowbridge IS. Identification of lymphocyte integral membrane proteins as substrates for protein kinase C. J Biol Chem 261:8334–8341, 1986.
34. Buxbaum JD, Gandy SE, Cicchetti P, et al. Processing of Alzheimer β/A4 amyloid precursor protein: Modulation by agents that regulate protein phosphorylation. Proc Natl Acad Sci USA 87:6003–6006, 1990.
35. Bancher C, Grundke-Iqbal I, Iqbal K, et al. Immunoreactivity of neuronal lipofuscin with monoclonal antibodies to the amyloid beta-protein. Neurobiol Aging 10:125–132, 1989.
36. Benowitz LI, Rodriguez PP, Mufson EJ, et al. The amyloid precursor protein is concentrated in neuronal lysosomes in normal and Alzheimer disease subjects. Exp Neurol 106:237–250, 1989.
37. Cole GM, Tuan HV, Saitoh T. Evidence for lysosomal processing of amyloid beta-protein precursor in cultured cells. Neurochem Res 14:933–939, 1989.
38. Chen W-J, Goldstein JL, Brown MS. NPXY, a sequence often found in cytoplasmic tails, is required for coated pit-mediated internalization of the low density lipoprotein receptor. J Biol Chem 265:116–123, 1990.
39. Sisodia SS, Koo EH, Beyreuther K, et al. Evidence that β-amyloid protein in Alzheimer's disease is not derived by normal processing. Science 248:492–495, 1990.
40. Esch FS, Keim PS, Beattie EC, et al. Cleavage of amyloid β peptide during constitutive processing of its precursor. Science 248:1122–1124, 1990.
41. Selkoe DJ. Molecular pathology of amyloidogenic proteins and the role of vascular amyloidosis in Alzheimer's disease. Neurobiol Aging 10:387–395, 1990.
42. Wolf D, Quon D, Wang Y, et al. Identification and characterization of C-terminal fragments of the β-amyloid precursor produced in cell culture. EMBO J 9:2079–2084, 1990.
43. Glenner GG, Mehlhaff P. Proteolysis in the formation of amyloid fibrils in Alzheimer's disease. Neurobiol Aging 11:300, 1990.
44. Glenner GG. Amyloid deposits and amyloidosis: The β-fibrilloses. N Engl J Med 302:1283–1292; 1333–1343, 1990.
45. Joachim CL, Mori H, Selkoe DJ. Amyloid beta-protein deposition in tissues other than in brain in Alzheimer's disease. Nature 341:226–230, 1989.
46. Schlossmacher MG, Podlisny MB, Ostaszewski BL, et al. Detection of circulating forms of the amyloid β-protein precursor (APP) in human plasma. Neurobiol Aging 11:332, 1990.
47. Van Nostrand WE, Schmaier AH, Farrow JS, et al. Protease nexin-II (amyloid β-protein precursor): A platelet α-granule protein. Science 248:745–748, 1990.

48. Schultz AM, Henderson LE, Oroszlan S. Fatty acylation of proteins. Ann Rev Cell Biol 4:611-647, 1988.
49. Dice JF. Molecular determinants of protein half-lives in eukaryotic cells. FASEB J 1:349-357, 1987.
50. Sternberger NH, Sternberger LA, Ulrich J. Aberrant neurofilament phosphorylation in Alzheimer disease. Proc Natl Acad Sci USA 82:4274-4276, 1985.
51. Grundke-Iqbal I, Iqbal K, Tung Y-C, et al. Abnormal phosphorylation of the microtubule-associated protein τ (tau) in Alzheimer cytoskeletal pathology. Proc Natl Acad Sci USA 83:4913-4917, 1986.
52. Selkoe DJ. Biochemistry of altered brain proteins in Alzheimer's disease. Ann Rev Neurosci 12:463-490, 1989.
53. Baudier J, Cole RD. Phosphorylation of tau proteins to a state like that in Alzheimer's brain is catalyzed by a calcium/calmodulin-dependent kinase and modulated by phospholipids. J Biol Chem 262:17577-17583, 1987.
54. Mattson MP. Antigenic changes similar to those seen in neurofibrillary tangles are elicited by glutamate and Ca^{2+} influx in cultured hippocampal neurons. Neuron 4:105-117, 1990.
55. McKee AC, Kosik KS, Kennedy MB, et al. Hippocampal neurons predisposed to neurofibrillary tangle formation are enriched in type II calcium/calmodulin-dependent protein kinase. J Neuropathol Exp Neurol 49:49-63, 1990.
56. Saitoh T, Iimoto DS. Altered protein kinase and amyloid beta-protein precursor in Alzheimer's disease: Which comes first? In Boller F, Katzman R, Rascol A, et al. (eds): Biological markers of Alzheimer's disease, Springer Verlag, New York, 105-117, 1989.
57. Goldgaber D, Harris HW, Hla T, et al. Interleukin 1 regulates synthesis of amyloid β-protein precursor mRNA in human endothelial cells. Proc Natl Acad Sci USA 86: 7606-7610, 1989.
58. Goldgaber D, Schmechel DE, Odenwald WF. Hox 1.3, amyloid β-protein and aging. Soc Neurosci Abst 15:23, 1989.
59. Fienberg AA, Belting H-G, Nordstedt C, et al. Unpublished observations.
60. Liebow C, Reilly C, Serrano M, et al. Somatostatin analogues inhibit growth of pancreatic cancer by stimulating tyrosine phosphatase. Proc Natl Acad Sci USA 86: 2003-2007, 1989.
61. Hammond KD, Cloutman LJ, Gilbert DA. Cancer reversal: regulation of phosphotyrosine phosphatase. Biochem Soc Trans 6:1048-1049, 1989.
62. Hunter T, Cooper JA. Protein-tyrosine kinases. Ann Rev Biochem 54:897-830, 1985.

14

Phosphomonoesters, Phospholipids, and High-Energy Phosphates in Alzheimer's Disease: Alterations and Physiological Significance

Jay W. Pettegrew, William E. Klunk, Richard J. McClure, Kanagasabai Panchalingam, and Sandra Strychor
University of Pittsburgh School of Medicine, Pittsburgh, Pennsylvania

Phosphorus-31 nuclear magnetic resonance (^{31}P NMR) spectroscopy can be used both in vitro and in vivo to study membrane turnover, energy metabolism, and phospholipid content. Membrane turnover is assessed by determining steady-state levels of phospholipid precursors, the phosphomonoesters (PME), and breakdown products, the phosphodiesters (PDE) (Fig. 1). Energy metabolism can be determined by observing phosphocreatine (PCr) and adenosine triphosphate (ATP) resonances, as well as a final product of energy utilization, inorganic phosphate. Individual phospholipid types can be distinguished and quantified in lipid extracts of brain tissue. Application of these techniques to the study of Alzheimer's disease (AD) brain revealed several abnormalities in phospholipid and energy metabolism. Subsequent studies demonstrated the physiologic relevance of several of these abnormalities. This chapter describes the abnormalities in PME, phospholipids, and energy metabolism observed in AD and discusses the possible role of these changes in the pathophysiology of this dementing illness.

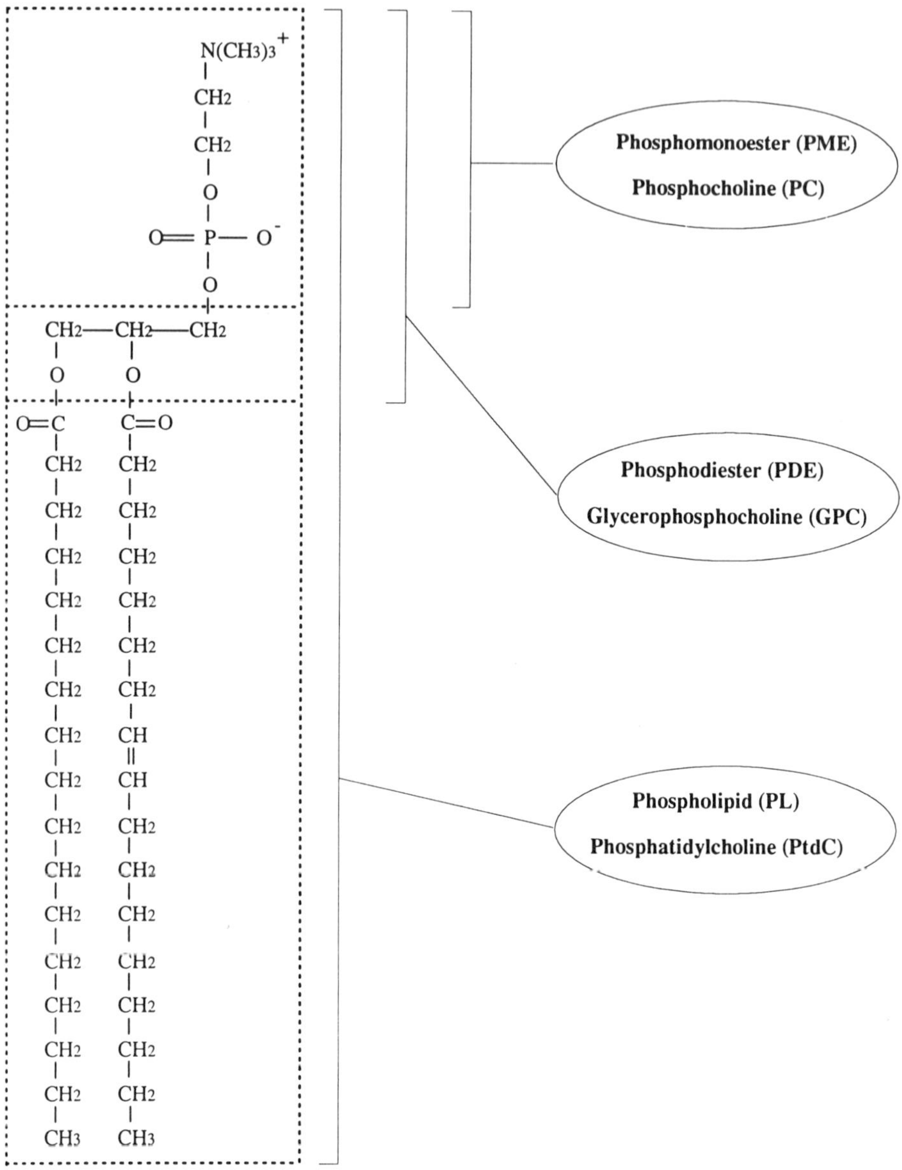

Figure 1 Schematic of a phosphatidylcholine phospholipid demonstrating the component parts of phosphomonesters (PME) and phosphodiesters (PDE).

I. ALTERED PHOSPHOMONOESTERS

PME are precursors of membrane phospholipids and products of phospholipase C and glycerol phosphodiesterase activity (1). The PME (phosphoethanolamine, L-phosphoserine, and phosphocholine) are normally found in abundance (1-2 mM) in brain in contrast to other organs (2). In developing brain, PME concentrations are normally elevated (5-7 mM) during the period of neuritic proliferation (3). This also coincides with the occurrence of normal programmed cell death and synaptic pruning in developing brain (4-7). Phosphodiesters (PDE) are breakdown products of membrane phospholipids which result from the action of phospholipase A_2 and B (8). PDE concentrations are low during development and gradually increase throughout life (3). Recent ^{31}P NMR spectroscopic studies from this laboratory reveal alterations in both membrane phospholipid and energy metabolism in AD patients (1,8-13). These findings have now been supported by in vivo studies of AD brain (14,15). Both in vitro and in vivo studies have shown that PME levels are elevated in AD brain. The abnormal elevation of PME levels in AD brain (5-7 mM) is similar to those observed in developing brain (3). This elevation appears to occur early in the course of the disease because the PME levels inversely correlate with the numbers of senile plaques (SP) (8). PDE levels are unchanged in AD overall, but PDE levels do show a positive correlation with numbers of SP, suggesting that PDE levels reflect later degenerative events (8,13). The elevation of PME is one of many metabolic derangements in AD, but the significance of this particular metabolic alteration becomes apparent when the physiologic activity of the PME is considered. The sections below describe the structural characteristics and physiologic actions of the PME.

II. MOLECULAR STRUCTURE OF PHOSPHOMONOESTERS

L-phosphoserine differs structurally from the amino acid neurotransmitter, L-glutamate, only in the substitution of a phosphate group for the terminal carboxylate of L-glutamate and an oxygen for the γ-methylene group (Fig. 2). Phosphoethanolamine shows exactly the same relationship to GABA. Furthermore, L-phosphoserine and phosphoethanolamine differ from each other structurally in the same way that L-glutamate differs from GABA, i.e., the lack of the α-carboxylic acid on phosphoethanolamine and GABA. All of these molecules are conformationally mobile, and each of the molecules can exist in a number of different conformations. This is best illustrated by the existence of three subtypes of receptors for L-glutamate and the two stable conformations found in the crystal structures of L-glutamate (16,17). In a molecular mechanics study (18), the crystal structures of L-glutamate, L-phosphoserine, GABA, and phosphoethanolamine [obtained from the Cambridge Structural Database System (19)] were used as the starting

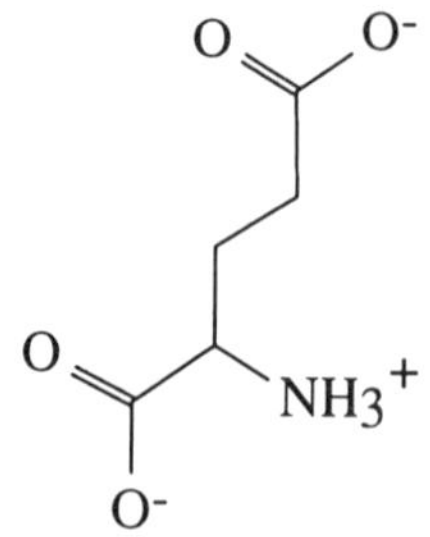

L-Glutamate

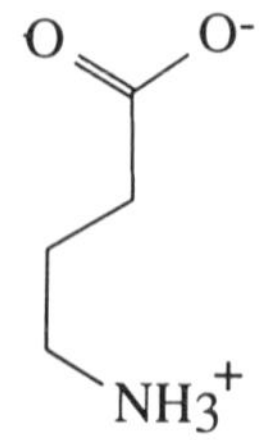

GABA

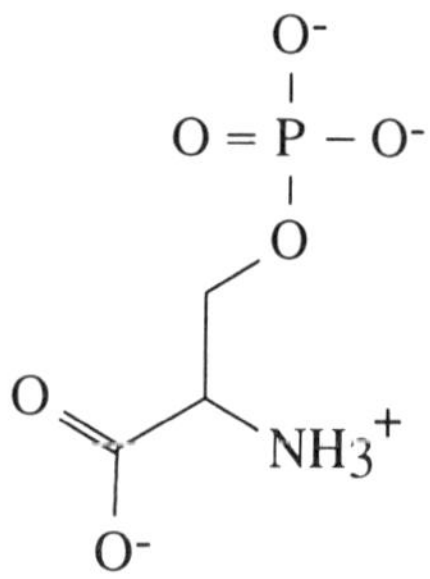

L-Phosphoserine

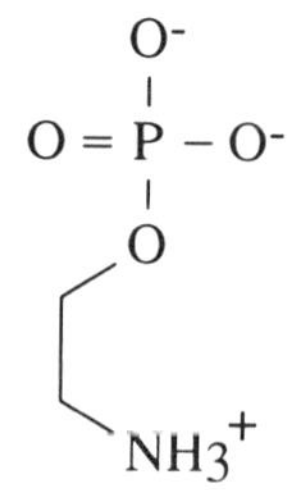

Phosphoethanolamine

Figure 2 Chemical structures of the neurotransmitters, L-glutamate and GABA, and the PME, L-phosphoserine and phosphoethanolamine.

point for energy minimization using the MacroModel (Version 2.5, Copyright Columbia University) suite of programs. The energy-minimized structure of L-phosphoserine has a molecular shape similar to L-glutamate (1); likewise, phosphoethanolamine is similar to GABA, as seen in Figure 3. The functional groups of the minimized conformers of L-glutamate and L-phosphoserine were superimposed on each other in three-dimensional space by a least squares procedure and found to overlap with less than 0.2 Å average deviation per atom. Similarly, the overlap of the minimized structures of GABA and phosphoethanolamine was excellent. The charge-charge interactions of the amino groups and the terminal acidic groups was the predominant energy term affecting the above minimiza-

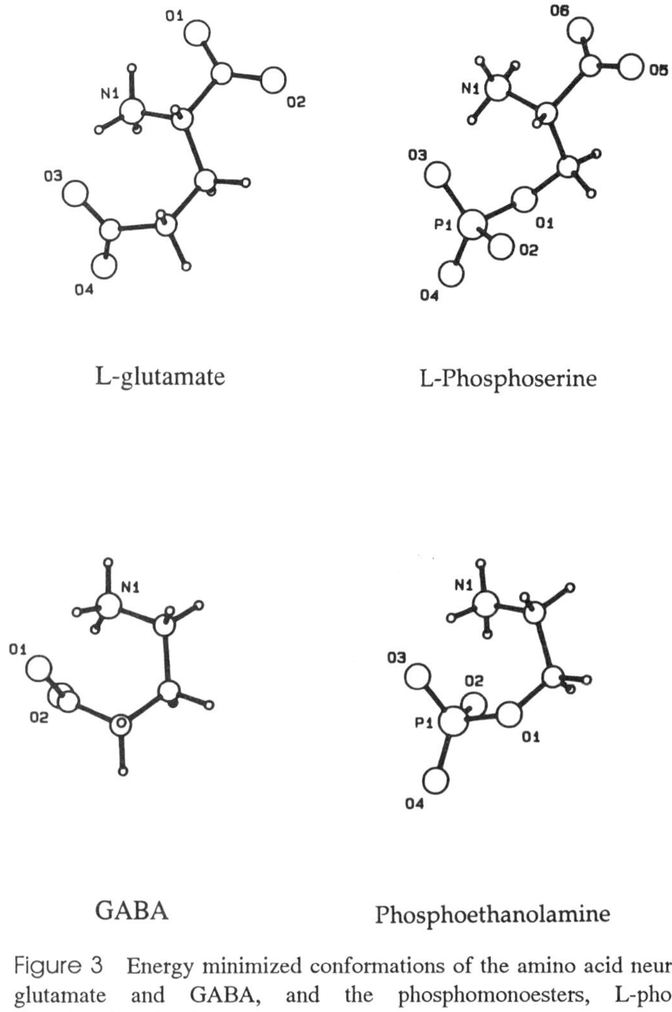

Figure 3 Energy minimized conformations of the amino acid neurotransmitters, L-glutamate and GABA, and the phosphomonoesters, L-phosphoserine and phosphoethanolamine.

tions. These interactions may be overestimated because the calculations were done without the dampening of solvation effects. However, the similarity of both the crystal structures and the minimized structures indicate that L-phosphoserine and phosphoethanolamine can adopt conformations that have a shape and charge topology comparable to those of L-glutamate and GABA respectively.

III. PHYSIOLOGIC ACTIVITY OF PHOSPHOMONOESTERS

In hippocampal slice preparations, the two abundant PME, phosphoethanolamine and L-phosphoserine, reliably alter properties of synaptic transmission at the Schaffer collateral/commissural-CA1 cell synapse. Phosphoethanolamine (1–5 mM) reversibly decreases the population excitatory postsynaptic potential (EPSP) amplitude of CA1 pyramidal cells in a concentration-dependent fashion. There is no effect on levels of phosphocreatine or ATP in the slices. L-phosphoserine initially decreases the EPSP; then, after 30 minutes of incubation, it increases the EPSP in the same preparation. These effects are not reversible. The increase in EPSP is mirrored by a decrease in both phosphocreatine and ATP (20).

Electrophysiologic and structural studies suggest that PME could act at L-glutamate sites. To explore this further, we have investigated the ability of PME to compete for binding with markers of several specific amino acid receptor subtypes. There are at least three L-glutamate receptor subtypes—commonly referred to as the AMPA/Quis, kainic acid, and NMDA receptors, since these ligands preferentially label the respective receptor subtypes (21,22). PME have specific interactions with these receptor subtypes, dependent on the PME tested and the receptor subtype studied (23). None of the PME, at concentrations up to 10 mM, are able to compete for binding with [^{3}H]-AMPA, which labels the AMPA/Quis site. L-Phosphoserine is able to compete for binding sites with [^{3}H]-kainic acid with an IC_{50} (concentration which inhibits 50% of the basal response) of approximately 1 mM. Phosphoethanolamine showed no significant inhibition of [^{3}H]-kainic acid binding at concentrations up to 10 mM. Phosphocholine could not be tested in this assay, since it is only available as the calcium salt, and calcium alone inhibits [^{3}H]-kainic acid binding (24). L-Phosphoserine also proved to be unique among the PME in its ability to inhibit the binding of [^{3}H]-CGS-19755, a selective NMDA competitive antagonist (25). L-Phosphoserine inhibited [^{3}H]-CGS-19755 binding with an IC_{50} of 0.7 mM; phosphoethanolamine and phosphocholine showed no inhibition at 10 mM. While this would suggest activity at the NMDA receptor site, it does not differentiate between agonist and antagonist activity. This differentiation can be made by studying the effects of L-phosphoserine on the binding of the noncompetitive NMDA antagonist, [^{3}H]-MK-801 (26). NMDA stimulates basal levels of [^{3}H]-MK-801 binding and further augments glycine-stimulated, but not L-glutamate-stimulated, [^{3}H]-MK-801 binding (Fig. 4a, b).

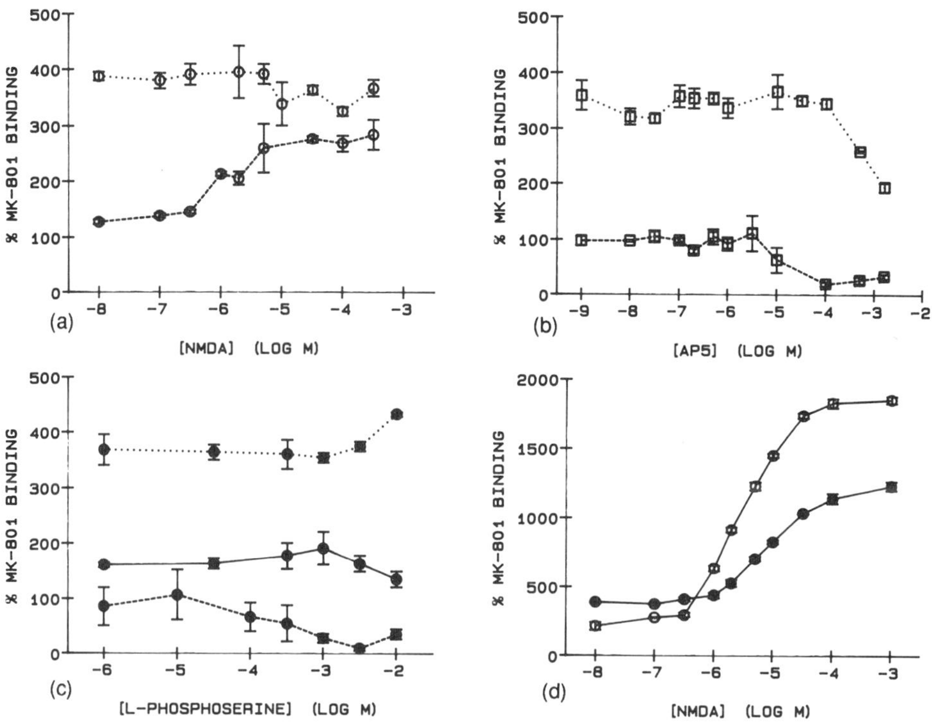

Figure 4 Binding curves. (See Reference 23 for methodologic details.) (a) The effect of NMDA (open circles) on basal (dashed line) and L-glutamate-stimulated (dotted line) [^{3}H]-MK-801 binding. (b) The effect of AP5 (open squares) on basal (dashed line) and L-glutamate-stimulated (dotted line) [^{3}H]-MK-801 binding. (c) The effect of L-phosphoserine (closed circles) on basal (dashed line), glycine-stimulated (solid line) and L-glutamate-stimulated (dotted line) [^{3}H]-MK-801 binding. The L-glutamate stimulated curve goes up at high L-phosphoserine concentrations due to L-serine impurities (23), a glycine agonist. (d) The effect of NMDA on glycine-stimulated [^{3}H]-MK-801 binding (open circles) and the inhibition of this effect by 10 mM L-phosphoserine (closed circles). The shift in IC_{50} indicates a competitive antagonism, while the decrease in maximal response indicates noncompetitive antagonism.

The competitive NMDA antagonist, 5-amino-phosphopentanoic acid (AP5), inhibits basal [^{3}H]-MK-801 binding as well as L-glutamate-stimulated binding (Fig. 4b). L-phosphoserine shows AP5-like antagonist activity (Fig. 4c, d), though it is less potent than AP5. L-Phosphoserine (10 mM) did not inhibit [^{3}H]-MK-801 binding stimulated by 100 μM L-glutamate (a supramaximal concentration), but it does shift the dose-response curve of NMDA-stimulated [^{3}H]-MK-801 binding in a manner that indicates both competitive and noncompetitive antagonism at the NMDA recognition site (23). The competitive actions are most prominent, and the noncompetitive effects may be mediated through the glycine regulatory site of the NMDA receptor complex (26) (Fig. 4d).

These binding studies support the hypothesis that L-phosphoserine can assume a shape and charge topology similar to L-glutamate; however, the replacement of the carboxylic acid function with phosphate has changed the action at this site to that of an antagonist. This may be due to the increased negative charge of the phosphate group (27), or the addition of two more potential hydrogen bond acceptors in the oxygens of the phosphate groups (28).

L-Phosphoserine also has been reported to have relatively potent effects on the ibotenic acid–stimulated hydrolysis of inositol phospholipids (29,30). Hydrolysis of membrane inositol phospholipids may serve as a transduction mechanism for several neurotransmitters, including the excitatory amino acid system stimulated by ibotenic acid and inhibited by L-AP4 (29–31). Other studies (30) imply that the actions of L-phosphoserine may be mediated through binding to a calcium/chloride and L-AP4-sensitive uptake site for L-glutamate; this is presently under investigation. Also under investigation is the elucidation of the action of phosphoethanolamine at GABA receptors.

There are important implications of these neuropharmacological activities of L-phosphoserine for AD. The direct NMDA receptor antagonism of L-phosphoserine could play a role in the memory difficulties, since the NMDA receptor has been implicated in basic mechanisms of memory and learning, such as long-term potentiation (32). However, if L-phosphoserine has more prominent effects on the uptake of L-glutamate, then its predominant action could be as an indirect L-glutamate agonist and thereby a potential neurotoxin.

IV. MEMBRANE BIOPHYSICS

The PME region of phospholipids (Fig. 1) forms the polar head groups of membrane bilayers. When exogenous PME are added to biological or synthetic membranes, they most likely insert in this same region. This would effectively separate the surface membrane proteins and the fatty acyl chains, allowing more molecular motion in these areas. It may also pack the polar head region more tightly, reducing molecular motion in this region. Preliminary data support this hypothesis. L-Phosphoserine, phosphoethanolamine, and phosphocholine increase molecular motion in the hydrocarbon core of normal human erythrocytes (Fig. 5) after brief incubation (30 minutes) at concentrations observed in AD brain (1-5 mM) (33). Erythrocytes obtained from probable AD patients [ADRDA-NINCDS criteria (34)] have the same increased molecular motion in the hydrocarbon core as observed in normal erythrocytes incubated with the PME. Age-matched control erythrocytes do not demonstrate this increased motion (35). These results suggest that the PME could cross the brain-blood barrier and insert into the plasma membrane of circulating erythrocytes. After inserting into the erythrocyte membrane, the molecular dynamics of the hydrocarbon core are altered. Similar membrane changes have been observed in platelets from AD patients (36). These results suggest that circulating erythrocytes and platelets might be used as "reporter cells" for molecular changes occurring in the brain of AD patients.

The PME also have structural effects on membranes. Both L-phosphoserine and phosphoethanolamine significantly alter the phase and structure of model membranes made from phosphatidylserine (PtdS) and phosphatidylethanolamine (PtdE) (Fig. 6), but not phosphatidylcholine (PtdC). This effect may also be explained by altered packing in membrane headgroup and fatty acid regions caused by insertion of the PME. The changes induced in the model membranes are those that underlie the formation of vesicles (micellar phase) and the fusion of vesicles to membrane bilayers (hexagonal II phase)—i.e., exocytosis of vesicle content as observed in neurotransmitter release. Therefore, the PME could enhance their own delivery into the extracellular space, where they may be active against receptors such as the L-glutamate receptor (1,37).

V. MEMBRANE PHOSPHOLIPIDS

The mole ratios of bilayer/nonbilayer membrane phospholipids are normally tightly controlled (38). The phospholipid composition of membranes is an important determinant of membrane structure and dynamics; in addition, phospholipids are important modulators of membrane protein structure, dynamics, and function (39-57). Therefore alterations in the phospholipid composition of brain cellular membranes could have important consequences for neuronal function. For example, a recent study suggests that altered membranes could account for the altered binding affinity of D_1 dopamine receptors in AD brain (58). Levels of the building blocks (PME) and breakdown products (PDE) of membrane phospholipids are altered during the course of AD. For this reason, studies were initiated to determine if the levels of the membrane phospholipids themselves were altered in AD, and if so, how the phospholipid levels might correlate with the numbers of SP and neurofibrillary tangles (NFT).

Previous work in our laboratory demonstrated a reduction in AD brain phospholipids measured by high-performance liquid chromatography (HPLC) (59). As compared to non-AD diseased controls (60 samples, nine brains), AD brain

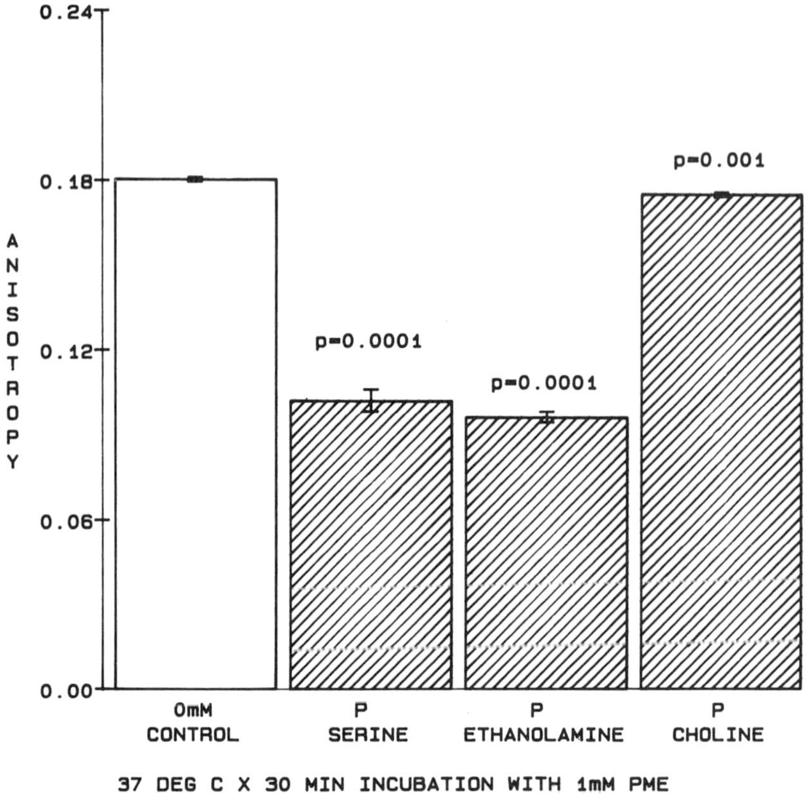

(a)

Figure 5 Effect of PME on anisotropy of RBC membranes. (a) The effect of PME on human erythrocyte membranes labeled with fluorescamine to monitor membrane surface motion. (b) The effect of PME on human erythrocyte membranes labeled with 12(9)AS to monitor motion at the hydrocarbon core.

(131 samples, 17 brains) has decreased levels of PtdC ($p = 0.001$), PtdE ($p = 0.003$), cholesterol ($p = 0.01$), and PtdS ($p = 0.04$). From this perspective, there is a fundamental degeneration of brain membranes in AD that is not observed in the other non-AD diseases studied.

The quantitation of the phospholipids by high-resolution ^{31}P NMR provides an important independent technique, which complements the results obtained by HPLC analysis and provides quantitation of some phospholipids not separated by HPLC analysis (60). Twenty-two samples from 10 AD brains and 22 samples from nine non-AD neurological control brains were analyzed. High-resolution

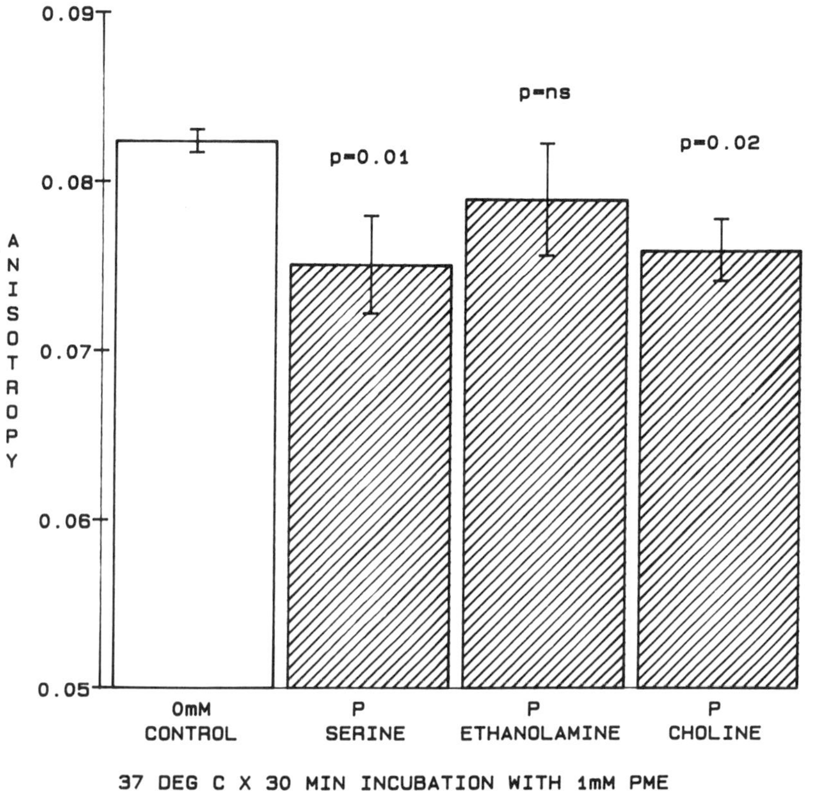

(b)

^{31}P NMR spectra allowed quantitation of lyso-PtdE, cardiolipin, an unknown resonance, PtdE-plasmalogen, PtdE, PtdS + sphingomyelin, phosphatidylinositol (PtdI), PtdC-plasmalogen, PtdC, and phosphatidic acid (PtdA). In AD brain compared to non-AD controls, there were no significant differences in the mean levels of PtdC-plasmalogen, PtdI, PtdS, sphingomyelin, PtdE-plasmalogen, cardiolipin, or PtdA. There was, however, a decrease in the mean levels of PtdE ($p < 0.03$) and PtdC, but the decrease in PtdC was not significant at the 0.05 level ($p = 0.07$) in AD brain.

As a way of comparing phospholipid levels to a measure of disease severity, the levels of PtdC, PtdE, PtdS, and cholesterol as determined by HPLC were compared with the number of senile plaques per $\times 200$ magnification (SP $\times 200$) between cortical layers II and IV in the same brain regions (Fig. 7). This comparison

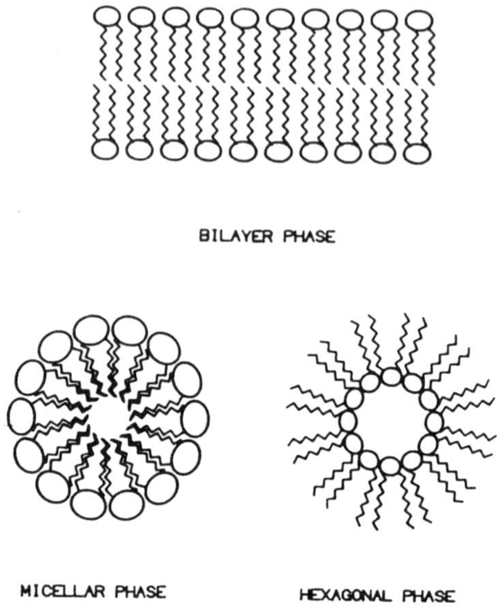
BILAYER PHASE
MICELLAR PHASE
HEXAGONAL PHASE

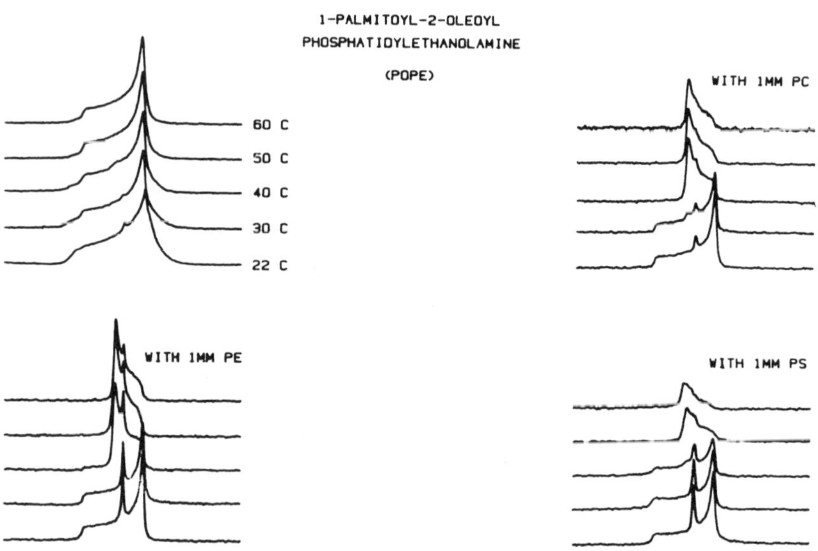
1-PALMITOYL-2-OLEOYL
PHOSPHATIDYLETHANOLAMINE
(POPE)
60 C
50 C
40 C
30 C
22 C
WITH 1MM PC
WITH 1MM PE
WITH 1MM PS

revealed a nonlinear correlation for PtdC which peaked around 10 SP × 200 and declined with increasing SP numbers ($p = 0.0001$, $r = 0.9$). Linear negative correlations were observed for PtdE ($p = 0.02$, $r = 0.6$) and PtdS ($p = 0.003$, $r = 0.8$) and no correlation for cholesterol ($p = 0.5$, $r = 0.08$) (59). When the levels of the individual phospholipids as determined by ^{31}P NMR were compared to the numbers of SP and NFT, the only significant correlations were between the levels of PtdC and cardiolipin and the numbers of SP. Again there was a nonlinear correlation between the levels of PtdC and SP which peaked at approximately 15–20 SP × 200 and then decreased ($p = 0.007$, $r = 0.65$). These results are quite similar to those obtained by HPLC. The cardiolipin levels have a nonlinear correlation with SP; the levels of cardiolipin increase with the numbers of SP ($p = 0.0006$, $r = 0.75$). The levels of phospholipids in AD and non-AD diseased controls, as determined by HPLC or ^{31}P NMR, showed no correlation between the levels of PtdS, PtdE, PtdC, or cholesterol and the postmortem interval.

Several other significant correlations were found between various metabolites or between metabolites and measures of disease severity. In the same tissue samples, there were significant correlations between the levels of PtdC-plasmalogen and the levels of both PME ($p = 0.01$, $r = 0.81$) and PDE ($p = 0.01$, $r = 0.81$). The levels of PtdA and Blessed scores correlated significantly ($p = 0.05$, $r = 0.63$), as did the levels of cardiolipin and the Mini-Mental Status scores ($p = 0.01$, $r = 0.74$).

By both HPLC and ^{31}P NMR analyses, the levels of PtdC initially increase, then decrease with increasing numbers of SP. These findings suggest an increase in PtdC synthesis early in the pathogenesis of AD at a time when PME levels are high. In theory, the augmented synthesis of PtdC could shunt available choline from acetylcholine synthesis (1) producing a functional cholinergic deficit which is observed clinically (61).

VI. INTERACTIONS BETWEEN MEMBRANE AND ENERGY METABOLISM

Studies in the Fischer 344 rat demonstrate that brief anoxia produces decreased levels of phosphocreatine and increased levels of the PME without changes in the levels of ATP. These results suggest a metabolic linkage between high-energy phosphate and membrane phospholipid metabolism (Pettegrew and Panchalingam, unpublished observations). This is of considerable interest, since a recent in vivo ^{31}P NMR spectroscopy study demonstrates a linear correlation between the

Figure 6 Effect of PME on membrane phase and conformation of synthetic phospholipid POPE. Transformation from bilayer to micellar and hexagonal II phases is demonstrated.

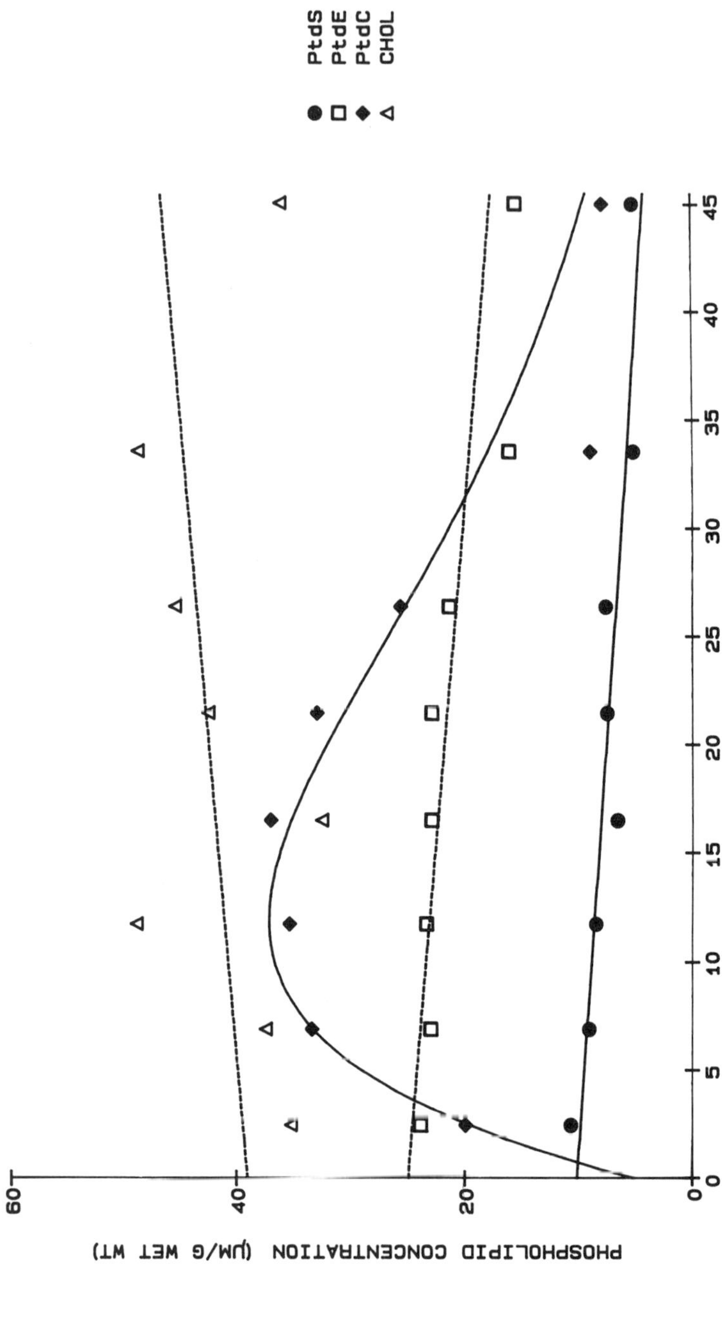

Figure 7 Number of senile plaques versus phospholipid concentration in AD brain.

levels of brain phosphocreatine and Mini-Mental Status scores [$p = 0.006$, $r = 0.8$ (Pettegrew et al. unpublished results)]. In keeping with this suggestion of an association between AD and compromised energy metabolism is the recent report of increased incidence of AD in elderly females with a history of myocardial infarction (62).

^{31}P NMR studies show that the levels of cardiolipin appear to rapidly increase with increasing numbers of SP. Cardiolipin is found predominantly in the inner mitochondrial membrane of the cell (63). In the inner mitochondrial membrane, complex IV (cytochrome c oxidase) has a predilection for phospholipids (64-66) and cardiolipin in particular (67). Cardiolipin is thought to be an important modulator of complex IV activity (68), but this has been disputed (67). The increase in cardiolipin levels with increasing numbers of SP could reflect a compensatory mechanism to maintain normal electron transport chain function and ATP production. PET findings reveal decreased glucose uptake in areas of association cortex of AD brain (69); these areas characteristically also have the greatest numbers of SP (70,71).

VII. DISCUSSION

Alzheimer's disease has been frequently described as a degenerative disorder. While it is true that the ultimate outcome is profound degeneration, the critical, early events may be not so much degenerative as they are reactivations of developmental processes. One finding that supports this notion is the expression of a fetal form of tau protein in AD (72). In this and previous reports (1,8-13), we describe another abnormality in AD that resembles a normal occurrence in developing brain, i.e., a transient elevation of a group of compounds collectively referred to as PME. In developing brain, the elevation in PME is temporally correlated with the period of neuritic proliferation, synaptic pruning, and normal programmed cell death (4-7). It is possible that PME are inherently involved in these processes which are crucial for development to proceed normally. This may involve action at L-glutamate sites, as suggested by structural, electrophysiologic, and binding studies. The PME also alter the dynamics, phase, and structure of model and cellular membranes. The induced changes in phase and structure provide a mechanism for the packaging and release of the PME into the extracellular space. If this process is reactivated in AD, it could result in the prominent early memory loss and the later loss of pyramidal cells which contain L-glutamate receptors. Additionally, PME alter the biophysical properties of membranes, which are essential for information storage, retrieval, and transfer. AD brain also shows abnormalities in phospholipid composition as compared to normal and diseased control. This abnormality also could lead to membrane dysfunction. Furthermore, early elevations in PtdC may cause choline to be shunted away from acetylcholine synthesis.

Changes in membrane metabolism appear to be coupled to changes in energy metabolism which, in turn, correlates with disease severity by in vivo studies.

In addition, erythrocytes from AD patients show strikingly similar changes in membrane dynamics, as observed in normal erythrocytes incubated with the PME. This suggests that erythrocytes might provide a "cellular reporter" on molecular changes occurring in the brain of AD patients. This phonemenon could be exploited in developing a relatively simple, inexpensive diagnostic test for AD.

REFERENCES

1. Pettegrew JW. Molecular insights into Alzheimer's disease. In Khachaturian Z, Cotman C, Pettegrew JW (eds): *Calcium Membranes, Aging, and Alzheimer's Disease.* New York Academy of Sciences, New York, 1989, pp 5-28.
2. McIlwain H, Bachelard HS. *Biochemistry and the Central Nervous System*, Churchill Livingstone, New York, 1985, pp 41-43.
3. Pettegrew JW, Panchalingam K, Withers G, et al. Changes in brain energy and phospholipid metabolism during development and aging in the Fisher 344 rat. J Neuropathol Exp Neurol 49:237-249, 1990.
4. Pittman R, Oppenheim RW. Cell death of motoneurons in the chick embryo spinal cord. IV. Evidence that a functional neuromuscular interaction is involved in the regulation of naturally occurring cell death and the stabilization of synapses. J Comp Neurol 187:425-446, 1979.
5. Cowen WM, Fawcett JW, O'Leary DDM, et al. Regressive events in neurogenesis. Science 225:1258-1265, 1984.
6. Oppenheim RW. Naturally occurring cell death during neural development. Trends Neurosci. 8:487-493, 1985.
7. Clarke PG. Neuronal death in the development of the vertebrate nervous system. Trends Neurosci. 8:345-349, 1985.
8. Pettegrew JW, Panchalingam K, Moossy J et al. Correlation of phosphorus-31 magnetic resonance spectroscopy and morphologic findings in Alzheimer's disease. Arch Neurol 45:1093-1096, 1988.
9. Pettegrew JW, Minshew NJ, Cohen MM, et al. P-31 NMR changes in Alzheimer's and Huntington's disease brain. (Abstract). Neurology 34 (Suppl 1):281, 1984.
10. Pettegrew JW, Kopp SJ, Minshew NJ, et al. 31PNMR Studies of phospholipid metabolism in developing and degenerating brain. (Abstract). Neurology 35 (Suppl 1): 257, 1985.
11. Pettegrew JW, Kopp SJ, Minshew NJ, et al. 31P Nuclear Magnetic Resonance studies of phosphoglyceride metabolism in developing and degenerating brain: Preliminary observations. J Neuropathol Exp Neurol 46:419-430, 1987.
12. Pettegrew JW, Withers G, Panchalingam K, et al. 31P nuclear magnetic resonance (NMR) spectroscopy of brain in aging and Alzheimer's disease. J Neural Transm 24 (suppl):261-268, 1987.
13. Pettegrew JW, Moossy J, Withers G, et al. 31P Nuclear Magnetic Resonance study of the brain in Alzheimer's disease. J Neuropathol Exp Neurol 47:235-248, 1988.

14. Brown GG, Levine SR, Gorell JM, et al. In vivo 31P NMR profiles of Alzheimer's disease and multiple subcortical infarct dementia. Neurology 39:1423–1427, 1989.
15. Gdowski JW, Brown GG, Levine SR, et al. Patterns of phospholipid metabolism differ between Alzheimer and multi-infarct dementia (Abstract). Neurology 38 (Suppl 1):268, 1988.
16. Bernal JD. The crystal structure of the natural amino acids and related compounds. Z Kristallogr 78:363-365, 1931.
17. Hirokawa S. A new modification of L-glutamic acid and its crystal structure. Acta Cryst 8:637–641, 1955.
18. McClure RJ, Pettegrew JW. Computer molecular modeling of L-glutamate agonists and antagonists. (Abstract). Neurology 39 (Suppl 1):398, 1989.
19. Allen FH, Bellard SA, Brice MD, et al. The cambridge structural data base. Acta Crystallogr B35:2331-2339, 1979.
20. Bradler JE, Barrionuevo G, Panchalingam K, et al. Intermediates of phospholipid metabolism elevated in Alzheimer's disease have neurophysiological and metabolic action in hippocampus. Synapse 1991 (in press).
21. Watkins JC, Krogsgaard-Larsen P, Honore T. Structure-activity relationships in the development of excitatory amino acid receptor agonists and competitive antagonists. Trends Pharmacol Sci 11:25-33, 1990.
22. Lodge D, Johnson KM. Noncompetitive excitatory amino acid receptor antagonists. TIPS 11:81–86, 1990.
23. Klunk WE, McClure RJ, Pettegrew JW. L-Phosphoserine, a metabolite elevated in Alzheimer's disease, interacts with specific L-glutamate receptor subtypes. J Neurochem 56:1997-2003, 1991.
24. Braitman DJ, Coyle JT. Inhibitionof [3H]kainic acid receptor binding by divalent cations correlates with ion affinity for the channel. Neuropharmacology 26:1247–1251, 1987.
25. Murphy DE, Hutchison AJ, Hurt SD, et al. Characterization of the binding of [Hydrogen-3]- CGS 19755: a novel N-methyl-D-aspartate antagonist with nanomolar affinity in rat brain. Br J Pharmacol 95:932-938, 1988.
26. Reynolds IJ, Miller RJ. Multiple sites for the regulation of the N-methyl-D-aspartate receptor. Mol Pharmacol 33:581-584, 1988.
27. Fagg GE, Foster AC, Harris EW, et al. Structure-activity relationships of L-glutamate receptor ligands: Role of the ω-acidic terminal. Neurosci Lett 31:59-64, 1982.
28. Freund RK, Crooks SL, Koerner JF, et al. Antagonist activity of phosphorus-containing glutamate analogs in the perforant path. Brain Res 291:150–153, 1984.
29. Nicoletti F, Wroblewski JT, Iadarola MJ, et al. Serine-O-phosphate, an endogenous metabolite, inhibits the stimulation of inositol phospholipid hydrolysis elicited by ibotenic acid in rat hippocampal slices. Neuropharmacology 25:335-338, 1986.
30. Schoepp DD, Johnson BG. Comparison of excitatory amino acid-stimulated phosphoinositide hydrolysis and N-[3H]acetylaspartylglutamate binding in rat brain: Selective inhibition of phosphoinositide hydrolysis by 2-amino-3-phosphonopropionate. J Neurochem 53:273-278, 1989.
31. Nicoletti F, Meek JL, Iadarola MJ, et al. Coupling of inositol phospholipid metabo-

lism with excitatory amino acid recognition sites in rat hippocampus. J Neurochem 46:40–46, 1986.

32. Brown TH, Chapman PF, Kairiss EW, et al. Long-term synaptic potentiation. Science 242:724–728, 1988.
33. Pettegrew JW, McKeag D, Strychor S. Metabolites elevated in Alzheimer's brain alter membrane properties. (Abstract) Soc Neurosci Abs 15:1110, 1989.
34. McKhann G, Drachman D, Folstein M, et al. Clinical diagnosis of Alzheimer's disease: Report of the NINCDS-ADRDA work group under the auspices of the Department of Health and Human Services Task Force on Alzheimer's disease. Neurology 34:939–944, 1984.
35. Pettegrew JW, Strychor S, Tretta M, et al. Membrane molecular alterations in Alzheimer's erythrocytes. (Abstract). Neurology 40 (Suppl 1):404, 1990.
36. Zubenko GS, Cohen BM, Reynolds CF, et al. Platelet membrane fluidity in Alzheimer's disease and major depression. Am J Psychiatry 144:860–868, 1987.
37. Pettegrew JW, Panchalingam K. Solid State ^{31}P and ^{27}AL NMR studies of model membranes and mammalian brain: Possible implications for Alzheimer's disease. In: Pettegrew JW, ed. NMR: Principles and Applications to Biomedical Research. Springer-Verlag, New York, 1989, pp. 310–354.
38. Wieslander A, Rilfors L, Johannson L, et al. Reversed cubic phase with membrane glucolipids from achaleplasma laidlawii. 1H, 2H, and diffusion nuclear magnetic resonance measurements. Biochemistry 20:730–735, 1981.
39. Storch J, Kleinfeld A. The lipid structure of biological membranes. Trends Biochem Sci 10:418–421, 1985.
40. Benga G, Holmes RP. Interactions between components in biological membranes and their implications for membrane function. Prog Biophys Mol Biol 43:195–257, 1984.
41. Carruthers A, Melchior D. How bilayer lipids affect membrane protein activity. Trends Biochem Sci 11:331–335, 1986.
42. Cullis PR, DeKruijff B. Lipid polymorphism and the functional roles of lipids in biological membranes. Biochim Biophys Acta 559:399–420, 1979.
43. DeKruiiff B. Polymorphic regulation of membrane lipid composition. Nature 329:587–588, 1987.
44. Carruthers A, Melchior D. A rapid method of reconstituting human erythrocyte sugar transport proteins. Biochemistry 23:2712–2718, 1984.
45. Cohen CM. The molecular organization of the red cell membrane skeleton. Semin Hematol 20:141–158, 1983.
46. Connolly T, Carruthers A, Melchior D. Effects of biolayer cholesterol of human erythrocyte hexose transport protein activity in synthetic lecithin bilayers. Biochemistry 24:2865–2873, 1985.
47. DeLisle R, Williams J. Regulation of membrane fusion in secretory exocytosis. Annu Rev Physiol 48:225–238, 1986.
48. Farmer BT, Harmon TM, Butterfield DA. ESR study of the erythrocyte membrane skeletal protein network: Influence of the state of aggregation of spectrin on the physical state of membrane proteins, bilayer lipids, and cell surface carbohydrates. Biochim Biophys Acta 821:420–430, 1985.

49. Fong TM, McNamee MG. Correlation between acetylcholine receptor function and structural properties of membranes. Biochemistry 25:830-840, 1986.
50. Froehner S. The role of the postsynaptic cytoskeleton in AChR organization. Trends Neurosci 9:37-41, 1986.
51. Hirokawa N. Quick-freeze, deep-etch visualization of the axonal cytoskeleton. Trends Neurosci 9:67-71, 1986.
52. Maksymiw R, Sui SF, Gaub H, et al. Electrostatic coupling of spectrin dimers to phosphatidylserine containing lipid lamellae. Biochemistry 26:2983-2990, 1987.
53. Nelson W, Veshnock PJ. Ankyrin binding to 9(Na^+ + K^+)ATPase and implications for the organization of membrane domains inpolarized cells. Nature 328:533-536, 1987.
54. Foster AC, Gill R, Woodruff GN. Neuroprotective effects of MK-801 in vivo: Selectivity and evidence for delayed degeneration mediated by NMDA receptor activation. J Neurosci 8:4745-4754, 1988.
55. Avdonin PV, Men'shikov MY, Svitina-Ulitina IV, et al. Blocking of the receptor-stimulated calcium entry into human platelets by verapamil and nicardipine. Thromb Res 52:587-597, 1988.
56. Peng H, Poo M. Formation and dispersal of acetylcholine receptor clusters in muscle cells. Trends Neurosci 9: 125-129, 1986.
57. Prives H, Fulton A, Penman S, et al. Interaction of the cytoskeleton framework with acetylcholine receptors on the surface of embryonic muscle cells in culture. J Cell Biol 92:231-236, 1982.
58. Keyser JD, Ebinger G, Vauquelin G. D1-dopamine receptor abnormality in frontal cortex points to a functional alteration of cortical cell membranes in Alzheimer's disease. Arch Neurol 47:761-763, 1990.
59. Pettegrew JW, Moossy J, Panchalingam K, et al. Correlation of phospholipids and senile plaques in Alzheimer's Brain. (Abstract). Neurology 39 (Suppl 1):396, 1989.
60. Meneses P, Glonek T. High resolution 31P NMR of extracted phospholipids. J Lipid Res 29:679-690, 1988.
61. Bartus RT, Dean RL, Beer B, et al. The cholinergic hypothesis of geriatric memory dysfunction. Science 217:408-417, 1982.
62. Aronson MKI, Ooi WL, Morgenstern H, et al. Women, myocardial infarction, and dementia in the very old. Neurology 40:1102-1106, 1990.
63. Daum G. Lipids of mitochondria. Biochim Biophys Acta 822:1-42, 1990.
64. Griffith OH, McMillen DA, Keana JFW, et al. Lipid-protein interactions in cytochrome c oxidase. A comparison of covalently attached phospholipid photo-spin-label with label free to diffuse in the bilayer. Biochemistry 25:574-584, 1986.
65. Knowles PF, Watts A, Marsh D. Spin-label studies of lipid immobilization in dimyristoylphosphatidylcholine-substituted cytochrome oxidase. Biochemistry 18:4480-4487, 1979.
66. Marsh DA, Watts A, Pates RD, et al. ESR spin label studies of lipid-protein interactions in membranes. Biophys J 37:265-274, 1982.
67. Powell GL, Knowles PF, Marsh D. Association of spin-labeled cardiolipin with dimyristoylphosphatidylcholine-substituted bovine heart cytochrome c oxidase. A generalized specificity rather than highly specific binding sites. Biochim Biophys Acta 816:191-194, 1985.

68. Seelig A, Seelig J, Phospholipid composition and organization of cytochrome c oxidase preparations as determined by ^{31}P-nuclear magnetic resonance. Biochim Biophys Acta 815:153–158, 1985.
69. Haxby JV, Grady CL, Duara R, et al. Neocortical metabolic abnormalities precede non-memory cognitive deficits in early Alzheimer's-type dementia. Arch Neurol 43:882–885, 1986.
70. Brun A, Gustafson L. Distribution of cerebral degeneration in Alzheimer's disease. A clinico-pathological study. Arch Psychiatr Nervenkr 223:15–33, 1976.
71. Pearson RCA, Esiri MM, Hiorns RW, et al. Anatomical correlates of the distribution of the pathological changes in the neocortex in Alzheimer disease. Proc Natl Acad Sci USA 82:4531–4534, 1985.
72. Kosik KS, Orecchio LD, Bakalis S, et al. Developmentally regulated expression of specific tau sequences. Neuron 2:1389–1397, 1989.

15

Abnormal Phospholipid Metabolism and the Pathophysiology of Alzheimer's Disease

Jan Krzysztof Blusztajn and He-Chong Lee
Boston University School of Medicine, Boston, Massachusetts

John H. Growdon and Mary Logue
Massachusetts General Hospital, Boston, Massachusetts

Mordechai Liscovitch
Weizmann Institute of Science, Rehovot, Israel

Ignacio Lopez G-Coviella, Charlotte Mauron, U. Ingrid Richardson, and Richard J. Wurtman
Massachusetts Institute of Technology, Cambridge, Massachusetts

Ismail Ulus
Uludag University Medical School, Bursa, Turkey

All cells incorporate choline into phosphatidylcholine (PC), a structural component of biological membranes, but cholinergic neurons also use choline for acetylcholine (ACh) synthesis (1). Disorders in which membrane phospholipid turnover is abnormal may especially affect cholinergic neurons because they would use the choline liberated from PC to synthesize ACh (2,3), thus limiting the amount of choline available for resynthesis of membranes (3). In brains of AD patients, the activity of choline acetyltransferase (the ACh-synthesizing enzyme) is decreased (4). The cholinergic deficit strongly correlates with both the cell loss (5) and senile plaques (6) characteristic of AD, and may contribute to the amnesia in this disorder.

Here we summarize the results of studies on in vitro model systems, which demonstrate that PC serves as presursor of choline for ACh synthesis. Based on studies of human brain tissue postmortem, we also show that abnormal phospholipid turnover may be a feature of AD brain.

I. PHOSPHATIDYLCHOLINE AS A RESERVOIR OF CHOLINE FOR ACETYLCHOLINE SYNTHESIS: IN VITRO STUDIES

Direct evidence that the PC in neuronal membranes is a "reservoir" of choline which could be used to make ACh was provided by investigating the cholinergic human neuroblastoma cell line LA-N-2 (7). Using a radioisotopic approach, we specifically labeled the PC prior to labeling of other choline-containing compounds by incubating the cells with [^{3}H-methyl]methionine. The cells used the [^{3}H-methyl]-S-adenosylmethionine produced from the labeled amino acid to methylate endogenous phosphatidylethanolamine (PE) in a reaction catalyzed by PE N-methyltransferase; the [^{3}H]PC formed from PE via the methylation pathway was isotopically labeled in its choline moiety. Radioactivity from this source was then followed into free [^{3}H]choline, and into [^{3}H]ACh. The specific radioactivities of the [^{3}H]PC, [^{3}H]choline, and [^{3}H]ACh (12, 6, and 1.2 dpm/pmol, respectively) were compatible with a precursor-product relationship, i.e., with the conversion of PC to choline to ACh. More recent studies (8) showed that the predominant labeled PC-degradation product which accumulates in LA-N-2 cells is glycerophosphocholine (GPC), suggesting that it may be the intermediate of PC degradation to free choline. GPC is produced from PC by the combined actions of phospholipase A_2 (PLA_2) and lysophospholipase. The possibility that the pathway from PC to choline involves these two enzymes is currently being explored.

In a series of separate studies performed on superfused, electrically stimulated rat striatal slices, we tested the hypothesis that prolonged release of ACh (during superfusion with choline-free medium, in the presence of a cholinesterase inhibitor) was, in fact, associated with depletion of membrane PC (3). In these studies, the slices were stimulated electrically for one to eight 20-minute periods, separated by 20-minute intervals without stimulation. The superfusion media contained either no choline (except that released from the hydrolysis of PC and other choline-containing tissue phospholipids) or choline concentrations within the range observed in human plasma (10, 20, or 40 μM).

ACh release from the slices superfused with choline-free medium did not deteriorate, even after more than 2 hours of electrical stimulation; this release was enhanced in a dose-dependent manner when choline was added to the superfusion medium. In the absence of exogenous choline, membrane levels of PC (expressed per tissue DNA) declined, in proportion to the number of stimulation periods; however, tissue ACh and free choline levels did not change. Moreover, levels of the other two major membrane phospholipids—PE and phosphatidylserine (PS)—also declined stoichiometrically, suggesting that the absolute amount of membrane had decreased. (Protein levels per DNA also fell significantly, but not by as great a proportion as the phospholipids. This probably is due to the different distributions of phospholipids and proteins within the cell: phospholipids are confined almost entirely to membranes, while proteins are also present in the cells' cytoplasm.) Addition of exogenous choline to the medium caused a dose-related preservation of membrane PC levels for up to six periods (2 hours) of stimulation; the choline also blocked the declines in tissue PE, PS, and protein. In similar experiments performed on slices of rat cerebellum (a brain region which contains very few cholinergic structures), electrical stimulation did not cause changes in the tissue phospholipid content. Taken together, these data indicate that membrane PC can be used as a storage pool of choline for ACh synthesis and that membrane breakdown may be enhanced when more choline than can be supplied by the circulation is necessary to sustain ACh synthesis and release.

II. ABNORMAL PHOSPHOLIPID TURNOVER IN ALZHEIMER'S DISEASE BUT NOT IN DOWN'S SYNDROME

To determine the indices of membrane phospholipid turnover in AD, we measured the levels of major metabolities of PC and PE: GPC and glycerophosphoethanolamine (GPE), respectively, in several brain regions obtained at autopsy from AD and control subjects. As an additional control, we used brains of patients with Down's syndrome (DS), because they exhibit pathological features similar to those characteristic of AD by the fourth decade of life (ref. 9, for a recent review) and develop cholinergic deficits similar to those seen in AD (10,11).

Fifteen AD cases with a characteristic clinical course of dementia and which met histopathological criteria for AD (12) were assayed. Eight control brains were obtained from subjects who died without clinical evidence of neurological or psychiatric illness and whose brains were normal upon neuropathological examination. Five DS brains used had confirmed histopathological characteristics of AD. The ages at death [(years, mean ± SEM) were similar among the groups: controls, 74±3; AD, 76±3; and DS, 64±4]. Times from death to brain collection [(hours, mean ± SEM) were also similar among the groups: controls, 15±3; AD, 12±2; and DS, 10±2].

We analyzed tissue from the temporal cortex (area 20/21), parietal cortex (area 40), lateral cerebellar cortex, and caudate nucleus. The temporal and parietal neocortices were selected because they contain abundant senile plaques characteristic of AD; these regions are thought to be involved in some of the behavioral manifestations of AD. The caudate nucleus and cerebellum were selected because these regions generally lack AD-type pathology. The number of samples assayed in each region varied according to tissue availability. GPC was purified by HPLC (13) and determined by a radioenzymatic assay (14) after acid hydrolysis to free choline. GPE was determined as its 9-fluorenylemethyl chloroformate derivative by HPLC with fluorimetric detection (15).

Comparison of the postmortem concentrations of the metabolites of the two major brain phospholipids, PC and PE, in control subjects, AD, and DS patients revealed dramatic differences. Levels of two catabolic intermediates, GPC and GPE, were increased in AD relative to controls or DS patients (Tables 1 and 2). The increase of GPC levels in AD relative to controls was 1.7–2.3-fold (Table 1), and the increase in GPE levels was 20–50% relative to controls (Table 2). [Since the amounts of phosphodiesters (GPC, GPE) have been reported as stable in human brain tissue postmortem (16,17), the changes described here most likely reflect antemortem conditions.]

These data, obtained with biochemical assays, confirm and extend previous observations based upon 31-phosphorus nuclear magnetic resonance (^{31}P NMR)

Table 1 Glycerophosphocholine in Human Brain

	Glycerophosphocholine (nmol/g weight)		
	Control	Alzheimer's disease	Down's syndrome
Temporal cortex	585 ± 370 n=5	1464 ± 607 n=10	786 ± 309 n=5
Parietal cortex	619 ± 186 n=6	1269 ± 442 n=8	700 ± 204 n=4
Caudate/putamen	1014 ± 422 n=5	1698 ± 552 n=6	891 ± 224 n=5
Cerebellar cortex	707 ± 327 n=6	1574 ± 530 n=10	773 ± 344 n=5

The results are reported as means ± SD. Two-way analysis of variance showed significant differences between groups ($p<0.001$), and no significant effect of brain regions or interaction between groups and brain regions. Additional one-way analyses of variance were performed on each brain region separately. Using these analyses, contrast computations were then performed to determine the statistical significance of differences between groups. There were significant differences between controls and Alzheimer's disease patients at $p=0.005$, $p=0.003$, $p=0.022$, and $p=0.001$ in the temporal cortex, parietal cortex, caudate/putamen, and cerebellar cortex, respectively, and between Alzheimer's disease and Down's syndrome patients in the same regions at $p=0.024$, $p=0.014$, $p=0.009$, and $p=0.004$. No significant differences between controls and Down's syndrome were found. (Reprinted from Reference 48.)

Table 2 Glycerophosphoethanolamine in Human Brain

	Glycerophosphoethanolamine (nmol/g weight)		
	Control	Alzheimer's disease	Down's syndrome
Temporal cortex	658 ± 173 n=4	1003 ± 337 n=16	522 ± 155 n=5
Parietal cortex	679 ± 105 n=5	1008 ± 236 n=14	790 ± 224 n=4
Caudate/putamen	872 ± 171 n=8	1060 ± 216 n=12	785 ± 212 n=5
Cerebellar cortex	888 ± 182 n=8	1154 ± 307 n=13	740 ± 178 n=5

The results are reported as means ± SD. Statistical analyses were performed as described in Table 1. Two-way analysis of variance showed significant differences between groups ($p<0.001$), and no significant effect of brain regions or interaction between groups and brain regions. There were significant differences between controls and Alzheimer's disease patients at $p=0.047$, $p=0.007$, and $p=0.029$, in the temporal, parietal, and cerebellar cortices, respectively, but not in the caudate/putamen ($p=0.056$). Significant differences were found between Alzheimer's disease and Down's syndrome patients in the caudate ($p=0.0219$), temporal ($p=0.004$), and cerebellar ($p=0.005$) cortices, but not in the parietal cortex ($p=0.083$). No significant differences between controls and Down's syndrome were found. (Reprinted from Reference 48.)

in vitro spectroscopic determinations in which we (18,19) and others (17,20–23) showed elevated levels of phosphodiesters, including GPC and GPE, in AD. Our data regarding GPE are at variance with the report of Perry et al. (24), who found normal levels of GPE in AD brain. Explanations for this discrepancy are not clear but may include the fact that different brain regions were examined and different assay techniques were used. Pettegrew et al. (17,22,23) found increased levels of phosphomonoesters including the PC and PE precursors, phosphocholine and phosphoethanolamine, in AD, especially in patients with low senile plaque counts (which they regarded as an indication of early AD). Perhaps because the cases we examined by ^{31}P NMR (18,19) had severe AD there were no increases in phosphomonoesters. The elevations in GPC levels were found in brain regions rich in senile plaques and neurofibrillary tangles (cortex) as well as in regions normally devoid of this overt AD-pathology (caudate, cerebellum). Recent studies, which utilized immunohistochemical techniques, showed, however, that accumulation of β-amyloid occurs in the latter regions of AD brains as well (25,26). Thus, our observations suggest that abnormal phospholipid metabolism may be quantitively similar in many brain regions while accumulation of abnormal proteins is more prominent, but not limited to, cortex. Since neuronal degeneration appears to be less pronounced in caudate or cerebellum as compared to the cortical areas in AD, our data may indicate that accumulations of GPC and GPE are not an epiphenomenon of cell death, but rather a fundamental aspect of pathophysiology of AD.

Concentrations of GPC and GPE in DS brains were similar to those of age-matched, elderly controls, indicating that despite similar cerebral pathological manifestations of AD and DS, the properties of phospholipid metabolism *distinguish* these diseases. The data also suggest that the AD-like changes in DS brain are more appropriately viewed as similar to normal aging but occurring at an earlier age, as postulated by Rumble et al. (27), who reported that deposition of amyloid protein in DS occurs at a rate similar to that noted for normal aging but that it begins at a younger age. It remains possible that there are other abnormalities of phospholipid turnover in DS that measures of GPC and GPE do not detect.

Increased levels of GPC might be due to decreased activity of phospholipase D, which catalyzes release of choline from PC (28), concomitant with increased rates of PC hydrolysis via a PLA_2 and a lysophospholipase-mediated pathway, which generates GPC and GPE. Consistent with this hypothesis are the reports by Farooqui et al. (29) that lysophospholipase activity is increased many-fold, and by Kanfer and McCartney (30) that phosphocholine hydrolysis is diminished in AD brains.

Other membrane abnormalities affecting various cell types in the body have been reported in AD and raise the possibility of a systemic defect in phospholipid metabolism. Phosphoinositide levels in temporal cortex were lower in AD patients than in controls (31), and brain [^{3}H]inositol 1,4,5-trisphosphate binding was diminished (32). Changes in membrane fluidity in the hippocampus and in the platelets of AD patients have been extensively characterized (33–38). The changes in platelets have been associated with a lower phospholipid to cholesterol ratio (37). The pattern of this abnormality within families of the AD probands was consistent with a fully penetrant autosomal dominant trait (38,39). Other evidence for membrane abnormalities in tissues outside of the brain includes: lack of the normal age-related decline in platelet adenylate cyclase activity (40); increases in erythrocyte choline concentrations, accompanied by reductions in choline uptake (41); reductions in colchicine-induced concanavalin A capping in lymphocytes (42); and increases in total cell calcium, associated with decreases in cytosolic free calcium and with reduced spreading in cultured skin fibroblasts (43,44).

Taken together, the data indicate a general involvement of cellular membranes in the pathophysiology of AD, and suggest that the disease process is widespread and not confined to a subset of CNS neurons which actually degenerate in the disease. Whether abnormalities in phospholipid turnover are the primary lesion or represent secondary manifestations of the disease is presently unknown. [Recent reports that some of these abnormalities are detectable in living patients by noninvasive spectroscopic techniques (45,46) raise the possibility that they may be used as an antemortem marker for AD.] In either case, cholinergic neurons would be especially vulnerable to damage because they alone use choline for both PC and ACh synthesis. Under normal conditions, phospholipid turnover in cholinergic cells may be faster than in other neurons because they hydrolyze some of their PC to supply choline for ACh synthesis (2,3,7). Under abnormal conditions in AD, phospholipid degradation mediated via PLA_2 and lysophospholipase may be increased. This accelerated catabolism may transcend the neurons' ability to resynthesize membranes and eventually compromise their structural and functional integrity. As cholinergic cells die, some of the surviving neurons may fire faster to maintain cholinergic transmission, perhaps accelerating the hydrolysis of their PC to supply choline for ACh synthesis (47) and thereby causing irreversible changes.

ACKNOWLEDGMENTS

Supported by grants from the National Institute of Aging P50AG05134, R01AG07906, the National Institute of Mental Health MH-28783, and NSF BNS8808942.

REFERENCES

1. Blusztajn JK, Wurtman RJ. Choline and cholinergic neurons. Science 221:614–620, 1983.
2. Maire JC, Wurtman RJ. Effect of electrical stimulation and choline availability on the release and contents of acetylcholine and choline in superfused slices from rat striatum. J Physiol (Pairs) 80:189–195, 1985.
3. Ulus IH, Wurtman RJ, Mauron C, et al. Choline increases acetylcholine release and protects against the stimulation-induced decrease in phosphatide levels within membranes of rat corpus striatum. Brain Res 484:217–227, 1989.
4. Bowen DM, Smith CB, White P, et al. Neurotransmitter related enzymes and indices of hypoxia in senile dementia and other abiotrophies. Brain 99:459–496, 1976.
5. McGeer PL, McGeer EG, Suzuki J, et al. Aging, Alzheimer's disease, and the cholinergic system of the basal forebrain. Neurology 34:741–745, 1984.
6. Perry EK, Tomlinson BE, Blessed G, et al. Correlation of cholinergic abnormalities with senile plaques and mental test scores in senile dementia. Br Med J 11:1457–1459, 1987.
7. Blusztajn JK, Lisovitch M, Richardson UI. Synthesis of acetylcholine from choline derived from phosphatidylcholine in a human neuronal cell line. Proc Natl Acad Sci USA 84:5475–5477, 1987.
8. Lee HC, Blusztajn JK. Glycerophosphocholine is the prdominant metabolite of phosphatidylcholine in a human cholinergic cell line, LA-N-2. FASEB J 4(7):2655, 1990.

9. Coyle JT, Oster-Granite ML, Reeves RH, et al. Down syndrome, Alzheimer's disease and the trisomy 16 mouse. TINS 11:390-394, 1988.
10. Yates CM, Simpson J, Gordon A, et al. Catecholamines and cholinergic enzymes in pre-senile and senile Alzheimer-type dementia and Down's syndrome. Brain Res 280:119-126, 1983.
11. Kish S, Karlinsky H, Becker L, et al. Down's syndrome individuals begin life with normal levels of brain cholinergic markers. J Neurochem 52:1183-1187, 1989.
12. Khachaturian Z. Diagnosis of Alzheimer's disease. Arch Neurol 42:1097-1105, 1985.
13. Liscovitch M, Freese A, Blusztajn JK, et al. High performance liquid chromatography of water soluble choline metabolites. Anal Biochem 151:187, 1985.
14. Goldberg AM, McCaman RE. The determination of picomole amounts of acetylcholine in mammalian brain. J Neurochem 20:1-8, 1973.
15. Cunico R, Anton G, Mayer C, et al. High sensitivity amino acid analysis using a novel automatted precolumn derivatization system. BioChromatography 1:6-14, 1986.
16. Perry TL, Hansen S, Gandham SS. Postmortem changes of amino compounds in human and rat brain. J Neurochem 36:406-412, 1981.
17. Pettegrew JW, Kopp SJ, Minshew NJ, et al. ^{31}P nuclear magnetic resonance studies of phosphoglyceride metabolism in developing and degenerating brain: preliminary observations. J Neuropathol Exp Neurol 46:419-430, 1987.
18. Miatto O, Gonzalez G, Buonanno F, et al. In vitro ^{31}P NMR spectroscopy detects altered phospholipid metabolism in Alzheimer's disease. Can J Neurol Sci 13:535-539, 1986.
19. Miatto O, Blusztajn JK, Logue M, et al. Detection of phospholipids in brain tissue using ^{31}P NMR spectroscopy. In Bazan NG, Horrocks LA, Toffano G (eds): *Phospholipids in the Nervous System: Biochemical and Molecular Pathology*. Liviana Press, Padua, Italy, 1989, pp 243-250.
20. Barany M, Chang YC, Arus C, et al. Increased glycerol-3-phosphorylcholine in postmortem Alzheimer's brain. Lancet 1:517, 1985.
21. Pettegrew JW, Minshew NJ, Cohen MM, et al. ^{31}P NMR changes in Alzheimer's and Huntington's disease brain. Neurology 34 (suppl 1):281, 1984.
22. Pettegrew JW, Moossy J, Withers G, et al. ^{31}P nuclear magnetic resonance study of the brain in Alzheimer's disease. J Neuropathol Exp Neurol 47:235-248, 1988.
23. Pettegrew JW, Panchalingam K, Moossy J, et al. Correlation of phosphorus-31 magnetic resonance spectroscopy and morphologic findings in Alzheimer's disease. Arch Neurol 45:1093-1096, 1988.
24. Perry TL, Yong VW, Bergeron C, et al. Amino acids, glutathione, and glutathione transferase activity in the brains of patients with Alzheimer's disease. Ann Neurol 21:331-336, 1987.
25. Selkoe D. Biochemistry of altered brain proteins in Alzheimer's disease. Ann Rev Neurosci 12:463-490, 1989.
26. Ogomori K, Kitamoto T, Tateishi J, et al. β-Protein amyloid is widely distributed in the central nervous system of patients with Alzheimer's disease, Am J Pathol 134: 243-251, 1989.

27. Rumble B, Retallack R, Hilbich C, et al. Amyloid A4 protein and its precursor in Down's syndrome and Alzheimer's disease. N Engl J Med 320:1446-1452, 1989.
28. Kanfer JN, Hattori H, Oribel D. Reduced phospholipase D activity in brain tissue samples from Alzheimer's disease patients. Ann Neurol 20:265-267, 1986.
29. Farooqui AA, Liss L, Horrocks LA. Neurochemical aspects of Alzheimer's disease: Involvement of membrane phospholipids. Metabol Brain Dis 3:19-35, 1988.
30. Kanfer JN, McCartney DG. Reduced phosphorylcholine hydrolysis by homogenates of temporal regions of Alzheimer's brain. Biochem Biophys Res Commun 139:315-319, 1986.
31. Stokes CE, Hawthrone JN. Reduced phosphoinositide concentrations in anterior temporal cortex of Alzheimer's-diseased brains. J Neurochem 48:1018-1021, 1987.
32. Young LT, Kish Sj, Li PP, et al. Decreased brain [3H]inositol 1,4,5-trisphosphate binding in Alzheimer's disease. Neurosci Lett 94:198-202, 1988.
33. Zubenko GS, Cohen BM, Growdon JH, et al. Cell membrane abnormality in patients with Alzheimer's disease. Lancet 2:235, 1984.
34. Zubenko GS. Hippocampal membrane alteration in Alzheimer's disease. Brain Res 385:115-121, 1986.
35. Zubenko GS, Malinakova L, Chojnacki B. Proliferation of internal membranes in platelets from patients with Alzheimer's disease. J Neuropathol Exp Neurol 46:407-418, 1987.
36. Hicks N, Brammer MJ, Hymas N, et al. Platelet membrane properties in Alzheimer and multi-infarct dementias. Alzheimer Disease and Associated Disorders 1:90-97, 1987.
37. Cohen BM, Zubenko GS, Babb, SM. Abnormal platelet membrane composition in Alzheimer's-type dementia. Life Sci 40:2445-2451, 1987.
38. Zubenko GS, Wusylko M, Cohen Bm, et al. Family study of platelet membrane fluidity in Alzheimer's disease. Science 238:539-542, 1987.
39. Zubenko GS, Ferrell RE. Monozygotic twins concordant for probable Alzheimer disease and increased platelet membrane fluidity. Am J Med Genet 29:431-436, 1988.
40. Ebstein RP, Oppenheim G, Zlotogorski Z, et al. Age-post-receptor changes in cyclic AMP second messenger signal amplification in normal aging and dementia of the Alzheimer type. Life Sci 39:1167-1175, 1986.
41. Miller BL, Jenden DJ, Cummings JF, et al. Abnormal erythrocyte choline and influx in Alzheimer's disease. Life Sci 38:485-490, 1986.
42. Dujindan-Van den Berge Mr, Goekoop JG. Lymphocyte concanavalin A capping: A similarity between Down's syndrome and early onset primary degenerative dementia. J Neurol Neurosurg Psychiatr 49:595-598, 1986.
43. Peterson C, Goldman JE. Alterations in calcium content and biochemical processes in cultured skin fibroblasts from aged and Alzheimer's donors. Proc Natl Acad Sci USA 83:2758-2762, 1986.
44. Peterson C, Ratan RR, Shelanski ML, et al. Cytosolic free calcium and cell spreading decrease in fibroblasts from aged and Alzheimer's donors. Proc Natl Acad Sci USA 83:7999-8001, 1986.
45. Brown GG, Levine Sr, Gorell JM, et al. In vivo ^{31}P NMR profiles of Alzheimer's disease and multiple subcortical infarct dementia. Neurology 39:1423-1427, 1989.

46. Fujimoto T, Nakano T, Noguchi S, et al. Study of dementia of Alzheimer's type using ^{31}P chemical shift imaging and ^{31}P NMR spectroscopy. Jpn J Psychaitr Treat 4:1249–1257, 1989.
47. Wurtman RJ, Blusztajn JK, Maire J-C. "Autocannibalism" of choline-containing membrane phospholipids in the pathogenesis of Alzheimer's disease. Neurochem Int 7:369–372, 1985.
48. Blusztajn, JK, Lopez Gonzalez-Coviella, I, Logue, M, Gowdon, JH and Wurtman, RJ (1990). Levels of phospholipid catabolic intermediates, glycerophosphocholine and glycerophosphoethanolamine are elevated in brains of Alzheimer's disease but not in Down's syndrome patients. Brain Res 536:240–244.

16

Acetyl-L-Carnitine: Its Role in Neuronal Metabolism

Menotti Calvani and Angelico Carta
Sigma Tau Pharmaceutical Industries, Rome, Italy

Alteration of calcium homeostasis undoubtedly plays a key role in neurodegenerative processes of several different types (1). Indeed dysfunction of NMDA receptors, which directly affect the entry of calcium into neurones which have these receptors, represents an established mechanism of neurotoxicity (2). According to some hypotheses, in Alzheimer's disease (AD) aluminum accumulation might be relevant in starting the cascade of pathophysiological events causing dementia. Interestingly, aluminum has been proposed to act through NMDA receptors, eventually altering calcium homeostasis (3). Biological studies have claimed a gross alteration of calcium balance in AD cells (4). Apart from NMDA receptors, the fate of calcium is tightly controlled by mitochondrial functions. There is also evidence that uncoupling of mitochondrial activity does occur in Alzheimer's dementia cells (4,5). Therefore, it could be worthwhile to investigate more carefully mitochondrial functions in neurodegenerative diseases, and drugs eventually acting at the mitochondrial site should merit consideration for therapeutic efforts. Among these molecules, a naturally occurring family of substances, the carnitines seem quite intriguing.

I. BACKGROUND

Carnitine is a betaine synthesized from protein-bound lysine in the liver, and basically constitutes the carrier for free fatty acids (6,7). Carnitine is synthesized mainly in the liver, but all body tissues contain it in different concentrations—particularly the heart, brain, adipose tissue, skeletal muscle, testes, kidney, and brain (8–11). Without the presence of carnitine fatty acids are not able to transverse the mitochondrial membrane to be oxidized (12–14). For this purpose, two enzymatic systems are employed: acetyl-L-carnitine transferase-1 and acetyl-L-carnitine transferase-2 (15,16).

Once inside the mitochondria, acetylcarnitine (ALC), the compound derived from oxidation of long-chain fatty acids, releases its acetyl group to start beta oxidation (17). The acetyl groups can serve as a pool from which to regenerate acetyl-CoA and acetylcholine. It has to be borne in mind that acetyl-CoA is not able to pass directly through the inner membrane of mitochondria.

Conversely, acetyl-CoA can donate its acetyl group to carnitine to form acetylcarnitine again. The ratio between acetyl-CoA and CoA is a limiting factor for the activity of the pyruvate dehydrogenase complex. When acetylcholine reaches high concentrations, pyruvate dehydrogenase activity is lowered (11). Another relevant issue to be considered is that lipid accumulation, i.e., accumulation of long-chain fatty acids, can block ATP/ADP translocation, thereby causing a reduction of cell energy production (14). Di Mauro (18) found that in carnitine deficiencies cyclic AMP function is also impaired.

Acetylcarnitine also has metabolic effects. In experimental models—i.e., during anoxia, MPTP-lesion, or ethanol intoxication—ALC consistently reduced free radical production as measured by malonaldehyde production (19–21), while carnitine was ineffective. An enhancement of the actions of some antioxidizing agents, such as reduced glutathione and ubiquinol, has been also detected after chronic administration of ALC (22,23). In this respect, the observations that ALC is able to sustain complex I mitochondrial respiratory chain activity (Jenner, personal communication), and to reverse an age-related impairment of DNA/RNA transcription, again inside the mitochondria, might be relevant (24). These data match well with previous evidence of a positive ALC effect on the activity of cytochrome-oxidase, the mitochondrial complex IV of the electron transport chain (25) and with modification in the turnover of mitochondiral membrane proteins (26,27). Carnitine by itself was not effective—probably because it has a relatively small capability of getting into the cells. Acetylcarnitine, which is transported by specific carriers, easily crosses biological membranes (28).

And what of the brain content of carnitines? In aging rats, the total carnitine balance remains substantially unchanged for the whole family of molecules. The free carnitine amount is quite stable, while a progressive age-related increase of long-chain acylcarnitines is evident (29). This could mean that in aged brain the enhancement of long-chain fatty acids is coming from the catabolism of membrane phospholipids. Interestingly, these data were reproduced in human muscle samples (30).

II. EXPERIMENTAL RESULTS

What are the effects of long-chain acylcarnitines? A number of types of evidence suggest that palmitylcarnitine is a potent time-dependent inhibitor of calcium transport into the endoplasmic reticulum (31). Long-chain acylcarnitines are tightly involved in the pathophysiology of myocardial ischemic injury, disturbing and altering calcium homeostasis inside the mitochondria and the delicate equilibrium of acetyl CoA and CoA as well (32,33). Interestingly, an inverse ratio does exist between long-chain acylcarnitine and the maximum calcium uptake rate (34). In fact, increasing experimentally the amount of long-chain acylcarnitine leads to a decrease of calcium uptake rate. This finding is very important, because both long-chain acylcarnitine and long-chain acylCoA exert a sort of detergent activity on membranes (35) and block calcium exchange inside mitochondria and other organelles (36). Preliminary data on synaptosomal calcium exchange, in which carnitine and free carnitine prevent this effect, seem indirectly to confirm such a hypothesis (Arduini, personal communication).

Chronic administration of ALC in rats for as long as 6 months and 20 months led to an increase of carnitine and aceylcarnitine, but a decrease of long-chain acetylcarnitine (29). Furthermore, morphological studies performed on aged rats demonstrated that ALC can ameliorate, to a certain extent, the characteristic loss of pyramidal neurons in hippocampus and frontal cortex (37,38) and the loss of Nissl staining and mossy fibers (39) in the same areas. ALC also affects the function of different receptors. A quantitative enhancement of glucocorticoid receptors in aged hippocampus has been found, perhaps ameliorating the response to stress (40); an increase in nerve growth factor binding, which appears to be decreased in certain brain areas during aging, was also detected (41), together with a reduction of NMDA receptor sensitivity (42). Moreover, ALC influences even the choline acetyltransferase activity in PC-12 cells (43).

CONCLUSIONS

Human clinical correlates of chronic administration of ALC are quite promising so far, although an established mechanism of action of this compound is still unclear. A number of different controlled trials agree in indicating possible efficacy in ameliorating progression in demented patients, together with remarkable safety (44). According to the most recent findings, such efficacy would be interpreted as a possible capacity to slow the progression of the neurodegeneration, perhaps acting on aging processes per se, perhaps restoring depleted energy sources of the surviving neurons, or perhaps detoxifying the cell environment from free radicals or other endogenous toxins (accumulation long-chain acylcarnities ?). The potential clinical ability to slow the disease course is a fascinating possibility for a naturally occurring molecule such as ALC. Symptomatic benefit to demented patients does not seem to be the sole hope in the clinical administration of ALC. For antidementia drugs, having a compound which might interfere with the critical pathophysiologic mechanisms of the disease and therefore with progressive cell deterioration and death, could represent an encouraging hope for the future. Further basic and clinical studies on ALC seem justified.

REFERENCES

1. Khachaturian ZS, Monjan AA, Radebaugh TS. The future of Alzheimer's Disease Research. In *Alzheimer Disease and Related Disorders.* Iqbal K, Wisniewski HM, Winbald B (eds): Alan P. Liss, New York, 1989, pp 13–21.
2. Pettegrew JM. Molecular insights into Alzheimer's disease. Ann NY Acad Sci 568:5–28, 1989.
3. McLachlan DR, Lukiw NJ, Kruck TP. New evidence for an active role fo aluminum in Alzheimer's Disease. Can J Neurol Sci 16(4):490–497, 1989.
4. Sims NR, Finegan JM, Blass JP. Alterated metabolic properties of cultured skin fibroblasts in Alzheimer's disease. Ann Neurol 21:451–457, 1987.
5. Sims NR, Finegan JM, Blass JP, et al. Mitochondrial function in brain tissue in primary degenerative dementia. Brain Tes 436:30–38, 1987.
6. Fritz IB, Yue KTM. Effects of carnitine of acetyl-CoA oxidation by heart muscle mitochondria. Am J Physiol 206:531, 1964.
7. Marquis NR, Fritz IB. The distribution of carnitine, acetylcarnitine, and carnitine acetyltransferase in rat tissues. J Biol Chem 240(5):2193–2196, 1965.
8. Montgomery JA, Mamer OA. Measurement of urinary free and acylcarnitines: Quantitative acylcarnitine profiling in normal humans and in several patients with metabolic errors. Anal Biochem 176:85–95, 1989.
9. Normann PT, Flatmark T. Long-chain Acyl-CoA synthetase and "outer" carnitine long-chain acetyltransferase activities of intact brown adipose tissue mitochondria. Biochim Biophys Acta 530:461–473, 1978.
10. Valkner KJ, Bieber LL. Short-chain acetylcarnitines of human blood and urine. Biochem Med 28:197–203, 1982.
11. Shug AL, Schmidt MJ, Golden GT, et al. The distribution and role of carnitine in the mammalin brain. Life Sci 31:2869–2874, 1982.
12. Bieber LL, Lewin M. Measurement of carnitine and O-acylcarnitines. Meth Enzymol 72:276–287, 1981.
13. Siliprandi N, Siliprandi D, Ciman M. Stimulationof oxidation of mitochondrial fatty acids and of acetate by acetylcarnitine. Biochem J 96:777–780, 1965.
14. Christiansen En, Davis EJ. The effects of coenzyme A and carnitine on steady-state ATP/ADP ratios and the rate of long-chain free fatty acid oxidation in liver mitochondria. Biochim Biophys Acta 502:17–28, 1978.

15. Farrel S, Vogel J, Bieber LL. Entry of acetyl-L-carnitine into biosynthetic pathways. Biochem Biophys Acta 876:175-177, 1986.
16. Bieber LL. Carnitine. Ann Rev Biochem 57:261-283, 1988.
17. Murray WJ, Reed KW, Roche EB. Conformations of carnitine and acetylcarnitine and the relationship to mitochondrial transport of fatty acids. J Theo Biol 82:559-572, 1980.
18. Di Mauro S, Di Mauro PM. Muscle carnitine palmityltransferase deficiency and myoglobinuria. Science 182:929-931, 1973.
19. Fariello RG, Calabrese V. Prevention of ischemia-induced increase of malonaldehyde by acetyl carnitine. Ann Neurol 24:154, 1988.
20. Fariello RG, Ghirardi O, Peschechera A, et al. Transient nigral ubiquinone depletion after single MPTP administration in mice. Neuropharmacology 26:1799-1802, 1987.
21. Calabrese V, De Bernardis E, Rizza V. Acetyl-L-carnitina nello stress ossidativo del tessuto cerbrale. (Personal communication.)
22. Fariello RG, Ferraro TN, Golden GT. Systemic acetyl-L-carnitine elevates nigral levels of glutahione and GABA. Life Sci 43:289-292, 1988.
23. Fariello RG, Ghilardi O, Peschechera A, et al. Regonal distribution of ubiquinones and tocopherols in the mouse brain: Lowest content of ubiquinols in the substantia nigra. Neuropharmacology 27(10):1077-1080, 1988.
24. Gadaleta MN, Petruzzella V, Renis M. Reduced transcription of mitochondrial DNA in senescent rat: tissue dependence and effect of acetyl-L-carnitine. Eur J Biochem, 1990 (in press).
25. Curti D, Dagani F, Galmozzi MR, Marzatico F. Effect of aging and acetyl-L-carnitine on energetic an cholinergic metabolism in rat brain regions. Mech Aging Dev 47:39-45, 1989.
26. Villa RF, Gorini A, zanada F, et al. Action of acetylcarnitine on different cerebral mitochondrial populations from hippocampus. Arch Internat Pharmaco Ther 279:195-211, 1986.
27. Villa RF, Turpeenoja L, Benzi G, et al. Action of L-acetylcarnitine on age-dependent modifications of mitochondrial membrane proteins from rat cerebellum. Neurochem Res 13(10):909-916, 1988.
28. Burlina AP, Sershen H, Debler EA, et al. Uptake of acetyl-L-carnitine in the brain. Neurochem Res 14:489-493, 1989.
29. Maccari F, Arseni A, Ghiodi P, et al. Levels of carnitines in brain and other tissues of rats of different ages: Effect of acetyl-L-carnitine
30. Costell M, O'Connor JE, Grisolia S. Age-dependent decrease of carnitine content in muscle of mice and humans. Biochim Biophys Res Comm 161:1135-1143, 1989.
31. Watanabe H, Kobayashi A, Hayashi H, et al. Effects of long-chain acylcarnitine on membrane fluidity of human erythocytes. Biochim Biophys Acta 980:315-318, 1989.
32. Branca D, Toninello A, Scutari G, et al. Involvement of long-chain Acyl CoA in the antagonistic effects of halothane and L-carnitine on mitochondrial energy-linked processes. Biochim Biophys Res Comm 139:303-307, 1986.
33. Cho KS, Proulx P. Lysis of erythrocytes by long-chain acyl esters of carnitine. Biochim Biophys Acta 193:30-35, 1969.

34. Black SC, McNeill JH, Katz S. Sarcoplasmic reticulum Ca^{2+} transport and long chain acylcarnitines in hyperthyroidism. Can J Physiol Pharmacol 66:159–165, 1988.
35. Lopaschuk GD, Katz S, McNeill JH. The effect of alloxan and streptozotocin-induced diabetes on calcium transport in rat cardiac sarcoplasmic reticulum. The possible involvement of long chain acylcarnitines. Can J Physiol Pharmacol 61:439–448, 1983.
36. De Villiers M, Lochner A. Mitochondrial Ca^{2+} fluxes: Role of free fatty acids, acyl CoA and acylcarnitine. Biochim Biophys Acta 876:309–317, 1986.
37. Badiali De Giorgi L, Bonvicini F, et al. Ultrastructural aspects of aging rat hippocampus and effects of L-acetyl-carnitine treatment. Drugs Exp Clin Res 13(3):185–189, 1987.
38. Ramacci MT, De Rossi M, Lucreziotti MR, Mione MC, Amenta R. Effects of long-term treatment with acetyl-L-carnitine on structural changes of aging rat brain. Drugs Expt Clin Res 14, 1988.
39. Ricci A, Ramacci MT, Ghirardi O, Amenta F., Age-related changes of the mossy fibers in rat hippocampus: effect of long term acetyl-L-carnitine treatment. Gerontol Geriatr 8:63–71, 1989.
40. Agnelucci L, Amenta F, Ghirardi O, Lorentz G, Ramacci MT. The hippocampus as a site of integration of morphological endocrine and behavioral markers of aging in the rat: an experimental model for acetyl-L-carnitine. In *Neurodegenerative Disorders: The Role Played by Endotoxins and Xenobiotics*. Nappi G. et al., Eds. 23–31, Raven press, 1988.
41. Angelucci L, Ramacci MT, Taglialatela G, Hulsebosch C, Morgan B, Weirbach-Perez K, Perez-Polo R. Nerve growth factor binding in aged rat central nervous system: effect of acytl-L-carnitine. J Neurosci Res 20:491–496, 1988.
42. Fiore L, Rampello L. L-Acetylcarnitine attenuates the age-dependent decrease of NMDA-sensitive glutamate receptors in rat hippocampus. Acta Neurol. (In press).
43. Perez-Polo JR, Weirbach-Perez K, Yang R, Angelucci L. Effects of acetylcarnitine on PC12 cells and aged rat hippocampus. Trans Am Soc Nuerochem 19:(1), 1988.
44. Calvani M, Jannuccelli M, Orfalian Z, Marchionni A, Benedetti R, Colonna V, Caruso G, Marchionni M. Acetyl-L-carnitine: an anti-aging agent for the treatment of dementia? In *Aging Brain and Dementia: New Trends in Diagnosis and THerapy, Neurology and Neurobiology,* (*Vol. 54*), Battistin L, gesterbrandt F, Eds. Alan Liss New York 603–622, 1990.

Index

Abnormal phospholipids metabolism, 213-222
  abnormal phospholipid turnover in AD but not in Down's syndrome, 215-219
  phosphotidylcholine as a reservoir of choline for acetylcholine synthesis (in vitro studies), 214-215
Acetylcholinersterase (AChe) activity, 94
Acetyl-L-carnitine in neuronal metabolism, 223-228
  background, 224-225
  experimental results, 225
Acidic fibroblast growth factor (aFGF), 89-90
Adenosine triphosphate (ATP), 193
Aging, NGF and, 108
Agitation, 10
Altered phosphomonoesters, 195
Alzheimer β/A4 amyloid precursor protein (APP)
  cell biological approach to therapy of, 175-192
  NGF and, 108-111
  presumed pathway for synthesis of, 176, 177
  processing pathway of, schematic representation of, 185
Animal models of Alzheimer's disease, 126
Antibodies, 137-145, 148
  complement proteins and, 155-157
  production of, 154-155
Antibody independent complement activation, 157-159
Anti-inflammatory drugs, 165-171

Antigen presentation:
- activation and proliferation of B-lymphocytes by, 153–154
- activation of T-lymphocytes by, 152–153
- scavenger cells involved in, 148–151

Antilipidemic drugs, 74
Anxiety, 10
Arecholine, 58–59

β-amyloid protein (BAP), 69–72
- background, 69
- mechanistic understanding of Congo red binding, 69–71
- searching for new molecules that bind to, 71–72

Basal forebrain cholinergic system:
- as focus of AD therapies, 15–16
- chronic NGF infusion on neurons of, 103–123
- future directions, 114–116
- grafting of genetically modified cells, 114
- NGF and aging, 108
- NGF and amyloid protein precursor mRNA, 108–111
- NGF and fimbria-fornix lesions, 105–107
  - NGF and its receptor, 104–105
  - recombinant human β-NGF, 111–113

Basic fibroblast growth factor (bFGF), 89–90, 92
Behavioral disturbances, 10
Bethanechol, 58–59
Bezafibrate (BZF), 74
Blessed Information-Memory-Concentration Test (BIMC), 11
Blood-brain barrier (BBB), 37

[Blood-brain barrier (BBB)]
- ability of redox-based chemical delivery system to penetrate, 41–43
- drug penetration of, 38

B-lymphocytes, 147–148
- antigen presentation by, 153–154

Brain-derived neurotrophic factor (BDNF), 127
- in cortex cerebri and claustrum, 128
- made by neurons in the hippocampal formation, 127–128

Brain-enhanced drug delivery, 37–55
- Alzheimer's specific pharmacotherapy considerations, 38–39
- general pharmacotherapy considerations, 37–38
- problems of drug delivery to the brain, 39–40
- strategies for delivery of drugs to the brain, 41–51
  - delivery of steroids with redox chemical delivery systems, 43–51
  - prodrugs, 41
  - redox-based chemical delivery systems, 41–43
- use of steroid delivery systems to deliver neuroactive peptide to the brain, 51–52

Brain levels of neurotrophic factors, strategies to increase, 129–130
- administration of purified NGF, 129
- regulation of endogenous trophic factor production, 129–130

[Brain levels of neurotrophic factors]
transplantation of cells that make NGF, 129

Carnitine, 224-225
Cell biological approach to therapy of Alzheimer's disease, 175-192
experimental results, 182-186
future directions, 186-189
mechanisms, 176-182
Choline actyltransferase (ChAT), 94
Cholinergic agonists, 57-66
cholinergic therapeutic strategies, 57-59
development and testing of new agonists, 61-63
information which helps to constrain choice of therapeutic agents, 59-61
research issues and factors requiring greater emphasis, 63-64
Cholinergic neurons, 16
Cholinergic toxins in the development of molecular modeling, 67-69
Cholinesterase inhibitors, 12, 24-25
Chronic nerve growth factor infusions, 103-123
future directions, 114-116
grafting of genetically modified cells, 114
NGF and aging, 108
NGF and amyloid protein precursor mRNA, 108-111
NGF and fimbria-fornix lesions, 105-107
NGF and its receptor, 104-105
recombinant human β-NGF, 111-113
Ciliary neurotrophic factor (CNTF), 89
Claustrum, BDNF in, 128
Clinical trials in AD, 15-21
basic research, 15-17
clinical studies, 17-19
drug trials, 9-14
inherent problems, 9-10
societal perspective, 19-20
Clofiric acid, 74
Complement proteins, antibodies (Ig) and, 155-157
Cortex cerebri, BDNF in, 128
Cytokines, 154
Cytoskeletal proteins, percentage of cell line supernatants reactive to, 142-143

Delusions, 10
Dementia Rating Scale of Mattis (DRS), 11
Depression, 10
Down's syndrome, abnormal phospholipid turnover in AD but not in, 215-219
Drugs tested, 2-5, 11-13
Dysgnosia, 125
Dysphasia, 125
Dyspraxia, 125

Endogenous trophic factor production, regulations of, 129-130
Energy metabolism, interactions between membrane metabolism, 205-207
Enzyme-linked immunosorbent assay (ELISA), 142-143
Epidermal growth factor (EGF), 90, 92
Epidermal growth factor receptor (EGFR), 179

Estradiol-chemical delivery system (E_2–CDS), 43
effects on cholinergic function, 49–51
pharmacodynamic evaluation of, 46–49
pharmacokinetic studies, 43–46

Fimbria-fornix lesions, NGF and, 105–107

GABA (γ-aminobutryic acid), 16, 196
energy minimized conformations by, 197
L-Glutamate, 196
energy minimized conformations by, 197
Glycerophosphocholine (GPC), 214, 215–216
in human brain, 216–219
Glycerophosphoethanoline (GPE), 215
in human brain, 216, 217
Glycine, activation of the NMDA receptor by, 80
Grafting of genetically modified cells, 114
Growth factors acting on neurons, 89–90

HeLa cells, 139
antibodies reactive with, 142
Hemoglobin:
As a model for NMDA ion channel, 78–79
structure and function of, 72–74
Hemopoietic system, relationship of neurotrophic factors to, 90–91
Hippocampal-derived neurotrophic factor (HDNF), 127
made by neurons in the hippocampal formation, 127–128

Immune-related mechanisms, 147–163
future directions, 160–161
immunologic parallels in AD pathogenesis, 148–160
activated immune cells express cytokines, 154
antibody independent complement activation, 157–159
antibody (Ig) is produced, 154–155
B-lymphocytes are present, 153–154
complement binds to Ig mediating inflammation, 155–157
phagocytic chemotoxis to complement dependent lesion sites, 159–160
scavenger cells phagocytize the products of pathology, 148
scavenger cells process and present antigens, 148–151
T-lymphocytes are present and are activated by antigen presentation, 152–153
overview of the immune response and inflammation, 147–148
significance of immune related phenomena to AD pathogenesis, 160
Insomnia, 10
Insulin, 90

Insulin-like growth factor I (IGF-I), 90, 92
Insulin-like growth factor II (IGF-II), 90, 92
Interleukin-2 receptor (IL-2R), 179

Lesioned central cholinergic neurons, pharmacological actions of rhNGF on, 93-97
Lymphocytes, 147-148

Membrane metabolism, interactions between energy metabolism and, 205-207
Membrane phospholipids, 201-205
Memory, 11
Memory impairment, 125
Metabolic alterations in AD, 193-212
  altered phosphomonoesters, 195
  interactions between membrane and energy metabolism, 205-207
  membrane biophysics, 199-201
  membrane phospholipids, 201-205
  molecular structure of phosphomonoesters, 195-198
  physiologic activity of phosphomonoesters, 198-199
Molecular modeling, 67-84
  cholinergic toxins in the development of an animal model, 67-69
  modeling of agents of diagnose early deposits or inhibit polymerization of β-amyloid filament proteins, 69-72
  NMDA receptor modeling, 72-81
    background, 72
    glycine activation of the NMDA receptor, 80
    hemoglobin as a model for the NMDA ion channel, 78-79
    hemoglobin structure and function, 72-74
    phencyclidine (PCP)-binding site, 80-81
    summary of the NMDA-binding proposal, 81
Multi-neurotransmitter deficits, 23-33
Muscarinic receptors in the brain, 59

Nerve growth factor (NGF), 16
  aging and, 108
  amyloid protein precursor mNRA, 108-111
  fimbria-fornix lesions and, 105-107
  purified, administration of, 129
  and its receptor, 104-105
Neurofibrillary tangles (NFT), 139
  antibodies reactive with, 141
Neuronal metabolism, acetyl-L-carnitine in, 223-228
  background, 224-225
  experimental results, 225
Neuropeptides, 11-12
  delivery to the brain of, via steroid delivery systems, 51-52
Neurotrophic factors, 87-101
  neurotrophins, 88-89
  other growth factors acting on neurons, 89-90
  pharmacological actions of recombinant human nerve growth factor on lesioned central cholinergic neurons, 93-97
  pharmacology of, 92-93

[Neurotrophic factors]
possible involvement in pathophysiology of Ad, 91
potential use of, 125–134
animal models of AD, 126
functional considerations, 130
the NGF family of growth factors, 126–128
rationale for clinical trials with NGF in patients with AD, 130–131
treatment strategies based on neurotrophic factors, 128–130
proteases and protease inhibitors, 91
relationship to factors of the hemopoietic system, 90–92
Neurotrophins, 88–89
Nicotinic acetylcholine receptors in the brain, 59
NMDA receptor modeling, 72–81
background, 72
glycine activation of the NMDA receptor, 80
hemoglobin as a model for the NMDA ion channel, 78–79
hemoglobin structure and function, 72–74
phencyclidine (PCP)-binding site, 80–81
summary of the NMDA-binding proposal, 81
Noradrenergic lesions, 28–29

Oxotremorine, 58–59

Paranoid delusions, 10
Pathogenesis of Alzheimer's disease: immunologic parallels in, 148–160
activated immune cells express cytokines, 154
antibody independent complement activation, 157–159
antibody (Ig) is produced, 154–155
B-lymphocytes are present, 153–154
complement binds to Ig mediating inflammation, 155–157
phagocytic chematoxis to complement dependent lesion sites, 159–160
scavenger cells phagocytize the products of pathology, 148
scavenger cells process and present antigens, 148–151
T-lymphocytes are present and are activated by antigen presentation, 152–153
significance of immune related phenomena to, 160
Pathophysiology of Alzheimer's disease, possible involvement of neurotrophic factors in, 91
Phencyclidine (PCP)-binding site, 80–81
Phosphatidycholine (PC), 213–214
as a reservoir of choline for acetylcholine synthesis (in vitro studies), 214–215
Phosphocreatine (PCr), 193
Phosphodiesters (PDE), 193
components parts of, 194
Phosphoethanolamine, 196
energy minimized conformations by, 197

Phospholipid metabolism, abnormal, 213-222
  abnormal phospholipid turnover in AD but not in Down's syndrome, 215-219
  phosphatidylcholine as a reservoir of choline for acetylcholine synthesis (in vitro studies), 214-215
Phospholipids, membrane, 201-205
Phosphomonoesters (PME), 193
  altered, 195
  component parts of, 194
  molecular structure of, 195-198
  physiologic activity of, 198-199
Phosphorylatable residues in the putative cytoplasmic domains of APP, 179
Phosphorylation of the synthetic peptide APP, kinetics of, 178
L-Phosphoserine, 195-198
  energy minimized conformations by, 197
Physostigmine, 30-31
Pilocarpine, 58-59
Prodrugs, 41
Proteases and protease inhibitors, 91
Purified NGF, administration of, 129

Recombinant human β-NGF, 111-113
Recombinant human NGF (rhNGF), 93-97
Redox-based chemical delivery systems, 41-43
  brain-enhanced delivery of steroids with, 43-51
Research, basic, 15-17
RS-86, 58-59

Scavenger cell chemotaxis to complement dependent lesion sites, 159-160
Scavenger cells, 147
  antigen presentation and, 148-151
  products of pathology phagocytized by, 148
Senile dementia of the Alzheimer type (SDAT), 9
Societal perspectives of Alzheimer's disease, 19-20
Somatostatin depletion, 27-28
Steroids:
  brain-enhanced delivery of, with redox chemical delivery system, 43-51
  delivery of neuroactive peptides to the brain via steroid delivery system, 51-52
Symptom complexes in Alzheimer patients, 10-11

Tetrahydroaminoacridine (THA), 12
T-lymphocytes, 147-148
  activation of, by antigen presentation, 152-153
Transforming growth factor-α (TGF-α), 90, 92
Transplantation of cells that make NGF, 129
Treatment:
  current approaches to, 10-11
  strategies based on neurotrophic factors, 128-130

Vasodilators, 11

About the Editors

ZAVEN S. KHACHATURIAN is Associate Director, Neuroscience and Neuropsychology of Aging Program, and Director, Office of Alzheimer's Disease Research, National Institute on Aging, National Institutes of Health, Bethesda, Maryland. The author or coauthor of over 50 journal articles, book chapters, and abstracts, and coeditor of two books, he is a member of the Society for Neuroscience. Dr Khachaturian received the B.A. degree (1961) from Yale University, New Haven, Connecticut, and the M.A. (1966) and Ph.D. (1968) degrees in neurobiology from Case Western Reserve University, Cleveland, Ohio.

JOHN P. BLASS is Winifred Masterson Burke Professor of Neurology and Neurosciences and Medicine, Cornell University Medical College, and Director, The Dementia Research Service, Burke Medical Research Institute, White Plains, New York. The author or coauthor of over 325 journal articles, book chapters, and abstracts, and coeditor of three books, including *Familial Alzheimer's Disease* (Marcel Dekker, Inc.), he is a member of the American Society for Clinical Investigation, the Association for Research in Nervous and Mental Disease, the Alzheimer's Disease and Related Disorders Association, and the American Federation for Aging Research, among others. Dr. Blass received the A.B. degree (1958) in biochemistry from Harvard University, Cambridge, Massachusetts, the Ph.D. degree (1960) in neurochemistry from the University of London, England, and the M.D. degree (1965) from Columbia University, New York, New York.